Introduction to
Diagnosis in
Traditional Chinese Medicine

World Century Compendium to TCM

World Century Compendium to TCM – Vol. 2

Introduction to
Diagnosis in
Traditional
Chinese
Medicine

Hong-zhou Wu
Zhao-qin Fang
Pan-ji Cheng
Shanghai University of Traditional Chinese Medicine, China

translated by

Chou-ping Han

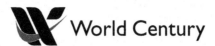

Published by

World Century Publishing Corporation
27 Warren Street
Suite 401-402
Hackensack, NJ 07601

Distributed by

World Scientific Publishing Co. Pte. Ltd.

5 Toh Tuck Link, Singapore 596224

USA office: 27 Warren Street, Suite 401-402, Hackensack, NJ 07601

UK office: 57 Shelton Street, Covent Garden, London WC2H 9HE

Library of Congress Control Number: 2013930711

British Library Cataloguing-in-Publication Data
A catalogue record for this book is available from the British Library.

World Century Compendium to TCM
A 7-Volume Set

INTRODUCTION TO DIAGNOSIS IN TRADITIONAL CHINESE MEDICINE
Volume 2

Copyright © 2013 by World Century Publishing Corporation

Published by arrangement with Shanghai Scientific & Technical Publishers.

Originally published in Chinese
Copyright © Shanghai Scientific & Technical Publishers, 2005
All Rights Reserved.

ISBN 978-1-938134-34-0 (Set)
ISBN 978-1-938134-13-5 (pbk)

Typeset by Stallion Press
Email: enquiries@stallionpress.com

Printed in Singapore

Contents

Preface

In the 21st century, people are starting to understand health and medical care in a new way. The conventional pattern of medical treatment alone cannot meet the demand of social development. It has become a trend to turn to natural therapies. Other than selecting Chinese medicine as a treatment option, more and more people hope to understand the principles and practice of Chinese medicine. That is exactly why we have compiled this book. It is our hope that the book will help readers get to know diagnosis in Chinese medicine and thus benefit their health.

PART A

CHAPTER 1

Introduction to Diagnosis in Chinese Medicine

DEVELOPMENT HISTORY

Diagnosis in Chinese medicine helps to diagnose medical conditions, identify specific patterns, predict the prognosis and thus provide the basis for treatment.

As early as the Zhou dynasty (1046–771 B.C.), *The Rites of Zhou: Offices of Heaven* (*Zhou Li: Tian Guan*, 周礼 • 天官篇) recorded, "A patient's prognosis can be predicted by five odors, five sounds and five colors, coupled with changes in the nine orifices (two eyes, two noses, two nostrils, mouth, urethra and anus) and the nine organs (heart, liver, spleen, lungs, kidneys, stomach, large intestine, small intestine and urinary bladder)." This indicates that inspection, olfaction and pulse-taking were employed at that time. Bian Que (410–310 BC), a legendary physician, was amazingly excellent in diagnosis via observation and pulse-taking. *The Records of the Grand Historian* (*Shi Ji*, 史记), completed in the Western Han dynasty (202 B.C.–9 A.D.), recorded the case studies of Bian Que and commented, "Bian Que is the very initiator of pulse-taking." In addition, Zhang Zhong-jing (150–219) mentioned in his preface to *Treatise on Cold Damage and Miscellaneous Diseases* (*Shang Han Za Bing Lun*, 伤寒杂病论), "Bian Que left a lasting admiration with his amazing diagnostic skills in observation and pulse-taking."

The Yellow Emperor's Inner Classic (*Huang Di Nei Jing*, 黄帝内经), completed during the Warring States Period (457–221 B.C.), contains texts on specific methods of observation, auscultation and olfaction, inquiry and palpation coupled with theoretical explanations. *Discussions on Yin and Yang with Natural Phenomena in the "Basic Questions" (Su Wen Yin Yang Ying Xiang Da Quan,* 素问阴阳应象大论) states, "Skillful physicians identify yin from yang first by observing the facial complexion and feeling the pulse, then identify the affected location by examining the five colors and be aware of the suffering by observing the breathing and listening to the voice. After that, they analyze the involved *zang–fu* organs by examining the colors and pulse conditions and further understand the causative factors by feeling the *cunkou* (radial artery) pulse (floating, deep, slippery or hesitant). In this way, they can make a correct diagnosis and subsequently an appropriate treatment plan."

Regarding observation, *The Yellow Emperor's Inner Classic* especially highlights the observation of spirit, color, shape and tongue conditions. For olfaction, the text initiated the theory on five notes (sounds) corresponding to the five *zang* organs. For inquiry, the text states, "It is necessary to inquire into the primary and current conditions." In addition, the text emphasizes the importance of pulse-taking. It covers the methods of three positions and nine subdivisions for pulse-taking, as well as more than 40 pulse conditions.

Classic of Difficult Issues (Nan Jing, 难经), completed in the Eastern Han dynasty (25–220), established the methods of "taking the *cunkou* pulse". If also discussed normal and abnormal pulses and their clinical significance.

Treatise on Cold Damage and Miscellaneous Diseases developed the principle of syndrome differentiation (or pattern identification) by combining diseases, pulse and symptoms—to differentiate the cold damage condition by the six meridians and differentiate miscellaneous diseases by the *zang–fu* organs. With treatment principles as well as formulas, the text has been influential even until today.

Pulse Classic (Mai Jing, 脉经) by Wang Shu-he (201–280) of the Jin dynasty (265–420), is considered the first monograph on the pulse. The text standardizes the terminology for the pulse conditions and summarizes them into 24 pulses. It clearly defines the six positions in both hands corresponding to the *zang–fu* organs. Also in that period, *Emergency Formulas to Keep up One's Sleeve (Zhou Hou Bei Ji Fang,* 肘后备急方),

by Ge Hong (283–363), recorded the method of 'urine staining on a piece of white paper' to diagnose jaundice.

Arcane Essentials from the Imperial Library (*Wai Tai Mi Yao*, 外台秘要) by Wang Tao (670–755) of the Tang dynasty (618–907), recorded the method of urine staining on white silk fabrics to test the urine color. The text mentioned that sweet urine is necessary for the diagnosis of diabetes. In addition, it recorded diagnosis and differentiation of typhoid, pulmonary tuberculosis, malaria, smallpox and cholera.

The Song (960–1279), Jin (1115–1234) and Yuan (1206–1368) dynasties witnessed a development in pulse studies. Other than books including *Cui's Verse on Pulse Diagnosis* (*Cui Shi Mai Jue*, 崔氏脉诀), *Verse on Pulse Diagnosis* (*Mai Jue*, 脉诀) and *Essential Points in Pulse Diagnosis* (*Zhen Jiao Shu Yao*, 诊家枢要), pulse graphs were also present to illustrate various pulse conditions. *Guide to Disease Examination* (*Cha Bing Zhi Nan*, 察病指南), completed in the year 1241 by Shi Fa of the Song dynasty, covered 33 types of pulses. *Ao's Golden Mirror Records for Cold Damage* (*Ao Shi Shang Han Jin Jing Lu*, 敖氏伤寒金镜录), completed in the year 1341 by Du Ben, a physician of the Yuan dynasty, remains the earliest monograph on tongue examination, including 36 types of tongue conditions. In addition, this era witnessed great progress in the diagnosis of pediatric conditions by observing the color and shape of the index finger. *Key to Diagnosis and Treatment of Children's Diseases* (*Xiao Er Yao Zheng Zhi Jue*, 小儿药证直诀), completed in the year 1119 by Qian Yi, also recorded the diagnosis by observing the face and eyes. The four masters in the Jin–Yuan period (115–1368) expressed distinctive points in diagnosis and treatment: Liu Wan-su emphasized the role of pathogenesis, Zhang Cong-zheng differential diagnosis, Li Dong-yuan combination of the four diagnostic methods and Zhu Dan-xi external manifestations.

Physicians in the Ming dynasty (1368–1644) favored combination of the four diagnostic methods, which had been mentioned in *[Li] Bin-hu's Teachings on Pulse Diagnosis* (*Bin Hu Mai Xue*, 濒湖脉学), completed in the year 1564 by Li Shi-zhen and *Simple and Concise Measures for Common Conditions* (*Jian Ming Yi Gou*, 简明医彀), completed in the year 1629 by Sun Zhi-hong. *Introduction to Medicine* (*Yi Xue Ru Men*, 医学入门), completed in the year 1575 by Li Chan, listed 55 questions for inquiry. *The Complete Works of [Zhang] Jing-yue* (*Jing Yue Quan Shu*, 景岳全书) completed in the year 1624 by Zhang Jing-yue, listed rhymes of 10 questions. These question items are still influential today.

Physicians in the Qing dynasty (1636–1922) valued the significance of diagnosis by inspection. *Tongue Inspection in Cold Damage* (*Shang Han She Jian*, 伤寒舌鉴), completed in the year 1699 by Zhang Deng, presented 120 tongue pictures. *Differentiation of Tongue Conditions* (*She Jian Bian Zhen*, 舌鉴辨证), by Liang Yu-yu, presented 149 tongue pictures. Additionally, Ye Tian-shi (1666–1745) paid much more attention to the tongue conditions in the diagnosis of externally contracted febrile conditions.

In regard to the syndrome differentiation of febrile conditions, Ye Tian-shi developed the method of examining the teeth, assuming that the luster of teeth is closely associated with the medical conditions. He also predicted the prognosis by observing the maculae or white patches. *Differentiation and Diagnosis by Inspection* (*Wang Zhen Zun Jing*, 望诊遵经), completed in the year 1875 by Wang Hong, collected the data of generations on inspection, including the color, luster and changes of sweat, blood, moustache and urine.

Numerous books on diagnosis have been published over the past hundred years. They include the *Guide to Tongue Diagnosis by Illustrations* (*Cai Tu Bian She Zhi Nan*, 彩图辨舌指南并), by Cao Bing-zhang, *Study on Tongue Diagnosis* (*She Zhen Yan Jiu*, 舌诊研究), by Chen Ze-lin, *Diagnosis Based on Signs and Symptoms* (*Zhong Yi Zheng Zhuang Jian Bie Zhen Duan Xue*, 中医症状鉴别诊断学) and *Syndrome Differentiation in Chinese Medicine* (*Zhong Yi Zheng Hou Jian Bie Zhen Duan Xue*, 中医证候鉴别诊断学), by Zhao Jin-duo; and *Diagnosis in Chinese Medicine* (*Zhong Yi Zhen Duan Xue*, 中医诊断学), by Fei Zhao-fu. These texts have greatly enriched diagnosis in Chinese medicine.

QUESTIONS

1. What are the two diagnostic methods Bian Que was especially excellent at?
2. When did the pulse graph and tongue pictures appear in history?

MAIN CONTENTS

Diagnosis in Chinese medicine mainly covers two aspects: collection of the signs, symptoms and case histories by inspection, auscultation and olfaction, inquiry and palpation; then evaluation and differentiation of the disease, syndrome and prognosis prior to treatment. This book will mainly focus on syndrome differentiation (or pattern identification), namely the pattern identification of the eight principles, etiology, *qi*, blood and blood fluids, *zang–fu* organs, meridians, and the six meridians, *wei* (defense), *qi*, *ying* (nutrients) and blood, and *Sanjiao*.

The four diagnostic methods are inspection, auscultation and olfaction, inquiry, and palpation. Inspection aims to understand a medical condition by observing the patient's spirit, color, shape, five sense organs, tongue and secretions or discharges. Auscultation and olfaction aims to identify a medical condition by listening to the patient's voice and breathing as well as smelling the patient's odor of the body, breathing and discharges. Inquiry aims to get an idea of the patient's health status, case history and symptoms by asking either the patient him/herself or his/her relatives. Palpation aims to understand the internal conditions by feeling the patient's pulse and palpating other body areas. The above four methods are always combined in the examination of a patient.

The pattern identification of the eight principles aims to generalize the data collected through the four diagnostic methods into eight principles. The eight principles are exterior, interior, cold, heat, deficiency, excess, yin and yang. Regarding a specific medical condition, cold and heat tell about the nature, exterior and interior tell about the location and depth, deficiency and excess tell about the strength between antipathogenic *qi* and pathogenic factors, and yin and yang tell about the general category.

The pattern identification of etiology aims to analyze causative factors and pathological changes. The causative factors mainly include six external pathogens, seven emotions, an improper diet and overexertion.

The pattern identification of *qi*, blood and body fluids aims to identify disorders of *qi*, blood and body fluids in specific conditions.

The pattern identification of the *zang–fu* organs aims to identify the involved *zang–fu* organs (locations), nature and strength between antipathogenic *qi* and pathogenic factors.

The pattern identifications of the six meridians, *wei*, *qi*, *ying* and blood, and *sanjiao,* are mainly indicated for acute externally contracted febrile conditions.

CHARACTERISTICS AND PRINCIPLES

Examining the Interior and Exterior

The interior refers to the five *zang* and six *fu* organs especially the former. The exterior refers to the external manifestations, such as mental activities, emotions, daily life activities, the five sense organs, the seven orifices, the torso and the extremities. Chinese medicine holds that the human body is an organic whole. The interior and the exterior are interconnected through the meridian system. The body and nature are interconnected through the five sense organs on the body surface. Environmental or natural changes can affect the five *zang* organs through the body surface and meridians. For example, seeing or hearing horrifying things may cause palpitations; a cold stimulus may cause nasal obstruction and sneezing. Likewise, disorders of the five *zang* organs may manifest in the exterior. For example, dysfunctions of the spleen and stomach may cause a foul breath and a greasy feeling in the mouth with a bitter taste; dysfunctions of the liver may cause chest or hypochondriac discomfort, blurred vision and tinnitus.

A local medical condition may affect the whole body, and a systemic condition may manifest in a specific area. An exterior condition may be transmitted into the interior, and an interior condition may manifest in the exterior. Mental stress may affect the functions of the *zang–fu* organs, and dysfunctions of the *zang–fu* organs may affect mental activities. As a result, for example, eye problems can be caused by a local lesion, such as a foreign body injury, but can also result from ascending of liver fire or heart fire.

In diagnosing medical conditions, it is important to evaluate the functions of the *zang–fu* organs by the external manifestations. It is also necessary to pay attention to the external environment, such as the season, geographical locations, life habits, living area and mental or social surroundings.

Identifying Patterns to Determine Causes

Patterns refer to the differentiation conclusions on the basis of signs and symptoms. Causes here can be causative factors, such as the six external pathogens, the seven emotions, an improper diet or overexertion, or pathological products, such as stagnant blood, phlegm fluid and *qi* stagnation. These factors can trigger or aggravate the patient's discomfort. Take a subjective fever, for example. Other than fever, the onset and accompanying symptoms need to be understood through the four examinations. Fever with a short duration and a history of contracting cold and chills is often caused by an external contraction. A floating pulse and a thin tongue coating indicate an exterior syndrome. A white and moistening tongue coating indicates cold, a dry scanty or yellow coating or a red tongue with a sore throat indicates heat, and a thick greasy yellow or brown tongue coating indicates other concurrent conditions.

Comprehensive Analysis of the Four Examinations

The four examinations are equally important in diagnosing medical conditions. Overexaggerating one method but neglecting the other methods can be misleading. For example, by observing the patient's constitution, age and gender, some physicians can get a general idea of deficiency, excess cold or heat. Then, by the local epidemic or seasonal conditions as well as the patient's external manifestations (such as coughing or the clothes he or she wears), they can make a preliminary diagnosis. After that, they just claim that they diagnosed by inspection or pulse-taking alone.

As far as the four examinations are concerned, some physicians may be more skillful at inspection, while others may be more skillful at pulse-taking. However, combination of the four examinations is always necessary for a complete and correct diagnosis.

RECOMMENDED LEARNING METHODS

Be Familiar with the Basic Theory of Chinese Medicine

As the basic theories of Chinese medicine run through the whole process in diagnosis, it is important to be familiar with theories such as yin, yang, the five elements, *qi*, blood, body fluids, *zang–fu* organs, meridians, etiology and pathogenesis. It is also necessary to learn clinical subspecialties so as to facilitate ability in diagnosis.

Participate in Practice

Diagnosis requires practice. Reading books alone is far from enough. For example, one can never understand a red or pale tongue without actually seeing it, and one can never experience a *wiry* or slippery pulse without actually feeling it.

Pay Attention to Details

As the saying goes, "Details determine outcomes." Only by attentive and rigorous examinations can one make a correct diagnosis.

Acquire Good Thinking Skills

Since diagnosis in Chinese medicine requires both theoretical foundation and actual practice, it is essential to equip oneself with substantial knowledge and good thinking skills.

QUESTIONS

1. What are the main principles of diagnosis in Chinese medicine?
2. Why is comprehensive analysis of the four examinations important?

CHAPTER 2

The Four Diagnostic Methods

The four diagnostic methods are inspection, auscultation and olfaction, inquiry, and palpation.

Since the human body is an organic whole, the physiology and pathology of the entire body and internal organs can manifest in the five sense organs, four extremities and body surface. The four diagnostic methods can be used to study the external manifestations of the physiology and pathology of the five *zang* and six *fu* organs by collecting the clinical signs and symptoms, thus providing the basis for diagnosis.

INSPECTION

Inspection aims to observe a patient's body, specific body parts, secretion and discharges to collect data for diagnosis.

It can be generalized into observation of the spirit (vitality), color, shape and movement.

Inspecting the Spirit

The spirit (*shen* in Chinese) is a basic, common concept in Chinese medicine. In a narrow sense, it refers to the mental/emotional activities. In a broad sense, it refers to the external manifestations of vital activities. By inspecting the spirit, we mean to inspect the spirit in a broad sense to understand the patient's abundance or insufficiency of essential *qi* and thus predict the prognosis.

Pattern	Clinical Manifestations	Remarks
Presence of spirit	Clear consciousness, clear speech, bright eyes, natural facial expressions, fast mental reactions, a moistening complexion, flexible body movement, normal breathing and normal muscles.	This pattern indicates a normal spirit, with abundant antipathogenic *qi* and a subsequent favorable prognosis.
Loss of spirit	Drowsiness or unconsciousness, incoherent speech, floccillation, slow mental reactions, awkward body movement, muscle wasting and dull eyes.	This pattern indicates failure of the spirit, with deficient antipathogenic *qi* and a subsequent unfavorable prognosis.
False spirit	Sudden bright eyes and talkativeness after an extended period of a critical condition, coupled with sudden clear loud speech, rosy cheeks and an increased appetite.	This pattern indicates a life-threatening condition, known as "the final momentary light before death."
Deficiency of spirit *qi*	A low spirit, lassitude, a weak voice, reluctance to talk and slow body movement.	This pattern is often seen in a deficiency syndrome.
Disorders of spirit	Mania, depression, epilepsy, restlessness, mental confusion or delirium.	This pattern is often seen in mental disorders or high fever.

Inspecting the Facial Complexion

The facial complexion involves the color and luster of the face. Since blood–*qi* of the 12 regular meridians and 365 collaterals ascend to the face, the abundance or deficiency of the *qi* and blood in the *zang–fu* organs as well as pathological changes can manifest in the face.

The projections of the zang–fu organs on the face

Midforehead — throat
Area between the two eyebrows — lungs

Area between the two eyes — heart

Area between the nasal bridge — liver with gallbladder (left or right side of the liver)

Nasal tip — spleen with stomach (left or right side of the spleen)

Area between the nose and the lips — urinary bladder and uterus

Area below the zygoma — large intestine and kidneys (lateral side of the large intestine)

Ten methods to observe the facial complexion

The ten types of facial complexion are floating, deep, clear, turbid, pale, dark, scattering, condensed, lustrous and withered.

Color	Indication
Floating: exposure of the luster on the surface	An exterior syndrome involving the *fu* organs
Deep: luster hidden subcutaneously	An interior syndrome involving the *zang* organs
Clear: clear bright luster	A yang syndrome
Turbid: dark dull complexion	A yin syndrome
Pale complexion	Deficiency of antipathogenic *qi*
Dark complexion	Excess of pathogenic factors
Scattering luster	An acute condition
Condensed luster	A chronic condition
Lustrous (moistening) complexion	*Qi* and blood remain undamaged
Withered complexion	Damage to essential *qi*

Normal color and morbid color

A normal facial complexion is characterized by a hidden mixed color of red and yellow, appearing bright and moistening. The normal color suggests the presence of spirit *qi* and stomach *qi*, along with abundant essential *qi*, blood and body fluids, and normal functions of the *zang–fu* organs.

Morbid color is characterized by loss of luster, manifesting as gray, dark, withered or floating–bright on the surface or incoordination of color. According to the disease severity, morbid color can be subdivided into benign color and malign color. A benign color is often bright and moistening, indicating that the essential *qi* remains undamaged. A malign color is often dull and dark, indicating deficiency of essential *qi*.

The five abnormal colors and indications are listed in the following table:

Color	Indications
Bluish	Cold or pain syndrome that can be caused by stagnant blood or high fever
Red	Heat syndrome. Dark red indicates excessive heat, while pale red indicates deficient heat. Pallor with rosy cheeks indicates a fatal floating yang syndrome.
Yellow	Deficiency or dampness syndrome. A lusterless pale yellow (sallow) complexion indicates *qi* deficiency of the spleen and stomach (insufficiency of *qi* and blood). A yellow complexion with facial puffiness indicates spleen *qi* deficiency with internal dampness. Yellow eyes and face indicates jaundice. A bright yellow indicates yang jaundice due to damp–heat, while a dark dull yellow indicates yin jaundice due to cold–dampness.
White	Deficiency or cold syndrome that can be caused by loss of blood or deprivation of *qi*
Dark	Kidney deficiency, cold syndrome, pain syndrome, water fluid retention or blood stasis

---

QUESTIONS

1. How do you understand "inspection"?
2. How do you understand the concept of the "spirit"? What are the focuses of inspecting the spirit?
3. List the manifestations of "presence of spirit" and "loss of spirit."
4. Describe the facial complexion showing the presence of spirit *qi* and stomach *qi*.
5. List the main indications of the five abnormal colors.

Inspecting the Body Shape and Posture

By observing the body shape and posture, a physician can tell about the abundance or deficiency of *qi* and blood in the *zang–fu* organs strength between yin and yang, the location of the pathogenic factors as well as the prognosis of a medical condition.

The body shape can manifest the functions of the *zang–fu* organs. Those with healthy *zang–fu* organs often have a strong physique: strong skeleton, wide thick ribcage, abundant muscles and lustrous moistening skin. The smoothness of the muscle can tell about the adequacy of the body fluids. The density of the skin striae can tell about the strength of *ying* (nutrients) and *wei* (defensive) *qi*. The firmness of the flesh can tell about the deficiency or excess of stomach *qi*. The thickness of the tendon can tell about the sufficiency of liver blood. The sizes of the bones can tell about the strength of kidney *qi*. Pathologically, obesity with less food ingestion indicates phlegm dampness due to spleen deficiency. Weight loss with an increased appetite indicates fire in the middle *jiao*. Underweight with a poor appetite indicates spleen *qi* deficiency. Deformities such as the pigeon chest or humpback are often caused by congenital kidney essence deficiency or acquired weakness of the spleen and stomach.

Abnormal postures and indications are listed in the following table:

Abnormal Postures	Indications
Occasional twitching of the lips and toes	Warning signs of convulsions in febrile conditions; malnourishment of the meridians due to deficiency of yin blood in internally damaged conditions
Tremors of the four extremities	Epilepsy, tetanus or rabies
Shivering	Episodes of malaria or pus toxins entering the interior
Floccillation	Life-threatening sign
Hemiplegia with deviated mouth and eyes	Wind stroke
Fainting in summer with red face and sweat	Sunstroke
Sleeping with frequent rolling over	Yang, heat, excessive syndrome
Sleeping with a general heavy sensation and difficulty in rolling over	Yin, cold, deficient syndrome
Sleeping with a curved body	Yang deficiency or severe abdominal pain
Sleeping supinely with a hot sensation	Heat syndrome
Sitting supinely	Lung excess
Sitting prone	Lung deficiency
Inability to lie flat (orthopnea)	Coughing and panting due to lung distension or water fluid retention
Inability to sit up, otherwise dizzy	Deficiency of *qi* and blood
Restlessness	Visceral agitation (hysteria)

Inspecting the Five Sense Organs

Since the five *zang* organs connect with the five sense organs through the meridians, functions of the *zang–fu* organs can manifest in the five sense organs.

Inspecting the eyes

The liver opens into the eyes. In addition, the essential *qi* of the five *zang* and six *fu* organs ascends to the eyes. As a result, inspecting the eyes can help one understand the states not only of the spirit and liver, but also of the other *zang–fu* organs. Inspecting the eyes is especially important for evaluating the spirit.

According to the five-wheel theory, there are correlations between the *zang* organs and parts of the eyes:

The inner and the outer canthus — heart (blood wheel)
The black part of the eyeball — liver (wind wheel)
The white part of the eyeball — lung (*qi* wheel)
The pupils — kidney (water wheel)
The upper and lower eyelids — spleen (flesh wheel)

Observing the eyes for spirit (in both the narrow and broad senses)

Presence of spirit: flexible eye movements with shining gleams.

Loss of spirit: slow eye movements with dull, listless expressions; a dilation of the pupil can be a fatal sign.

Observing the colors of the eyes

Redness in a specific wheel indicates fire or heat in the corresponding *zang* organ. Acute red eyes indicate wind–heat in the liver meridian. A pale white canthus (blood wheel) indicates blood deficiency. Bright edema in the upper eyelids indicates water or phlegm fluid retention. Gray dark circles of the eyes often indicate kidney deficiency.

Observing the movements of the eyeballs

Eyeball movements	Indications
Anopsia or staring blankly	Life-threatening sign
Strabismus (neither congenital nor trauma)	Internal stirring of liver wind
Sleep with open eyes	Weakness of the spleen and stomach in children
Preference for light (often open eyes)	Yang syndrome
Intolerance of light (often closed eyes)	Yin syndrome
Lacrimation	Wind–heat

Inspecting the ears

The kidneys open into the ears. The ears are the gathering places of all meridians. In addition, studies on ear acupuncture have further confirmed the close connection of the ears with the *zang–fu* organs and the four extremities.

According to the ancient literature, deficient conditions are often attributed to the kidneys, while excessive conditions are often attributed to *shaoyang* meridians. For example, dry thin ears indicate kidney yin deficiency; dark withered helices indicate extreme kidney water deficiency; small thin ears indicate kidney *qi* deficiency; redness and swelling of the helices indicate the ascending of liver fire or toxic fire transformed from damp–heat in the liver and gallbladder; pus discharge from the ear canal indicates the ascending of wind–heat in the kidney and *sanjiao* meridians, damp–heat in the liver and gallbladder or the ascending of liver fire due to kidney deficiency.

Inspecting the noses

The lung opens into the nose. The nose is associated with the spleen and stomach meridians. As a result, it can manifest the conditions of the lung, spleen and stomach. For example, nasal flaring in an acute febrile condition often indicates wind–heat accumulating in the lung, while nasal flaring in a chronic condition can be a fatal sign of the lung; the brandy nose indicates blood heat entering the lung. Nasal polyps indicate extreme lung heat. Nasal obstruction indicates heat attacking the *yangming* meridians. A dark yellow–withered nasal tip is a malignant sign due to severe damage to the fluids.

Inspecting the lips

The spleen opens into the mouth and its luster shows in the lips. Additionally, the stomach meridian winds around the lips. As a result, the lips can manifest the deficiency or excess of the spleen and stomach.

Conditions of the Lips	Indications
Pale lips	Blood deficiency, *qi* deficiency or cold
Red lips	Heat
Bluish	Cold or blood stasis
A dark circle around the mouth	Kidney failure
Dry cracked lips	Damage to fluids, contraction of dryness, spleen heat or febrile conditions damaging yin
Salivation	Internal dampness due to spleen deficiency, stomach heat or stroke
Lockjaw in children	Wind stirring
Inability to close the mouth	Deficiency of the lungs and spleen

Common mouth conditions also include painful mouth ulceration, sores and thrush (a yeast infection), which are often caused by heat accumulating in the heart and spleen or the damp–heat spleen meridian.

Inspecting the teeth and gums

The teeth are extensions of the bones. The kidneys dominate bones. Additionally, the stomach meridian enters the upper teeth and its collaterals reach the gums. As a result, the teeth and gums can tell about the conditions of the kidneys, intestines and stomach.

Observing the teeth

Loosened teeth with exposed roots indicate kidney deficiency. A delayed growth of teeth in children indicates kidney *qi* deficiency. Withered teeth indicate consumption of kidney essence. Teeth chattering most commonly indicates wind stirring. Teeth grinding during sleep indicates internal heat or indigestion.

Observing the gums

Pale gums indicate blood deficiency. Pale atrophic gums indicate deficiency of stomach yin or stomach *qi*. Red swollen gums indicate stomach fire. Bleeding of the gums coupled with redness and swelling indicates stomach heat damaging the collaterals. Bleeding of the gums with neither redness nor pain indicates *qi* deficiency alone or in combination with deficient fire.

Inspecting the skin

Inspecting the skin aims to observe the luster, moistening, sores, ulcers, maculae, white patches, carbuncles, gangrene or boils.

Erysipelas and fire flow (erysipelas of the shank) are often caused by internal accumulation of damp–heat.

Yang jaundice (bright yellow eyes and skin) is caused by damp–heat in the spleen and stomach, while yin jaundice (dull yellow eyes and skin) is caused by cold–dampness in the spleen and stomach.

Dry rough scaly skin is caused by stagnant blood.

Oval superficial vesicular skin rashes that can spontaneously resolve without left-behind marks are often caused by contraction of epidemic pathogens.

Yang maculae in a bright red color are caused by damp–heat entering the *ying* and blood, while yin maculae in a pale dark-purple color are caused by deficiency of *qi* and blood.

Measles in children are often secondary to a common cold, especially a fever of 3–4 days. Spots can be seen on the face, chest, abdomen and four extremities. Rubella is often caused by contraction of epidemic pathogens and characterized by intermittent tiny rashes with persistent itching. A mild fever may also be present. Urticaria is often caused by wind stirring due to blood deficiency.

Miliaria alba is commonly seen on the neck, nape, chest and abdomen, resulting from damp–heat affecting the skin. Gradually increased blisters indicate expulsion of damp–heat. Dry white blisters indicate insufficiency of fluids.

Red swollen elevated carbuncles are often caused by internal damp, heat and toxic fire. Diffuse swollen furuncles without discoloration, warmth or pain are often caused by deficiency of *qi* and blood with cold phlegm retention or wind and toxic heat in the five *zang* organs. Boils often start with small millets having a solid deep root and white tip. Scabies is often small and superficial. It may not cause redness, swelling or pain. It can resolve after rupture of the pus.

Inspecting the collaterals of the index fingers

This is a method for children under the age of three. It is also known as inspecting the three gates: wind gate (the proximal segment to the palm in the index finger), *qi* gate (the middle segment of the index finger) and vital gate (the distal segment to the palm in the index finger).

Examination method: gently hold the index finger using the left hand, and apply perpendicular pushing using the right hand from the fingertip to the palmar side a couple of times to expose the collaterals.

Regarding externally contracted febrile conditions, exposed collaterals in the wind gate indicate a mild condition after contracting pathogenic *qi*, exposed collaterals in the *qi* gate indicate pathogenic *qi* entering the meridians, and exposed collaterals in the vital gate indicate a critical condition where pathogenic *qi* enters the *zang–fu* organs. Furthermore, exposed collaterals on the tip of the index finger can be a fatal sign.

Inspecting the tongue (tongue diagnosis)

Tongue diagnosis is a key part of inspection and syndrome differentiation. A tongue condition can manifest the strength between antipathogenic *qi* and pathogenic factors, the depth and nature of the pathogens and disease progress in an objective way. It can also help to predict the prognosis and guide prescriptions. However, comprehensive analysis of the four examination methods is always necessary.

The heart opens into the tongue. The tongue can manifest the conditions of the spleen and stomach. In addition, the other *zang–fu* organs associate with the tongue through the meridians, divergent meridians or collaterals. Consequently, by observing the tongue, one can tell about the functions of the *zang–fu* organs.

The correlations between the *zang–fu* organs and the tongue are:
The root of the tongue — kidneys
The middle area of the tongue — spleen and stomach
The bilateral sides of the tongue — liver and gallbladder
The tip of the tongue — heart and lung

Examination methods and cautionary notes

Light. The light should be natural and clear. Colorful or reflected light should be avoided.

Posture. In a sitting position, open the mouth and naturally extend the tongue body. Tension, curve or strain should be avoided.

Diet. Food or medication may dye the tongue; for example, milk can leave a white coating; coffee, olive, soft drinks containing pigments or Chinese medicine decoctions may leave a brown coating; oranges and a powder of the Coptis root may leave a yellow coating; scraping or brushing the tongue coating may cause the coating to become thinner; spicy, cold or hot food can change the color of the tongue; and mouth breathing or drinking water can change the moistening of the tongue.

Additionally, geographic features, seasons, age and constitution may influence the tongue coating.

Contents of the tongue diagnosis

Normal tongue. A normal tongue appears pale red and moistening, coupled with flexible motility and a thin white coating.

Abnormal tongue colors and indications:

Colors of the Tongue	Indications
Pale white	Blood deficiency, *qi* deficiency, yang deficiency or cold syndrome
Red	Heat syndrome (excess or deficiency)
Crimson (dark red)	Heat entering the *ying* (nutrients) blood in externally contracted conditions; hyperactivity of fire due to yin deficiency in internally damaged conditions
Purple	Dark purple indicates heat damaging yin; bluish purple indicates cold retention, blood stasis or yang deficiency
Bluish	Cold retention or blood stasis

Abnormal tongue bodies and indications:

Tongue Bodies	Indications
Tough and old	Excess syndrome
Tender and delicate	Deficiency syndrome
Enlarged	Water, dampness and phlegm fluid
Swollen	Heat accumulating in the heart and spleen, excessive consumption of alcohol (often in a dark-purple color) or food poisoning (often in a dull bluish-purple color)
Thin	Deficiency of *qi* and blood (often in a pale color), yin deficiency (often in a red color) or hyperactivity of fire due to yin deficiency (often in a very red color)
Spotted and prickly	Heat syndrome
Fissured	Extreme heat damaging yin, blood deficiency or spleen deficiency
Mirrored	Yin deficiency or severe damage to stomach *qi*
Teeth-marked	Spleen deficiency with internal dampness

Abnormal tongue motilities and indications:

Tongue Motility	Indications
Stiff	Heat entering the pericardium, internal turbid phlegm or stroke
Flaccid	Damage to yin fluids or deficiency of *qi* and blood
Trembling	Deficiency or wind stirring
Deviated	Stroke
Protruding and waggling	Heat accumulating in the heart and spleen
Shortened	A critical condition

Abnormal coating colors and indications:

Color of the Tongue Coating	Indications
White	Exterior syndrome, cold syndrome
Yellow	Interior syndrome, heat syndrome
Gray or dark	Interior syndrome

Abnormal coating textures and indications:

Textures of the Tongue Coating	Indications
Thick	Interior syndrome or exuberant pathogenic factors
Slippery	Cold or dampness
Dry	Damage to fluids, heat or dryness
Greasy	Dampness, turbidity, phlegm fluid or food retention
Curdy	Food retention or phlegm turbidity
Peeling (complete or partial)	Damage to stomach *qi* and stomach yin

In summary, one can tell about the strength between antipathogenic *qi* and pathogenic factors, the depth and nature of the pathogens and disease progress by a comprehensive analysis of the aforementioned aspects of the tongue. For example, a pale swollen tongue with a thick greasy coating indicates spleen *qi* deficiency with internal phlegm dampness; a dark red trembling tongue with a dry peeling coating indicates heat entering the *ying* (nutrients) blood and damage to fluids.

QUESTIONS

1. What are the contents of tongue diagnosis?
2. What is a normal tongue like?
3. What are the clinical significances of a red tongue with a thick coating?
4. How do you differentiate an excess syndrome from a deficiency syndrome regarding a red tongue?
5. What are the tongue conditions of phlegm dampness?
6. What does a red tip of the tongue with a thin white coating indicate?

AUSCULTATION AND OLFACTION

Auscultation and olfaction aims to understand patients' conditions by listening to the sounds and smelling the odors. The sounds include speaking voices, speech, breathing, coughing, vomiting, hiccups, belching, sighing, sneezing and bowel sounds. The odors include a foul breath and offensive smells of the secretions and excretions.

Listening to the Sounds

Speaking voice

A high-pitched loud continuous voice indicates an excess syndrome, while a faint low intermittent voice indicates a deficiency syndrome.

Speech–abnormal speech and indications

Abnormal Speech	Indications
Reluctance to speak (silent, reserved)	Deficiency syndrome or cold syndrome
Restlessness with talkativeness	Excess syndrome or heat syndrome
Slurred speech	Wind phlegm obstructing the meridians or misting the brain
Paraphasia or soliloquy	Failure of heart *qi* to nourish the heart–mind
Manic raving	Yang heat excess syndrome
Delirium	Excess syndrome
Unconscious murmuring	Deficiency syndrome

Breathing

Fast breathing indicates an excess syndrome or heat syndrome, while faint slow breathing indicates a deficiency syndrome or cold syndrome. However, an excess syndrome may cause faint breathing and a deficiency syndrome may cause fast breathing. Other abnormal breathings include difficult breathing (in severe cases, breathing with an open mouth, raised shoulders, nasal flaring and an inability to lie flat may be present), shortness of breath and lack of *qi*. Except that lack of *qi* is caused by *qi* deficiency, other conditions in externally contracted or internally damaged conditions should be differentiated into cold, heat, deficiency and excess.

Coughing–abnormal coughs and indications

Abnormal Coughing Sounds	Indications
Unsmooth stuffy coughing	Wind–cold impairing lung *qi* or phlegm dampness with water fluid retention
Unproductive coughs or coughing with dyspnea	Insufficiency of fluids, contraction of dryness or yin damage in chronic conditions
Low faint coughing	Lung deficiency
Persistent coughing, especially at night	Kidney water deficiency
Severe coughing at dawn	Spleen deficiency with internal dampness

Other abnormal coughs include whooping coughs in children (characterized by a paroxysmal cough, an inspiratory whoop, and vomiting after coughing) and diphtheria (characterized by a barking cough).

Vomiting

Vomiting occurs when stomach *qi* ascends and forces the gastric contents, saliva or fluids out of the mouth. Some may experience only retching and nausea. This condition is known as *ou tu* in Chinese medicine ("*ou*" means concurrent vomiting sound and vomitus, while "*tu*" means vomitus coming out without vomiting sound).

Mild vomiting mixed with thin clear odorless vomitus indicates a deficiency, cold syndrome, while violent vomiting mixed with sticky foul-smelling vomitus indicates an excessive heat syndrome.

Regarding acid regurgitation, vomiting in the evening of food ingested in the morning and vice versa may also occur.

Hiccups

Hiccups occur as a result of adverse ascending of stomach *qi*. Acute loud hiccups are often caused by pathogenic factors attacking the stomach. Low faint hiccups in a chronic condition can be a fatal sign indicating depletion of stomach *qi*.

Generally, high-pitched frequent hiccups indicate an excess heat syndrome, while faint weak hiccups indicate a deficiency cold syndrome.

Hiccups with failure of *qi* to pass through the throat indicate *qi* deficiency of the spleen and stomach. Occasional hiccups in healthy people can resolve spontaneously.

Belching

Belching also occurs as a result of adverse ascending of stomach *qi*. Belching coupled with indigestion, gastric fullness and distension and a fetid breath indicates food retention, while loud belching that is associated with emotions indicates liver *qi* attacking the stomach.

Sighing

Sighing often indicates liver *qi* stagnation or fatigue.

Sneezing

Acute sneezing indicates external pathogens impairing the dispersing and descending of lung *qi*, while sneezing in a chronic condition is often a favorable sign of near-recovery.

Bowel sounds

Bowel sounds can be caused by disordered *qi* activity in the abdomen, phlegm fluid retention, contraction of external wind, cold or dampness, or deficiency of the spleen and stomach.

Smelling the Odor

A foul breath

A foul breath may indicate disharmony of stomach *qi* (due to stomach heat or food retention), dental caries, an unclean oral cavity or mouth ulceration.

Sweat odor

A foul-smelling sweat odor may indicate wind–damp–heat accumulating in the skin.

Sputum odor

Coughing with turbid foul-smelling sputum containing pus or blood indicates lung abscesses.

Stools

Stools that stink indicate heat, while stools with a fishy smell indicate cold. Flatus with a stinking odor indicates poor digestion.

Urine

Turbid yellow smelly urine often indicates damp–heat.

Menstruation or leukorrhea

Menstruation or leukorrhea that stinks indicates heat, while menstruation or leukorrhea with a fishy smell indicates cold.

A fetid body odor indicates dysfunction of the *zang–fu* organs. A blood-smelling body odor indicates loss of blood. A urine-smelling body odor often indicates uremia (later stages of edema). A rotten-apple-smelling body odor indicates a critical condition of diabetes.

In summary, loud, fast or heavy sounds often indicate an excess syndrome, while faint, slow or weak sounds often indicate a deficiency syndrome. A fetid odor often indicates an excess or heat syndrome, while an odorless or fishy smell often indicates a deficiency or cold syndrome.

Case Studies

Case 1

A 23-year-old male patient suffered from coughs for a couple of years, together with hoarseness. According to his family members, he never received treatment. Zhang Zi-he then prescribed formulas containing bitter medicinals, followed by *Zhōu Chē Jì Chuān Wán* (舟车济川丸, "Vessel and Vehicle Fluid–Replenishing Pill"). The patient recovered quickly.

Remarks. Based on the symptoms and case history, this patient should be diagnosed as having pathogenic factors impairing the dispersing and descending of lung *qi*. As a result, Zhang Zi-he prescribed formulas to remove pathogens and obtained a fast effect.

Case 2

A middle-aged male patient suffered from insomnia, fatigue, coughing with yellow purulent sputum and hoarseness. The physician prescribed four doses of *Xiǎo Qīng Lóng Tāng* (小青龙汤, "Minor Green Dragon Decoction"). After taking the prescribed decoction, the patient experienced blood-stained sputum, which was aggravated after a couple of days, along with bleeding from the mouth. The bleeding stopped after a while but recurred dozens of times. The pulse was wiry, big, scattering and weak, especially in the *chi* region of the right hand. Since overexertion and contraction of cold mainly contributed to this patient's condition, formulas containing pungent, sweet and dry-heat medicinals might cause bleeding or even subsequent lung atrophy. The physician then prescribed a formula containing *rén shēn* (人参, *Radix et Rhizoma Ginseng*), *huáng qí* (黄芪, *Radix Astragali*), *dāng guī* (当归, *Radix Angelicae Sinensis*), *bái zhú* (白术, *Rhizoma Atractylodis Macrocephalae*), *bái sháo* (白芍, *Radix Paeoniae Alba*), *chén pí* (陈皮, *Pericarpium Citri Reticulatae*), *gān cǎo* (甘草, *Radix et Rhizoma Glycyrrhizae*) and *má huáng* (麻黄, *Herba Ephedrae*). The patient was asked to drink the decoction with the juice of *ǒu jié* (藕节, *Nodus Nelumbinis Rhizomatis*). Two days later, the coughs stopped. The bleeding also stopped after he took an additional four doses of the same formula by removing *má huáng*. However, the pulse was still scattering, coupled with a poor appetite and severe fatigue. Then the formula was remodified by removing the juice of *ǒu jié* but adding *huáng qín* (黄芩, *Radix Scutellariae*), *shā rén* (砂仁, *Fructus Amomi*) and *bàn xià* (半夏, *Rhizoma Pinelliae*). After another two weeks, the patient made a full recovery.

Remarks. Based on the symptoms and case history, this patient should be diagnosed as having combined deficiency and excess. The first formula did not work well since it only acts to remove pathogenic factors. Despite the fact that both patients suffered from hoarseness, it is still necessary to make careful pattern identification.

QUESTIONS

1. What are the contents of auscultation?
2. What are the contents of smelling odors? How do you differentiate cold, heat, deficiency and excess?

INQUIRY

Inquiry aims to, by asking patients or the accompanying persons, collect information regarding the disease occurrence, development, treatment, present symptoms and other relevant data including life habits, hobbies and family histories, etc.

Cautionary Notes

First, focus on the chief complaints and try to obtain an overall understanding of the patient's condition.
Second, ask nicely and patiently.
Third, do not mislead the patient with hints.

Contents of Inquiry

Inquiry regarding the general information

This includes questions regarding the patient's name, age, gender, marital status, nationality, occupation and residential address. It is also necessary to note the date of the visit or the patient's telephone number for the future followup. This background information can help one to get a better understanding of the actual conditions. For example, women often have problems involving menstruation, leukorrhea, pregnancy or childbirth. Those working in humid places are more susceptible to contraction of dampness. Summer heat and dampness is more common in summer, and dryness is more common in autumn.

Inquiry regarding the lifestyle

This includes questions regarding life experience, food preferences, daily activities and lifestyles. Those who have been through adversities tend to have liver *qi* stagnation. Food preferences may impair the functions of the *zang–fu* organs. Occupations may also cause specific conditions. In addition, irregular lifestyles can contribute to numerous conditions.

Inquiry regarding the family history and past case history

This includes questions regarding the patient's genetic or contagious diseases. The past case history can probably indicate the inducing factor or primary causes of the present conditions.

Inquiry regarding the onset

This includes questions regarding the onset time, inducing factors, progression and treatment. These questions can help one to evaluate the causative factors of the disease, the pathogenic nature, the strength between antipathogenic *qi* and pathogenic factors, and the prognosis.

Inquiry regarding the present symptoms

Regarding the present symptoms, the following 10 questions are commonly asked, in sequence.

Inquiry regarding chills and fever

This question is especially indicated for patients who mainly present with fever and chills.

Chills and fever

Concurrent chills and fever indicate an exterior syndrome. Some physicians believe that severe chills with a mild fever indicate an exterior cold syndrome, while mild chills with a high fever indicate an exterior heat syndrome. This coupled with mild sweating can be diagnosed as disharmony between the *ying* and the *wei*.

Chills without fever

Chills without fever can be caused by either external contraction or interior cold. Chills that can be alleviated by warmth are known as intolerance of cold and ascribed to interior, deficiency cold. Chills that cannot be alleviated by warmth are known as aversion to cold and ascribed to exterior excess cold. An acute condition often results from external cold, while a chronic condition often causes interior cold.

Fever without chills

Fever without chills can be subdivided into three types: strong fever, tidal fever and mild fever.

Subtypes	Manifestations	Indications
Strong fever	A high-grade fever, a red face, a big surging pulse, thirst with desire to drink water and profuse sweating	Pathogenic factors transforming into heat after entering the interior (a fierce struggle between *wei* (defense) and pathogenic factors)
Tidal fever	Later afternoon tidal fever (3–5 p.m.), bloating and constipation	*Yangming* tidal fever (heat accumulating in the stomach and large intestine)
	Afternoon tidal (hidden) fever, coupled with dampness symptoms	Tidal fever due to warm–dampness
	A low-grade fever (especially in the afternoon or at night), rosy cheeks, night sweats, weight loss and a red tongue with a scanty coating	Tidal fever due to yin deficiency
Mild fever	A mild-grade fever	Recovery stage of internally damaged and externally contracted conditions

Alternating chills with fever

An alternating chill with fever is often seen in *shaoyang* disease or malaria.

Inquiry regarding the sweating

This includes questions about the presence or absence of sweating, profuse or scanty sweating, time and body parts of sweating, as well as other associated symptoms.

Sweating in an exterior syndrome

An exterior syndrome is characterized by an acute onset, a short duration, and concurrent chills and fever. A headache and a stuffy nose may also be present. Sweating in an exterior syndrome is often caused by disharmony between the *ying* and the *wei* (i.e. the *taiyang* wind invasion pattern). In addition, wind–heat or wind–dampness attacking the exterior may cause an exterior syndrome with sweating.

Sweating in an interior syndrome

Sweating in an interior syndrome can be seen either in pathogenic factors entering the interior in an externally contracted condition or in internally damaged conditions. It can be subdivided into four types: spontaneous sweating, night sweats, profuse sweating and shiver sweating.

Subtypes	Associated Symptoms	Indications
Spontaneous sweating	Sweating for no reason or after a mild exertion, mental fatigue, lassitude, intolerance of cold and susceptibility to the common cold	*Qi* or yang deficiency
Night sweats	Sweats during sleep, tidal fever and rosy cheeks	Yin deficiency
Profuse sweating	A strong fever, a red face, thirst and a big surging pulse	Excessive heat syndrome
	Pallor, cold limbs and a faint pulse	Yang depletion
Shiver sweating	Sweating following chills and shivering	Exuberant pathogenic factor with antipathogenic *qi* deficiency

Sweating in specific body areas

For sweating on the head, cold, heat, deficiency and excess should be differentiated.

Hemilateral sweating is often caused by blockage of the ipsolateral meridians.

For sweating on the soles and palms, deficiency and excess should be distinguished according to other systemic signs and symptoms.

Inquiry regarding the head and body

Headache

For headache, the questions will focus on the position and nature.

Position

Forehead headache — *yangming* meridians
Temporal headache — *shaoyang* meridians
Occipital headache — *taiyang* meridians
Parietal headache — *jueyin* meridians

Headache without specific positions should be differentiated according to other associated signs and symptoms.

Nature

An acute severe persistent headache — external contraction
Headache with a severe chill — wind–cold headache
Headache with a red face and sore throat — wind–heat headache
Headache with a sensation of being wrapped in a towel and heaviness of the extremities — wind–dampness headache
A chronic dull headache — internally damaged headache

Dizziness

Mild dizziness can be alleviated by closing the eyes, while severe dizziness may cause spinning, nausea and vomiting. The differentiation of deficiency and excess is similar to that for headache. It is also necessary to combine information collected by the four examination methods. Common contributing factors of dizziness are ascending of liver yang, internal phlegm dampness, deficiency of *qi* and blood, and insufficiency of kidney essence.

Inquiry regarding the chest, hypochondrium, epigastrium and abdomen

Since the heart and lungs reside in the chest, chest tightness and pain are often associated with the heart and lungs. Heart conditions may cause chest *bi* (impediment) and cardiac pain that are similar to angina pectoris. Patients may present with chest pain radiating to the shoulder and back, pallor and cold limbs. These symptoms (more commonly seen in middle-aged or elderly people) can be aggravated by fatigue or emotional fluctuations.

Chest pain due to lung conditions is often accompanied by coughing, sputum or dyspnea. Chest discomfort, breast distension and pain are often associated with *qi* stagnation.

Discomfort or pain in the hypochondriac regions is often associated with the liver.

The epigastrium is the upper central region of the abdomen. An epigastric discomfort is most commonly associated with the spleen and stomach. An epigastric pain with a cold sensation is often caused by cold, while a burning epigastric pain coupled with a foul breath and constipation is often caused by heat. An epigastric pain relating to emotions is caused by liver *qi* stagnation or liver *qi* affecting the stomach. A chronic epigastric pain is often associated with yin deficiency, yang deficiency or stagnant blood. An epigastric pain in children is often caused by indigestion or parasites.

Generally, the abdomen can be subdivided into three regions: central abdomen (periumbilical area), lower abdomen (below the umbilicus) and lateral lower abdomen. Disorders of the central abdomen are often associated with the spleen and stomach, disorders of the lower abdomen with the urinary bladder, and disorders of the lateral lower abdomen with the liver (meridian). The uterus is also located in the lower abdomen; it is, therefore, necessary to inquire regarding menstruation, leukorrhea, pregnancy and childbirth for lower abdominal discomfort in women.

Inquiry regarding the ears and eyes

Ears

Common ear problems include tinnitus, deafness and being hard of hearing.

Tinnitus

A sudden onset of loud ringing sounds within the ear is often seen in an excess syndrome, and chronic low ringing sounds within the ear in a deficiency syndrome. An excess syndrome is mainly caused by fire in the liver, gallbladder or *sanjiao*, and a deficiency syndrome by the failure of kidney essence to nurture the ears.

Deafness

Acute deafness is often seen in an excess syndrome, and chronic deafness in a deficiency syndrome. An excess syndrome can be caused by cold damage, febrile conditions or the common cold, and a deficiency syndrome by aging or deficiency of the heart and kidneys.

Being hard of hearing

Being hard of hearing (also known as hearing impairment) shares a similar pathogenesis with deafness.

Eyes

Common eye problems are dizzy vision, blurred vision and eye pain. Acute eye conditions are often seen in an excess syndrome, and chronic eye conditions in a deficiency syndrome. An excess syndrome can be caused by wind and phlegm, while a deficiency syndrome is often associated with the liver and kidneys.

Inquiry regarding the diet and taste

Thirst and drink

Thirst with desire to drink plenty of water is often caused by exuberant heat damaging fluids. It can be seen in an excessive heat syndrome in externally contracted conditions, diabetes or damage to fluids by profuse sweating, vomiting and diarrhea.

Thirst with no desire to drink water is often caused by yin deficiency, damp-heat, phlegm-fluid and stagnant blood.

Appetite

A poor appetite, reduced food ingestion and even loss of appetite: A poor appetite, reduced food ingestion and even loss of appetite in chronic conditions are often caused by deficiency of the spleen and stomach. In severe cases, these can be a fatal sign of stomach *qi* depletion. These symptoms in acute conditions are often caused by dampness obstructing the spleen, damp–heat in the liver and gallbladder, and food retention. Hunger with no appetite indicates stomach yin deficiency. Additionally, women during early pregnancy may experience these symptoms.

Fast hunger with an increased appetite: Fast hunger even with an increased appetite is often caused by hyperactivity of stomach fire.

Food preferences: Food preferences can be seen in special folk customs, pregnancy or intestinal parasites.

A sudden increased appetite in a critical condition: This can be a fatal sign of depletion of stomach *qi*.

Taste:

Tastes	Indications
Tastelessness (bland)	Spleen deficiency or dampness affecting the spleen and stomach
Sweet taste with a greasy sticky sensation	Indigestion or dampness affecting the spleen and stomach
Sour taste or acid reflux	Disharmony between the liver and the stomach
Sour fetid taste	Indigestion
Bitter taste	Heat syndrome
Salty taste	Kidney problems

Inquiry regarding sleep

Insomnia

Insomnia (also known as sleeplessness) can manifest as difficulty in falling asleep, waking up frequently during the night, interrupted sleep, sleeplessness throughout the night and dream(nightmare)-disturbed sleep.

Deficiency patterns of insomnia are often caused by yin blood deficiency of the heart, spleen and kidneys, and excess patterns of insomnia by fire, heat, phlegm and food retention affecting the heart, gallbladder and stomach.

Somnolence

Somnolence (or "drowsiness") is a state of near-sleep, a strong desire for sleep, or sleeping for unusually long periods. This is often caused by spleen deficiency, yang–qi deficiency or internal phlegm dampness. In addition, somnolence can be a fatal sign preceding a coma, caused by yang failure of the heart and kidneys or pathogenic factors entering the pericardium.

Inquiry regarding bowel movements and urination

Bowel movements

Constipation: Constipation refers to bowel movements that are infrequent and/or feces that are hard to pass. It is often caused by damage to fluids or deficiency of *qi* and fluids resulting from chronic conditions, aging or childbirth.

Diarrhea: Diarrhea is most commonly caused by cold, dampness, food retention, spleen deficiency or liver *qi* attacking the spleen.

Other abnormal bowel movements include diarrhea mixed with undigested food, loose stools, diarrhea alternating with constipation, stools containing mucus and blood (dysentery), tenesmus and fecal incontinence. For blood in the stools, a tarry color indicates distal bleeding, and a bright red color proximal bleeding.

Urination

Profuse urine: Profuse urine can be caused by deficiency and cold syndrome or diabetes.

Scanty urine: Scanty urine can be caused by damage to fluids, impaired *qi* transformation or water–dampness retention.

Other abnormal urination problems include urine retention and block-age, urine dribbling, urinary incontinence, enuresis and increased urina-tion at night (associated with kidney deficiency). Painful hesitant urination with urgency and a burning sensation is often caused by damp–heat in the urinary bladder.

Inquiry regarding menstruation, leukorrhea, pregnancy and childbirth

Menstruation

Menstruation is a woman's monthly bleeding. Starting from the age of 13–15, it often lasts 3–5 days, in the range of approximately 28 days apart. The menstruation appears red in color. Blood clots may be present. There is no menstruation during pregnancy or breastfeeding. Most women experience menopause around the age of 49. Irregular menstrua-tions include earlier (8–9 days) period, delayed (8–9 days) period, dys-menorrhea, amenorrhea (longer than 3 months), and metrorrhagia and metrostaxis.

Irregular menstruations are often associated with the liver, spleen and kidneys. Excess patterns can be caused by cold, heat, stagnant blood or phlegm dampness, and deficiency patterns by deficiency of *qi*, blood, yin or yang.

Leukorrhea

Physiological leukorrhea refers to leukorrhea due to estrogen stimulation. Pathological leukorrhea denotes a thick, whitish or yellowish vaginal dis-charge. Profuse white thin odorless leukorrhea indicates spleen deficiency with internal cold–dampness. Profuse yellow sticky foul-smelling leukor-rhea indicates downward flow of damp–heat. Red or red–white thick leukorrhea with a mild foul smell often indicates liver *qi* stagnation trans-forming into fire.

Pregnancy

Common pregnancy problems include morning sickness (characterized by loss of appetite, nausea, vomiting or even an inability to ingest food) and threatened miscarriage (characterized by a falling sensation of the lower abdomen, low back soreness and pain or vaginal bleeding).

Childbirth

Lochiorrhea refers to persistent profuse flow of the lochia for longer than 20 days after childbirth. It can be caused by *qi* deficiency, blood heat or blood stasis.

Inquiry regarding children's conditions

For neonatal (within one month cases), ask about the birth conditions. For infants, ask about the feeding and development (such as sitting, crawling, standing, walking, tooth growth and time to learn to talk). For babies older than six months, ask about the vaccination or contact histories of contagious diseases. It is often necessary to understand the causative factors for infantile conditions, such as feeding, fright, contraction of cold, fever, coughing, crying, vomiting and diarrhea.

QUESTIONS

1. What are the contents of inquiry?
2. What are the cautionary notes of inquiry?
3. How do you ask about the present symptoms?
4. Describe the contents of chills without fever and fever without chills.
5. How do you understand insomnia and somnolence?
6. How do you understand blurred vision and being hard of hearing?
7. What are the common symptoms of dietary disorders?
8. What are the common symptoms of abnormal bowel movements and urination?
9. What are the main inquiry contents for female patients?
10. What are the characteristics of inquiry regarding children?

PALPATION

Palpation is a method of touching, palpating or pressing the patient's body to obtain medical information. It includes two parts: feeling the pulse and palpating or pressing the body areas, such as the skin, hands, feet, chest and abdomen.

Feeling the Pulse (Pulse Diagnosis)

A systemic theory about pulse diagnosis can be traced back to over 2000 years ago. The human body is full of blood vessels. The *zang–fu* organs and tissues are nurtured by the nutrients absorbed by the spleen and stomach via the meridians. The vessels are the containers of blood and pathways for *qi* and blood to circulate. Consequently, the pulse conditions are closely related to the organs, *qi* and blood, and can manifest the disease location and nature as well as the strength between antipathogenic *qi* and pathogenic factors. However, other examination methods need to be integrated prior to diagnosis of a medical condition.

Three methods of pulse diagnosis

There are three methods of pulse diagnosis: three regions and nine positions of pulse-taking, three-region pulse-taking and *cunkou* pulse-taking.

Three regions and nine positions of pulse-taking

The three regions include the head, hands and feet. Each region has three positions: specifically, three positions on the head — frontal artery for *qi* of the forehead triangle, anterior auricular artery for *qi* of the ears and eyes, and buccal artery for *qi* of the mouth and teeth; three positions on the hands — *cunkou* (radial artery) for the lungs — *shenmen* (HT 7) point for the heart and *hegu* (LI 4) for chest *qi*; three positions on the feet — the area between *zuwuli* (LR 10) and *taichong* (LR 3) for the liver, the area between *jimen* (SP 11) and *chongyang* (ST 42) for the spleen and stomach, and *taixi* (KI 3) for the kidneys.

Three-region pulse-taking

The three regions include *renying* (ST 9), *cunkou* and *chongyang* (ST 42) (the dorsal artery of the feet).

Cunkou *pulse-taking*

The method of *cunkou* pulse-taking was initiated in the *Inner Classic* (*Nei Jing*, 黄帝内经) and further promoted in the *Pulse Classic* (*Mai Jing*, 脉经).

Cunkou refers to the pulsation area of the radial artery. The part slightly below the styloid process of the radius is the *guan* region, the part anterior to *guan* is the *cun* region and the part posterior to *guan* is the *chi* region.

The correlations between the *cunkou* regions and the *zang-fu* organs are as follows:

Cun region on the left hand — heart and chest
Guan region on the left hand — liver, gallbladder and diaphragm
Chi region on the left hand — kidneys and lower abdomen
Cun region on the right hand — lungs and chest
Guan region on the right hand — spleen and stomach
Chi region on the right hand — kidneys and lower abdomen

Methods of pulse-taking and cautionary notes

Time and length of pulse-taking

Traditionally, the best time for pulse-taking is in the morning. This is not necessary nowadays. It usually takes 3–5 min to feel the pulse.

Posture of pulse-taking

There are two requirements for posture in pulse-taking. One is to sit up or lie supinely with a fully relaxed state. The other is to extend the arms naturally at the same level as the heart. Place a cushion beneath the wrist to relax the wrist.

Finger technique

Generally, feel the patient's right hand using the left hand or vice versa. Place the middle finger on the *guan* region first, and then place the index finger on the *cun* region and ring finger on the *chi* region. Place the three fingers in an arc to feel the pulse, using the most sensitive sites of the finger pulps. The arrangement of the fingers depends on the height of the patient. The physician can press three fingers together or lift up two fingers and feel the condition of one specific region.

Touching, pressing and searching

Touching, pressing and searching are essential methods in pulse-taking. The subtle feeling of the pulse conditions can only be experienced through practice.

Case Studies

Case 1

A 23-year-old male patient came to Luo Qian-fu with complaints of fever, muscle wasting, heaviness and weakness of the four extremities, night sweats, loose stools, bowel sounds, a poor appetite, tastelessness and reluctance to talk for more than six months. The pulse was floating, rapid and weak upon pressing. The physician prescribed tonic formulas containing sweet and warm-property medicinals. The patient recovered.

Remarks. Despite a fever and a rapid pulse, the physician felt a weak pulse upon pressing, which indicates deficiency. As a result, Dr. Luo prescribed sweet and warm-property medicinals instead of bitter or cold-property ones.

Case 2

An elderly male patient came to Zhu Dan-xi with complaints of dizziness, blurred vision, a heavy sensation of the head, weakness of the hands and feet, and production of profuse sputum. The pulse was scattered, big and moderate on the left hand, and not so big and moderate on the right hand.

However, the pulse was weak on both hands upon pressing. In addition, the patient suffered from reduced ingestion, mild thirst, and one bowel movement every four days. Dr. Zhu prescribed a formula of condensed decoction containing *rén shēn* (人参, *Radix et Rhizoma Ginseng*), *huáng qí* (黄芪, *Radix Astragali*), *dāng guī* (当归, *Radix Angelicae Sinensis*), *bái sháo* (白芍, *Radix Paeoniae Alba*), *bái zhú* (白术, *Rhizoma Atractylodis Macrocephalae*) and *chén pí* (陈皮, *Pericarpium Citri Reticulatae*), coupled with 30 pills of *Lián Bǎi Wán* (连柏丸, Coptis and Cortex Phellodendri Chinensis Pill). After taking the formulas for one year, the patient completely recovered.

Remarks. The good effect of this patient was also attributed to the precise pulse diagnosis. If the pulse was deep, excessive and powerful (instead of being scattered), there was no way to prescribe the abovementioned formula.

QUESTIONS

1. Why can pulse conditions manifest the *qi* and blood of the five *zang* organs?
2. What are the three regions and nine positions for pulse-taking?
3. How do you understand the touching, pressing and searching in pulse-taking?

Contents of Pulse Diagnosis

A normal pulse

A normal pulse feels moderate and is approximately 72 times per minute, along with a regular rhythm. It is characterized by the presence of "stomach, spirit and root". The "stomach" and "spirit" here refer to the feeling of moderation. The "root" here refers to a powerful sensation upon pressing. The pulse can be influenced by seasons, climate, geographic locations, gender, age, constitution, emotions or diet; the characteristics of the "stomach, spirit and root" should always be present in a normal pulse.

Abnormal pulses

There are 28 abnormal pulses. Their descriptions and indications are listed in the following table:

Pulses	Descriptions	Indications
Floating	Feeling by mild touching, but weak upon pressing	An exterior syndrome. A floating, big and weak pulse indicates a deficiency syndrome.
Deep	Feeling only by pressing	An interior syndrome. A deep powerful pulse indicates excess, while a deep weak pulse indicates deficiency.
Rapid	Over 90 times/min	A heat syndrome. A rapid powerful pulse indicates excess, while a rapid weak pulse indicates deficiency.
Slow	Less than 60 times/min	A cold syndrome. A slow powerful pulse indicates cold accumulation, while a slow weak pulse indicates deficiency cold.
Surging (big)	Feeling like tidal waves	Exuberant heat in the *qi* phase. A surging weak pulse indicates deficiency.
	Wide pulse (big)	A big powerful pulse indicates excess, while a big weak pulse indicates deficiency.
Thready (small)	Thin like thread	A deficiency syndrome.
Faint	Thready and weak	Severe deficiency of yang *qi*
Scattered	Rootless and can hardly feel it by pressing	*Qi* collapse
Excessive (replenished)	Powerful by both touching and pressing	An excess syndrome
Deficient (feeble)	Weak by both touching and pressing	A deficiency syndrome
Slippery	Feeling like beads on a plate	Phlegm, food retention, excessive heat or pregnancy
Unsmooth (hesitant)	Feeling like scraping bamboo using a knife	Blood stasis or damage to the essence blood
Long	Extended pulse	A hyperactivity syndrome

(*Continued*)

(*Continued*)

Pulses	Descriptions	Indications
Short	Shortened pulse	A short powerful pulse indicates *qi* stagnation; a short weak pulse indicates *qi* damage
Wiry	Feeling like musical strings	Liver and gallbladder problems, pain or phlegm fluid retention
Tight	Feeling tense	Cold, pain or food retention
Tympanic	Feeling tight but empty	Loss of blood and essence, miscarriage or metrostaxis
Firm	Replenished, big, wiry and long	Internal yin cold, hernia or abdominal masses
Hidden	Feeling only by heavy pressing	Exuberant pathogens, syncope and intense pain
Hollow	Floating, big and hollow, feeling like a scallion	Loss of blood or yin damage
Soggy (soft)	Floating, thready and weak	Deficiency or dampness
Weak	Deep, thready and soft	Deficiency of *qi* and blood
Moderate	Approximately 60 times/min	Dampness or weakness of the spleen and stomach
Stirred (arterial pulsation)	Feeling like beans, slippery, rapid and powerful	Pain or fright
Swift	More than 120 times/min	Yin–yang exhaustion and *qi* collapse
Abrupt	Irregularly rapid	Excessive heat with exuberant yang, phlegm fluid, food retention or pain
Irregularly intermittent	Pulsation stops irregularly	Exuberant yin, *qi* stagnation, cold phlegm, blood stasis or abdominal masses
Regularly intermittent	Pulsation stops regularly	*Qi* deficiency of the *zang* organs

According to some scholars, the 28 pulses can be generalized into 6 categories:

Categories	Pulses
Floating pulses	Floating, surging, soggy (soft), scattered, hollow and tympanic
Deep pulses	Deep, hidden, firm and weak
Slow pulses	Slow, moderate, unsmooth (hesitant) and irregularly intermittent
Rapid pulses	Rapid, abrupt, swift and stirred
Feeble (deficient) pulses	Deficient, faint, thready, regularly intermittent and short
Replenished (excessive) pulses	Excessive, slippery, tight, long and wiry

In clinical practice, the above pulse conditions can occur in combination. Some pulses consist of multiple pulse conditions; for example, a weak pulse feels deficient, deep and small. Pulse diagnosis requires consistent practice.

Pulse-symptom consistency and preference

Generally, pulse-symptom consistency indicates a favorable prognosis, while pulse-symptom reversal (for example, a deficient pulse in an excess syndrome) often indicates an unfavorable one. Pulse-symptom reversal occurs when a medical condition is extremely complicated or when the pulse or symptoms are false. Under these circumstances, it is necessary to either prefer symptoms to pulse conditions or vice versa. For example, a thready pulse occurs along with abdominal pain, distension and fullness, tenderness, constipation and a red tongue with a yellow thick coating. The thready pulse here is caused by heat impairing the blood circulation. As a result, the treatment plan should be based on the symptoms instead of the pulse condition. For another example, take a high fever, a slippery rapid pulse and cold limbs. The symptom of cold limbs here is caused by heat blockage. The treatment should therefore be based on the pulse condition.

In summary, comprehensive analysis by the four examination methods is always necessary for a correct diagnosis.

Palpation

Palpating the skin can investigate cold, heat, dry, moistening or edema of the skin surface.

Palpating the hands and feet can investigate the cold or heat of the body.

Palpating the chest can investigate the strength of precordial *qi*. Pressing the abdomen can investigate cold, heat, pain, distension, masses, lumps or intestinal parasites.

Pressing specific acupuncture points can investigate the presence of nodules, sensitive reactions or tenderness, and thus provide understanding of the disorders of relevant *zang–fu* organs and meridians.

QUESTIONS

1. What are the common features of the 28 abnormal pulses?
2. How do you differentiate a floating pulse from surging, soft, scattered, hollow and tympanic pulses?
3. Describe the characteristics and indications of deficient (feeble), thready, faint, regularly intermittent and short pulses.

CHAPTER 3

The Eight Principles

CONCEPT

The eight principles include exterior, interior, cold, heat, deficiency, excess, yin and yang. Syndrome differentiation (pattern identification) of the eight principles is an essential paradigm in the Chinese medicine system.

Pattern identification of the eight principles aims to tell about the disease location, the pathogenic nature and the strength between antipathogenic *qi* and pathogenic factors, thus generalizing the condition into eight categories.

The eight principles can be divided into four pairs: interior/exterior for the depth of pathogens; cold/heat for the disease nature; deficiency/excess for the strength between antipathogenic *qi* and pathogenic factors; and yin/yang for the preponderance of yin and yang. However, yin and yang can also generalize the other six principles: exterior, heat and excess are ascribed to yang, and interior, cold and deficiency to yin.

Two or more principles may occur concurrently, such as an exterior cold syndrome and an interior deficiency cold syndrome. A combined deficiency and excess may also be present. The principles may transform into each other as well, such as cold transforming into heat, or the exterior entering the interior. Additionally, a true cold may sometimes manifest as a false heat or vice versa.

EXTERIOR SYNDROME AND INTERIOR SYNDROME

Differentiation of an exterior from an interior syndrome aims to tell about the disease location and is indicated for externally contracted febrile conditions.

Internally damaged miscellaneous conditions are not associated with contraction of external pathogens, and therefore do not have an exterior syndrome.

Generally, exterior and interior can be classified as follows: the body surface and meridians are ascribed to the exterior, and the *zang–fu* organs to the interior. Furthermore, the yang meridians and their attributed *fu* organs are ascribed to the exterior, and the yin meridians and their attributed *zang* organs to the interior. In terms of syndrome differentiation, the exterior mainly refers to the skin, skin hair and striae, and the interior to the *zang–fu* organs.

Exterior Syndrome

Overview

An exterior syndrome occurs when external pathogens attack the body through the skin, skin hair, mouth or nose. It often has a sudden onset, with a short duration.

Clinical manifestations

Fever, chills (or aversion to wind), headache, muscle ache, a thin white tongue coating and a floating pulse occur; a stuffy or runny nose, a sore or scratchy throat and coughing may also be present.

Analysis

Typically, an acute condition with concurrent fever and chills (or aversion to wind) can be diagnosed as an exterior syndrome. Pathogenic factors binding the *wei* (defense) may cause chills. The strength between *wei* (defense) and pathogens may cause a fever. The presence of other associated symptoms, such as headache, a general ache, a stuffy or runny nose or sneezing, can still be diagnosed as an exterior syndrome. However, a thin coating and a floating pulse are not necessarily the diagnostic basis for an exterior syndrome, except that they only mean that there is no interior syndrome.

Interior Syndrome

Overview

An interior syndrome occurs as a result of three conditions: external pathogens entering the interior; external pathogens directly attacking the *zang–fu* organs; and emotions, an improper diet or overexertion impairing the *zang–fu* organs.

Clinical manifestations

Unlike the exterior syndrome, there are no typical signs and symptoms for an interior syndrome due to complicated causative factors and extensive locations. External pathogens entering the interior may cause a strong fever, restlessness, unconsciousness, thirst, abdominal pain, constipation, diarrhea, vomiting, scanty dark-yellow urine, a yellow or white, thick, greasy tongue coating and a deep pulse. A history of an exterior syndrome is essential to diagnosing external pathogens entering the interior.

Analysis

Among the aforementioned symptoms, a strong fever, thirst, scanty dark-yellow urine and a yellow coating indicate a heat syndrome; restlessness and unconsciousness indicate pathogenic factors disturbing the heart–mind; abdominal pain, constipation, diarrhea and vomiting indicate pathogenic factors affecting the spleen and stomach; and a thick tongue coating and a deep pulse indicate an interior location.

Other than an exterior syndrome and an interior syndrome, the following syndromes may be present:

Half-Exterior Half-Interior Syndrome

This occurs when pathogenic factors remain between the exterior and the interior. Typical clinical manifestations include chills alternating with fever, fullness in the chest and hypochondrium, restlessness, vomiting, a poor appetite, a bitter taste, a dry throat, blurred vision and a wiry pulse. This syndrome can be seen in *shaoyang* disease.

Concurrent Exterior and Interior Syndrome

This occurs when an unresolved exterior syndrome enters the interior or externally-contracted and internally damaged conditions develop successively.

Inward Penetration of Exterior Pathogens to the Interior

This refers to the disease progression of an unresolved exterior syndrome affecting the interior.

Outward Penetration of Interior Pathogens to the Exterior

This refers to a favorable sign of outward penetration of interior pathogens. For example, a patient may present with fever, restlessness, coughing and chest tightness at first, but the fever may be subdued after sweating or eruptions.

Case Studies

Case 1

Due to a sudden weather change and subsequent contraction of a cold, a patient started (on the next day) to suffer from headache, chills, a stuffy runny nose, and soreness and pain on the neck, back and four extremities. The body temperature was 39.5°C. The pulse was rapid and the tongue coating was thin and white.

Remark. This case should be differentiated into an exterior syndrome. Diagnostic basis: concurrent chills and fever, a history of contracting colds and a short duration. Hidden phlegm and other associated symptoms cannot affect the clear diagnosis of an exterior syndrome. It is worth noting that an exterior syndrome is not necessarily correlated with the body temperature.

Case 2

A patient experienced a common cold last weekend. The symptoms did not respond to medications. The patient then started to have fever, thirst, a red face, a red tongue with a dry and slightly yellow coating, and a rapid pulse.

Remark. This case should be differentiated into an interior syndrome. Diagnostic basis: the patient had a history of contracting external pathogens, an absence of concurrent chills and fever, and interior heat syndrome symptoms (a red face, a red tongue with yellow coating).

QUESTIONS

1. How do you understand the concepts of "exterior," "exterior syndrome" and "interior syndrome"?
2. What is the key point to differentiate an exterior syndrome from an interior syndrome?

COLD SYNDROME AND HEAT SYNDROME

Differentiation of a cold syndrome from a heat syndrome aims to tell about the pathogenic nature. A cold syndrome occurs when yang becomes deficient or yin prevails over yang, while a heat syndrome occurs when yin becomes deficient or yang prevails over yin.

Cold Syndrome

Overview

A cold syndrome manifests conditions of yang–*qi* deficiency or yin prevailing over yang following contraction of a cold. More specifically, a cold syndrome can be caused by contraction of a yin cold (such as a cold attack, being caught in the rain or overingestion of cold food or medications) or by yang–*qi* deficiency and subsequent compromised warming function. A cold syndrome has the following characteristics: aversion to cold, white (color), and thin and clear (discharge).

Clinical manifestations

Aversion to cold with a preference for warmth, cold limbs, a bright pale complexion, a pale tongue with a white moistening slippery coating, tastelessness, production of thin clear sputum, salivation and nasal discharge, clear profuse urine, loose stools and a deep or tight pulse.

Analysis

Failure of yang–*qi* (either primary deficiency or secondary to a cold attack) to warm and push may cause the aforementioned cold, white, and thin and clear symptoms. Since yin cold has the property of contraction, a cold syndrome causes a tight pulse.

Heat Syndrome

Overview

A heat syndrome manifests conditions of external contraction of heat or hyperactivity of yang due to yin deficiency. Just like the cold syndrome, a heat syndrome can be caused by multiple factors. These include contraction of heat (for example, in a high-temperature working environment or hot weather), pathogenic cold transforming into heat after entering the interior or emotions (liver *qi* stagnation transforming into fire), an improper diet and hyperactivity of yang due to yin deficiency. A heat syndrome has the following characteristics: fever, red (color), dry and sticky (discharge), and restlessness.

Clinical manifestations

Red face and eyes, fever with a general hot sensation, restlessness, scanty dark-yellow urine, thirst with a preference to drink cold water, yellow thick nasal discharge, dry stools, a red tongue with a dry yellow coating, and a rapid pulse.

Analysis

Yang prevailing over yin may cause fever, a hot sensation and redness. Heat consuming fluids may cause dryness symptoms. Hyperactive yang may cause a rapid pulse and restlessness.

A cold syndrome and a heat syndrome may occur concurrently and transform mutually. Also, a cold syndrome may sometimes manifest as false heat, or vice versa.

Combined Cold and Heat Syndrome

A combined cold and heat syndrome has the following four patterns:

Upper heat with lower cold

This can be seen in patients presenting with restlessness, feverish sensations in the chest, and vomiting (upper heat) and abdominal pain with a preference for warmth and loose stools (lower cold).

Upper cold with lower heat

This can be seen in patients presenting with cold epigastric pain and vomiting of clear saliva (upper cold) and frequent painful passing of scanty dark-yellow urine (lower heat).

Exterior cold with interior heat

This can be seen in patients presenting with chills, fever, headache, muscle ache and a floating tight pulse (exterior cold), and restlessness, thirst and panting (interior cold).

Exterior heat with interior cold

This can be seen in patients presenting with fever, headache and a swollen sore throat (exterior heat), and loose stools, white clear urine and cold limbs (interior cold).

Mutual Transformation of Cold and Heat Syndromes

A cold syndrome transforming into a heat syndrome

This can be seen in patients presenting with an exterior cold syndrome first (chills, fever, a white moist tongue coating and a floating tight pulse), followed by an interior heat syndrome (a strong fever without chills, restlessness, thirst, a red tongue with a yellow coating and a rapid pulse).

A heat syndrome transforming into a cold syndrome

This can be seen in patients presenting with an excess heat syndrome first (a strong fever, profuse sweating, a red face and a rapid pulse), followed by a deficiency cold syndrome (dropped temperature, cold limbs, pallor and an extremely faint pulse).

True Cold with False Heat or True Heat with False Cold

True cold with false heat

This refers to internal exuberance of yin cold with false-heat symptoms. For example, patients with internal exuberance of yin cold may present with preference for warm drinks, intolerance of cold, a weak pulse, cold limbs, diarrhea mixed with undigested food, profuse clear urine and a pale tongue with a white coating; however, they may also present with false-heat symptoms, such as a hot sensation of the body, a red face, thirst and a big pulse. Actually, this is a critical syndrome known as exuberant yin repelling yang.

True heat with false cold

This refers to a heat syndrome with false-cold symptoms. For example, a heat syndrome can cause fever without chills, aversion to heat, and a deep rapid powerful pulse. Alternatively, restlessness, thirst with a desire to drink cold water, a dry throat, a foul breath, delirium, scanty dark-yellow urine, dry stools and a red tongue with a dry yellow coating may also be present. However, the patient may also present with cold limbs and a deep pulse. This is a severe heat syndrome known as exuberant yang repelling yin.

In summary, cold and heat can only be differentiated by an overall analysis of the disease course through the four examination methods.

Case Studies

Case 1

A patient suffered from a fever for two weeks. The temperature was 38.8°C but a little bit lower in the morning. The fever did not resolve after sweating or antibiotics. The patient later experienced restlessness, reduced food ingestion and unsmooth bowel movements. The tongue was red, with a yellow greasy coating. The pulse was rapid.

Remark. This case should be differentiated into a heat syndrome. Further analysis can conclude a damp–heat syndrome on the basis of a relatively long duration and symptoms due to dampness obstructing the spleen and stomach (reduced food ingestion and a greasy tongue coating).

Case 2

A patient suffered from abdominal discomfort, aversion to cold, and preferred warm food and more clothes. Since the weather was extremely hot, the patient drank a glass of cold beverage. After that, he started to experience epigastric pain with cold sensation, and diarrhea. The tongue was pale and swollen, with a thin white coating. The pulse was moderate.

Remark. This case should be differentiated into a cold syndrome. Further analysis can conclude a deficiency cold syndrome of the spleen and stomach, coupled with contraction of a cold (from the cold drinks).

QUESTIONS

1. How do you understand the concepts of "cold syndrome" and "heat syndrome"? List their clinical manifestations.
2. How do you understand a combined cold and heat syndrome? What are the common patterns of this syndrome?
3. How do you understand "true cold with false heat" and "true heat with false cold"?

DEFICIENCY SYNDROME AND EXCESS SYNDROME

Differentiation of a deficiency syndrome from an excess syndrome aims to tell about the strength between antipathogenic *qi* and pathogenic factors. Deficiency here refers to deficiency of antipathogenic *qi*. Excess here refers to exuberance of pathogenic factors. As a result, the treatment principle for an excess syndrome is to attack (remove) pathogenic factors, and the treatment principle for a deficiency syndrome to supplement or tonify antipathogenic *qi*. However, attacking (removing) pathogenic factors may damage antipathogenic *qi*, while supplementing or tonifying measures may facilitate pathogenic factors to some degree. Consequently, a correct diagnosis and an appropriate treatment are essential to the treatment effect.

Deficiency Syndrome

Overview

A deficiency syndrome manifests conditions of antipathogenic *qi* deficiency. The causative factors of a deficiency syndrome can be generalized as congenital deficiency and acquired malnutrition. Acquired malnutrition is of more clinical significance. It can be caused by an improper diet, emotional disturbance, overexertion, sexual indulgence, or delayed or inappropriate treatment of chronic conditions.

Deficiency syndromes include yang deficiency, yin deficiency, *qi* deficiency, blood deficiency, essence insufficiency, fluid insufficiency, deficiency of the *zang–fu* organs and concurrent patterns. Yang deficiency and yin deficiency will be focused on in this chapter, as the other patterns will be discussed in the later chapters regarding the pattern identification of *qi*, blood and body fluids as well as the *zang–fu* organs.

Yang Deficiency

Clinical manifestations

A pale white or sallow complexion, listlessness, mental fatigue, palpitations, shortness of breath, cold limbs, spontaneous sweating, fecal incontinence or diarrhea mixed with undigested food and urinary incontinence or profuse clear urine; the tongue is pale, swollen and tender, and the pulse is deficient, deep and slow.

Analysis

Failure of yang–*qi* to warm, push, transform *qi* and hold may cause the aforementioned signs and symptoms. Generally, a yang deficiency syndrome may not cause changes in the tongue coating.

Yin Deficiency

Clinical manifestations

Restlessness, feverish sensations on the palms, soles and chest, weight loss, rosy cheeks, a dry mouth and throat, night sweats and tidal fever; the tongue is red with a scanty coating and the pulse is deficient, thready and rapid.

Analysis

Clinically, yin deficiency does not include blood deficiency. Otherwise, a concurrent condition is called yin blood deficiency. Failure of yin to nourish and nurture may cause dry symptoms. Failure of yin to constrain yang may also cause heat symptoms. However, the heat here may not cause significant fever. Otherwise, the condition is called hyperactivity of fire (yang) due to yin deficiency. Generally, weight loss, a thin tongue with a scanty or peeling coating and a thready pulse can be diagnosed as yin deficiency.

Excess Syndrome

Overview

An excess syndrome manifests conditions of external pathogens attacking the body or retention of internal pathological products. External pathogens include wind, cold, summer heat, dampness, dryness, fire and epidemic *qi*. Internal pathological products include phlegm fluid, water–dampness, stagnant blood, etc.

Clinical manifestations

Fever, fast breathing, production of sputum and salivation, chest tightness and restlessness; unconsciousness, delirium, distending abdominal pain with tenderness, constipation, diarrhea, tenesmus, dysuria or hesitant dribbling urine may also be present; the tongue is tough and old with a thick greasy coating and the pulse is excessive and powerful.

Analysis

Exuberant heat may cause fever. Heat affecting the heart–mind may cause restlessness, unconsciousness or delirium. Heat attacking the lungs may cause fast breathing and production of sputum and salivation. Heat affecting the middle *jiao* may cause constipation, diarrhea or tenesmus. Heat affecting the urinary bladder may cause dysuria or hesitant dribbling urine. A tough old tongue with a thick greasy coating and an excessive powerful pulse indicate exuberant pathogenic *qi* and abundant antipathogenic *qi*.

A deficiency syndrome and an excess syndrome may occur concurrently and transform mutually. Also, a deficiency syndrome may sometimes manifest as false excess, or vice versa.

Combined Deficiency and Excess Syndrome

A combined deficiency and excess syndrome includes the following three patterns:

Excess syndrome mixed with deficiency

This refers to a predominantly excess syndrome containing mild deficiency of antipathogenic *qi*. It is often seen in conditions with a short duration or an excess syndrome without prompt, appropriate treatment. The primary treatment principle is to remove pathogenic factors.

Deficiency syndrome mixed with excess

This refers to a predominantly deficiency syndrome containing mild exuberance of pathogenic factors. It is often seen in chronic conditions or constitutional deficiency coupled with external contraction. The treatment principle is to supplement antipathogenic *qi* first, followed by removing pathogenic factors.

Concurrent deficiency and excess syndrome

This refers to concurrent presence of deficiency and excess syndromes. It occurs as a result of antipathogenic *qi* deficiency before the pathogenic factors are resolved or constitutional antipathogenic *qi* deficiency coupled with external contraction. For treatment, equal attention should be paid to supplementing *qi* and removing pathogenic factors.

Mutual Transformation of Deficiency and Excess Syndromes

This refers to the presence of an excess syndrome on top of the pre-existent deficiency syndrome, or vice versa. For example, on top of an excess syndrome (high fever), patients suddenly present with profuse sweating, pallor and a thready weak pulse due to yang–*qi* collapse, which requires emergent treatment measures.

True Deficiency with False Excess or True Excess with False Deficiency

This can be difficult for beginners to identify. For example, epigastric discomfort and pain (which can be alleviated by pressure), a lusterless complexion, a faint voice, a weak pulse, along with abdominal distension, an inability to eat and constipation actually indicate true deficiency with false excess. Abdominal masses with tenderness, a red face, fast breathing, a powerful pulse, along with reluctance to talk, lassitude, dizziness, blurred vision and loose stools actually indicate true excess with false deficiency.

In summary, the tongue and pulse conditions as well as the duration are essential for differentiation of deficiency from excess. A tough tongue often indicates excess, and a tender, swollen or thin tongue deficiency. A powerful pulse with spirit often indicates excess, and a weak pulse without spirit deficiency. An acute condition with a strong constitution can often be differentiated into excess, and a chronic condition with a weak constitution deficiency. Additionally, clinical data collected through the four examination methods are important for the final conclusion.

QUESTIONS

1. How do you understand the concepts of "deficiency syndrome" and "excess syndrome"? List their clinical manifestations.
2. How do you understand a combined deficiency and excess syndrome? What are the common patterns of this syndrome?
3. How do you understand "true deficiency with false excess" and 'true excess with false deficiency'?

CORRELATION INVOLVING COLD, HEAT, EXTERIOR, INTERIOR, DEFICIENCY AND EXCESS

The correlation involving cold, heat, exterior, interior, deficiency and excess includes the following 12 patterns:

Exterior Cold Syndrome

This syndrome is caused by cold attacking the exterior. The clinical manifestations include severe chills, mild fever, headache, general pain, no sweating, a thin white moist tongue coating.

Exterior Heat Syndrome

This syndrome is caused by warmth–heat attacking the exterior. The clinical manifestations include fever, mild intolerance of wind and cold, headache, a dry mouth, mild thirst, possibly sweating or a sore throat, redness on the tip of the tongue and a floating rapid pulse.

Remark. Sometimes it can be difficult to differentiate an exterior cold syndrome from an exterior heat syndrome, since both syndromes result from external pathogens attacking the exterior. Take the pulse, for example: exterior cold may also cause a rapid pulse. Alternatively, exterior heat may also cause severe chills. Some clinicians believe that a sore throat is indicative of exterior heat. Furthermore, a moist tongue, a tight pulse and the involved season are essential to differentiating exterior cold from exterior heat.

Interior Cold Syndrome

This syndrome can be caused by either yang–*qi* deficiency or cold directly attacking the interior. The clinical manifestations include cold limbs, a bright pale complexion, tastelessness, no thirst, preference for warm drinks, reluctance to talk, profuse clear urine, loose stools, a pale tongue with a white moist coating and a deep slow pulse; abdominal pain may also be present.

Interior Heat Syndrome

This syndrome is often caused by external pathogens transforming into heat after entering the interior. The clinical manifestations include a red face, fever, thirst with a preference for cold drinks, restlessness, talkativeness, dark-yellow urine, dry stools, a red tongue with a yellow coating and a rapid pulse.

Remark. An interior cold syndrome and an interior heat syndrome can both result from external pathogens entering the interior. The nature of pathogens (cold or heat) and individualized constitution play a role in causing interior cold or interior heat. For example, an interior heat syndrome tends to develop when pathogenic heat attacks a person with a strong or yang–heat constitution.

Exterior Deficiency Syndrome

An exterior deficiency syndrome can be further divided into two patterns:

Exterior deficiency due to cold damage

This originates from the *Guì Zhī Tāng* (桂枝汤, "Cinnamon Twig Decoction") syndrome in the *Treatise on Cold Damage* (*Shāng Hán Lùn*, 伤寒论). The clinical manifestations include aversion to wind, fever, sweating, headache, neck stiffness and a floating moderate pulse. This syndrome is seen in the early stage of an externally contracted condition and is characterized by unresolved fever after sweating.

Qi deficiency affecting the exterior

Qi deficiency can manifest as deficiency of antipathogenic *qi*, spleen *qi* deficiency and essential *qi* deficiency. One pattern of *qi* deficiency particularly manifests sweating and susceptibility to the common cold. The clinical manifestations include spontaneous sweating, sweating upon mild exertion, susceptibility to the common cold, fatigue, a poor appetite, a pale tongue, shortness of breath and a floating pulse.

Exterior Excess Syndrome

This syndrome also occurs in the early stage of an externally-contracted condition but is characterized by absence of sweating. The clinical manifestations include chills, fever, headache, muscle ache, absence of sweating and a floating tight pulse. It can be exterior cold or exterior heat.

Interior Deficiency Syndrome

This refers to the general deficiency syndrome. Due to its extensive contents and patterns the detailed information will be discussed in later chapters.

Interior Excess Syndrome

An interior excess syndrome can be seen in internally damaged miscellaneous conditions or occur as a result of external pathogens entering the interior.

Deficiency Cold Syndrome

This syndrome is caused by yang–*qi* deficiency. The clinical manifestations include mental fatigue, a pale white complexion, cold intolerance, cold limbs, a pale (or swollen, tender, tooth-marked) tongue and a weak (or deep, faint) pulse; abdominal pain with a preference for warmth and pressure and loose stools or profuse clear urine may also be present.

Deficiency Heat Syndrome

This syndrome is caused by insufficiency of internal yin fluids. The clinical manifestations include tidal fever, night sweats, weight loss, feverish sensations on the palms, soles and chest, a dry mouth and throat, a red tongue with a scanty coating and a thready rapid pulse.

Excess Cold Syndrome

This syndrome is caused by cold attacking the exterior and binding yang–*qi*. The clinical manifestations include chills, pallor, cold limbs, a white moist tongue coating and a deep (or tight) pulse; abdominal pain with tenderness, profuse clear urine, bowel sounds and diarrhea may also be present.

Excess Heat Syndrome

This syndrome is caused by warm-heat attacking the body or other pathogens transforming into heat after attacking the interior. The clinical manifestations include a strong fever, thirst with a preference for cold drinks, red face and eyes, restlessness, abdominal fullness and distension with tenderness, constipation, scanty dark-yellow urine, a red tongue with a yellow coating and a surging rapid slippery excessive pulse.

Case Study

A 58-year-old tall male patient has a bluish-purple complexion, a good appetite and likes eating meat. One year ago, after being caught in the rain, he ate some cold food on an empty stomach and then experienced distending abdominal pain and vomiting. Currently he complains of gastric pain after eating, loose stools and frequent waking during sleep. The pulse is soft, small and weak on the left hand, and deficient and hollow on the right hand.

Remark. This case should be diagnosed as an interior excess syndrome one year ago. However, the current pulse conditions indicate severe deficiency of antipathogenic *qi*. Also, the heart–mind in addition to the spleen and stomach is involved. There was no information regarding the tongue and coating as well as the gastric pain (whether or not it can be alleviated by pressure), and exuberance of pathogenic factors can still not be excluded. Gastric pain after eating and loose stools can be diagnosed as yang–*qi* deficiency. In conclusion, this case can be diagnosed as a deficiency cold syndrome mixed with partial exuberance of pathogenic factors.

It is also worth noting that a detailed medical record is extremely important in the four examination methods.

QUESTIONS

1. How do you understand the relationship between a deficiency syndrome and an excess syndrome?
2. List the clinical manifestations of deficiency cold, excess cold, deficiency heat and excess heat.

YIN SYNDROME AND YANG SYNDROME

Yin and yang are the general principle of the eight principles. Generally, yin prevailing over yang may cause yang disorder, while yang prevailing over yin may cause yin disorder. Yang deficiency causes external cold, yin deficiency causes internal heat, yang exuberance causes external heat, and yin exuberance causes internal cold.

Yin Syndromes

Yin syndromes include interior, cold and deficiency syndromes. Common clinical manifestations include listlessness, a low faint voice, a dull dark complexion, cold intolerance, cold limbs, a poor appetite, loose stools, profuse clear urine, a pale swollen tender tongue and a deep slow (or weak thready unsmooth) pulse.

Yang Syndromes

Yang syndromes include exterior, heat and excess syndromes. Common clinical manifestations include a red face, restlessness, a dry mouth with a desire to drink water, constipation, dark-yellow urine, a dark-red tongue with a dry yellow coating and a surging rapid (excessive) slippery pulse.

Differentiation of a Yin Syndrome from a Yang Syndrome

It is easy to differentiate a yin syndrome from a yang syndrome on the basis of identification of cold, heat, deficiency and excess. In terms of inspection, a yin syndrome often manifests as a pale dull complexion, lassitude, a low spirit and a pale swollen tender tongue; while a yang syndrome often manifests as a red face, restlessness and a dark-red tongue with a dry yellow coating. In terms of auscultation, a yin syndrome often manifests as a low voice and faint breathing, while a yang syndrome often manifests as a loud voice and fast breathing. In terms of inquiry, a yin syndrome often manifests as a poor appetite, tastelessness, no thirst, loose stools and profuse clear urine, while a yang syndrome often manifests as thirst with a desire to drink water, constipation and scanty dark-yellow urine. In terms of pulse-taking, a yin syndrome causes a deep slow (or weak thready unsmooth) pulse, while a yang syndrome causes a surging big slippery pulse. Generally, a yin syndrome is more difficulty than a yang syndrome to manage.

Exhaustion and depletion of yin and yang include the following four patterns:

Deficiency of Genuine Yin

This refers to insufficiency of yin essence, especially kidney yin. The clinical manifestations include a pale complexion with rosy cheeks, a dry mouth and throat, restlessness, dizziness, blurred vision, tinnitus, soreness and weakness of the low back and knee joints, night sweats, feverish sensations on the palms, soles and chest, constipation, scanty urine and a rapid weak pulse.

Deficiency of Genuine Yang

This refers to insufficiency of yang–*qi*, especially kidney yang. The clinical manifestations include a bright pale complexion, cold intolerance, cold limbs, soreness and weakness of the low back and knee joints, dizziness, blurred vision, listlessness, a pale swollen tongue with a white coating and a deep weak pulse. Infertility, impotence, diarrhea before dawn, edema and dyspnea may also be present.

Yin depletion and yang depletion can develop at the critical stages of medical conditions, often following high fever, profuse sweating, severe vomiting, diarrhea or bleeding. Since yin and yang are interdependent, yin depletion may cause scattering of yang–*qi*, while yang depletion may also cause loss of yin fluids.

Yin Depletion

This refers to a life-threatening sign following rapid severe loss of yin fluids and functional failure of the body. The clinical manifestations may include unconsciousness, restlessness, warm hands, feet and body, a dry mouth and thirst with a desire to drink cold water, profuse sweating, a dry dark-red tongue and a thready rapid weak pulse.

Yang Depletion

This refers to a life-threatening sign following rapid severe collapse of yang–*qi* and functional failure of the body. The clinical manifestations may include unconsciousness, cold limbs, cold sweating, no thirst or thirst with a preference for warm drinks, a white moist tongue coating and an extremely faint pulse.

Yin depletion can be differentiated from yang depletion by the sweating, thirst, temperature of the limbs, tongue and pulse. Both are fatal signs characterized by sudden unconsciousness and rapid progression.

QUESTIONS

1. How do you understand the concept of "yin syndrome" and "yang syndrome"? List the key differentiation points.
2. How do you understand "deficiency of genuine yin" and "deficiency of genuine yang"? Describe their clinical manifestations.
3. How do you understand "yin depletion" and "yang depletion"? How do you differentiate yin depletion from yin deficiency and yang depletion from yang deficiency?

CHAPTER 4

Syndrome Differentiation

CONCEPT

Syndrome differentiation, also known as pattern identification, is an approach to investigating the causative factors, identify the disease location and predict the disease progression and prognosis according to the clinical data collected through the four examination methods.

"Syndrome" is the term used to generalize the pathogenesis of a medical condition in specific stages.

There are numerous methods of pattern identification. In addition to pattern identification of the eight principles, other methods include: pattern identification of the etiologies; pattern identification of *qi*, blood and body fluids; pattern identification of the *zang–fu* organs; pattern identification of the meridians; pattern identification of the six meridians; pattern identification of *wei* (defense), *qi*, *ying* (nutrients) and blood; and pattern identification of *sanjiao*.

Pattern identification of etiologies aims to identify the causative factors of a medical condition. Pattern identification of the *zang–fu* organs is indicated for internally damaged miscellaneous conditions. The pattern identifications of *qi*, blood and body fluids as well as meridians are closely associated with and complementary to that of the *zang–fu* organs. The pattern identifications of the six meridians and *wei* (defense), *qi*, *ying* (nutrients) and blood are indicated for cold damage and febrile disease in externally contracted conditions. In addition, the pattern identification of *sanjiao* is indicated for febrile disease.

It is important to distinguish the concept of a syndrome from that of a disease (a medical condition associated with specific symptoms and signs resulting from specific causes, although patients may present with varying signs and symptoms; they do share common characteristics and pathology).

To date, common human diseases, particularly the contagious and hereditary diseases, have already been well understood at the molecular level. However, pattern identification in Chinese medicine is still of great significance, since it can provide the best available treatment options for individualized patients.

PATTERN IDENTIFICATION OF ETIOLOGIES

Many causative factors can contribute to the development of medical conditions. They include six external pathogens, pestilence, seven emotions, an improper diet, overexertion and trauma. Pattern identification of etiologies aims to identify the specific etiology according to the signs and symptoms and thus provide the basis for the treatment.

Six External Pathogens

The six external pathogens include wind, cold, summer heat, dampness, dryness and fire.

Wind syndrome

Overview

Wind usually invades the body by attacking the superficial muscles and skin first. It tends to open the striae of muscles. Conditions caused by wind are characterized by a sudden onset, fast changes and migratory symptoms.

Clinical manifestations

Fever, aversion to wind, sweating, headache, muscle ache, coughing with a stuffy and runny nose, a thin white tongue coating and a floating moderate pulse; alternatively, intermittent red intolerably itchy skin rashes, joint pain, facial numbness, and deviation of the mouth and eyes may also be present.

Analysis

Wind attacking the *wei* from the skin, skin hair and mouth or nose may cause a fever, aversion to wind, sweating, headache and muscle ache. Since the lungs dominate the skin and skin hair, wind attacking the exterior may cause coughs. Wind staying in the exterior may cause a thin white tongue coating and a floating moderate pulse. Wind affecting the skin may also cause intermittent red intolerably itchy skin rashes. Wind affecting the meridians and joints may cause joint pain, facial numbness or deviation of the mouth and eyes.

Cold syndrome

Overview

Cold is a yin pathogen in nature and tends to impair yang–*qi*. It has the property of coagulating, stagnating and contracting. As a result, it is liable to obstruct the circulation of *qi* and blood.

Clinical manifestations

Chills, fever, absence of sweating, headache, muscle ache, coughing, panting, a thin white tongue coating and a floating tight pulse; alternatively, contracture of the extremities, cold pain in the joints, abdominal pain, bowel sounds, diarrhea or vomiting may also be present.

Analysis

Cold binding the exterior may impair *wei qi*, causing fever, chills and an absence of sweating. Cold affecting the meridians may cause headache and muscle ache. Cold impairing the dispersing and descending of lung *qi* may cause coughing and panting. Cold attacking the body surface may cause a thin white tongue coating and a floating tight pulse. Cold impairing yang–*qi* may cause contracture of the extremities and cold pain in the joints. Cold entering the interior may damage yang of the spleen and stomach, resulting in abdominal pain, bowel sounds, diarrhea and vomiting.

Summer heat syndrome

Overview

Summer heat is a yang pathogen and tends to consume *qi* and body fluids. It has the property of ascending, scattering and scorching. In addition, it is liable to mix with dampness. Conditions caused by summer heat can be subdivided into summer heat damage and summer heat stroke.

Clinical manifestations

Aversion to heat, thirst, sweating, fatigue, dark-yellow urine, a red tongue with a yellow coating and a deficient rapid pulse (summer heat damage); sudden collapse, unconsciousness, fever, profuse sweating, thirst, panting, trismus, convulsions of the extremities, a dry dark-red tongue and a soft rapid pulse (summer heat stroke).

Analysis

Summer heat expelling body fluids may cause aversion to heat, thirst, sweating and dark-yellow urine. *Qi* scattering following sweating may cause fatigue and a deficient rapid pulse. Exuberant summer heat causes a red tongue with a yellow coating. Ascending of summer heat to disturb the mind may cause a sudden collapse and unconsciousness. Summer heat impairing the tendons and muscles may cause convulsions of the extremities and trismus. Summer heat scorching the *ying* yin may cause a dry dark-red tongue and a soft rapid pulse.

Dampness syndrome

Overview

Dampness is heavy, viscous and stagnant. It tends to consume yang–*qi* and obstruct the flow of *qi*. In addition, it often results in persistent lingering problems. Conditions caused by dampness can be further divided into dampness damage and dampness affection.

Clinical manifestations

Distending headache, chest tightness, absence of thirst, a general heaviness and pain, fever, lassitude, profuse clear urine, a white slippery tongue coating and a soft or moderate pulse (dampness damage); a heavy sensation of the head like being wrapped in a towel, heaviness of the extremities, a general discomfort and a soft weak pulse (dampness affection); alternatively, soreness, pain and impaired joint flexion and extension with restricted movement may also be present.

Analysis

Dampness obstructing the flow of *qi* and clean yang may cause distending headache, chest tightness, absence of thirst, a general heaviness and pain, and lassitude. Dampness suppressing *wei* yang may cause a fever. Dampness is a yin pathogen in nature, therefore causing an absence of thirst, profuse clear urine, a white slippery tongue coating and a soft or moderate pulse. It may impair the ascending of clean yang, resulting in a heavy sensation of the head like being wrapped in a towel. It is heavy and tends to descend, therefore causing a heaviness of the extremities and a general discomfort. It may block the circulation of *qi* and blood within the joints, leading to soreness, pain and impaired joint flexion and extension.

Dryness syndrome

Overview

Dryness tends to consume body fluids and attack the lungs through the mouth or nose. Conditions caused by dryness can be further divided into cool dryness and warm dryness.

Clinical manifestations

Fever, mild intolerance of wind and cold, headache, scanty sweating, thirst, dry mouth, nose, lips and throat, unproductive coughs or coughing with scanty sputum, restlessness, a dry tongue with a yellow coating and a floating rapid pulse (warm dryness); chills, an absence of sweating, mild headache, coughing with thin sputum, mild thirst, dry nose and throat, a dry white tongue and a wiry unsmooth pulse (cool dryness).

Analysis

Warm dryness is often seen in early autumn. Dry heat attacking the lungs may cause fever, mild intolerance of wind and cold, headache and scanty sweating. Dryness damaging the body fluids may cause thirst and dry mouth, nose, lips and throat. Dryness impairing the lung system may cause unproductive coughs or coughing with scanty sputum and restlessness. A dry tongue with a yellow coating and a floating rapid pulse are signs of dry heat. Cool dryness is often seen in late autumn. Cold dryness attacking the lung may cause chills, an absence of sweating and mild headache, coupled with cold-related symptoms including coughing with thin sputum, mild thirst, dry nose and throat, a dry white tongue and a wiry unsmooth pulse.

Fire syndrome

Overview

Fire and heat both arise from exuberant yang but differ in severity. Warmth is the smaller degree of heat, and fire is the maximum degree of heat. Warmth, fire and heat tend to damage yin fluids, stir wind and move blood.

Clinical manifestations

A strong fever, thirst, red face and eyes, restlessness, insomnia, unconsciousness, delirium, hematemesis, bleeding from the nostrils or at the gum, skin rashes, a dark-red tongue and a surging rapid or thready rapid pulse; mania and skin sores or ulcers may also be present.

Analysis

Fire, heat or warmth attacking the *qi* phase may cause a strong fever, thirst, red face and eyes, and a surging rapid pulse. Fire–heat entering the *ying* and blood may cause restlessness and insomnia. Fire–heat accelerating the circulation of the blood may cause hematemesis, bleeding from the nostrils or at the gum and skin rashes. Heat disturbing the heart–mind may cause unconsciousness, delirium or even mania. Persistent fire–heat may cause skin sores or ulcers. A dark-red tongue and a surging rapid or thready rapid pulse are signs of fire–heat entering the *ying* and blood.

QUESTIONS

1. How do you understand the concept of "syndrome differentiation"? List the methods of pattern identification.
2. How do you understand pattern identification of etiologies?
3. Describe the clinical manifestations of a wind syndrome and a cold syndrome.
4. Be familiar with the clinical manifestations of pathogenic summer heat, dampness, dryness and fire.
5. How do you distinguish warm dryness from cool dryness?

Pestilence

Pestilence is a toxic, contagious external pathogen. It may cause epidemic plague characterized by sudden onset, highly contagious and life-threatening conditions. Common conditions are plague, epidemic skin eruptions and pestilential jaundice.

Plague

Overview

Plague is an acute epidemic contagious condition after contraction of pestilential *qi*.

Clinical manifestations

Sudden onset of chills and fever, headache, muscle ache, chest discomfort, nausea and vomiting, followed by persistent fever (especially in the late afternoon) without chills, a white (appearing as a buildup of powder) tongue coating and a rapid pulse.

It can be deadly if not treated promptly.

Analysis

Epidemic pestilence attacking the membrane and the struggle between antipathogenic *qi* and epidemic pathogen in between the exterior and the interior may cause a sudden onset of chills and fever, headache and muscle ache. Epidemic pathogens coupled with turbidity obstructing the flow of *qi* may cause chest discomfort, nausea, vomiting and a white (appearing as a buildup of powder) tongue coating. Epidemic pathogens transforming into heat after entering the interior may cause persistent fever without chills and a rapid pulse.

Epidemic skin eruptions

Overview

Epidemic eruptions result from toxic heat entering the bloodstream.

Clinical manifestations

Fever, a general scorching sensation, a splitting headache, skin eruptions in a red, dark-red, purple or dark color and a rapid pulse; inactive skin eruptions may cause a thready rapid deep hidden pulse on the three regions of both hands, a bluish complexion, mental confusion, cold limbs, profuse sweating on the head, a splitting headache, abdominal colic, inability to vomit or diarrhea even with an urge, and frequent head shaking.

Analysis

Epidemic toxins attacking the blood may cause skin eruptions. Epidemic toxins affecting both the exterior and the interior may cause fever, a general scorching sensation and a splitting headache. Toxic heat in the blood may cause a rapid pulse. A floating big rapid pulse indicates that antipathogenic *qi* can prevail over the pathogens. A deep thready rapid pulse indicates pathogenic heat entering the interior. A rapid, neither floating nor deep pulse indicates toxic heat staying between the exterior and the interior. Toxic heat entering the deep interior may cause a thready rapid deep hidden pulse on the three regions of both hands. Exuberant heat disturbing the mind may cause mental confusion. Extreme heat may also cause cold limbs. Ascending of toxic fire causes profuse sweating on the head and a splitting headache. Abdominal colic, inability to vomit or diarrhea even with an urge, and head shaking are all signs of hidden epidemic toxins in the interior.

Pestilential jaundice

Overview

Pestilential jaundice is an acute condition resulting from epidemic toxins mixed with damp-heat.

Clinical manifestations

Fever, chills and sudden jaundice (yellow skin and eyes); in severe cases, fatal signs such as cold limbs, unconsciousness, delirium, staring blankly, enuresis, a curled tongue, retracted testicles and flocculation may be present.

Analysis

Epidemic toxins and dampness attacking the body may cause fever, chills and sudden jaundice. Epidemic toxins affecting the five *zang* organs may cause cold limbs. Toxic heat entering the pericardium may cause unconsciousness and delirium. Ascending of epidemic toxins may cause staring blankly. Epidemic toxins affecting the liver and kidneys may cause enuresis or retracted testicles. Epidemic toxins may exhaust kidney *qi* and result in a curled tongue and flocculation.

Seven Emotions

Overview

The seven emotions include joy, anger, worry, obsession, grief, fear and fright. Emotions are closely associated with the five *zang* organs. The five *zang* organs transform five *qi* and introduce seven emotions. Persistent extreme emotions may impair the bodily adaptability to maintain balance and affect the functions of the *zang–fu* organs. Emotional disturbance may affect the *qi* activity of the *zang–fu* organs, resulting in disharmony between *qi* and blood and yin–yang imbalance. The emotions are correlated with specific organs and may act on organs via the control cycle of the five elements. Additionally, clinical manifestations caused by emotions can be extremely complicated due to individualized life habits and temperaments.

Clinical manifestations

Extreme joy (overexcitability) damages the heart and causes restlessness, absent-mindedness, mental confusion, incoherent speech, crying or laughing for no apparent reason and abnormal behaviors. Extreme anger (rage) damages the liver and causes dizziness, distending headache, a red face and red eyes, a bitter taste, chest tightness, distending pain in the hypochondriac regions, restlessness and irritability; hiccups, vomiting, abdominal distension, diarrhea or sudden consciousness may also be present. Obsession (extreme worry) damages the spleen and causes dizziness, blurred vision, severe palpitations, a poor memory, a poor appetite, bloating, loose stools, weight loss and insomnia or dream-disturbed sleep; depression and mental fatigue may also be present. Grief (extreme sadness) damages the lungs and causes a pale complexion, frequent sighs and listlessness. Panic (extreme fear or fright) damages the kidneys and causes lower abdominal fullness and distension, nocturnal emissions, spermatorrhea, urinary or fecal incontinence, mood swings, mental confusion, and abnormal speech or behaviors.

Analysis

The representative emotion of the heart is joy. Moderate joy harmonizes the *ying* and *wei*, and produces a happy feeling. Extreme joy, however, can damage the heart and cause *qi* to slow down, resulting in restlessness, absent-mindedness, mental confusion, incoherent speech and abnormal behaviors.

The representative emotion of the liver is anger. Extreme anger can damage the function of the liver in maintaining the free flow of *qi*, causing *qi* stagnation and subsequent chest tightness, distending pain in the hypochondriac regions, restlessness and irritability. Liver *qi* may further affect the descending of stomach *qi* and result in hiccups, belching, bloating and diarrhea. The ascending of liver *qi* carrying blood may cause dizziness, headache, red face and eyes, and possibly a sudden collapse.

The representative emotion of the spleen is thinking or worry. Extreme worry damages the spleen and causes *qi* to stagnate, leading to a poor appetite, bloating and loose stools. Extreme worry may also consume heart blood, leading to severe palpitations, a poor memory, insomnia or dream-disturbed sleep, weight loss, dizziness and blurred vision.

The representative emotion of the lungs is grief. Extreme grief damages the lungs and affects the spleen, thus resulting in a poor appetite, a pale complexion and listlessness.

The representative emotion of the kidneys is fear or fright. Extreme fear or fright (panic) damages the kidneys and causes *qi* to descend, leading to lower abdominal fullness and distension, nocturnal emissions, spermatorrhea, and urinary and fecal incontinence. Sudden panic may also cause disorders of *qi* and blood, resulting in restlessness or mental confusion.

An Improper Diet and Overexertion

An improper diet, binge eating or ingestion of unclean or contaminated food may impair the functions of the spleen and stomach. Overexertion may affect the *qi*, blood, tendons and muscles.

Food injury

Overview

Food injury refers to spleen and stomach problems due to an improper diet.

Clinical manifestations

An improper diet damaging the stomach may cause stomachache, a foul breath, a poor appetite, chest or diaphragm fullness, acid reflux, belching, a thick greasy tongue coating and a slippery powerful pulse. An improper diet damaging the spleen may cause abdominal pain, diarrhea, a thick greasy or yellow tongue coating and a slippery swift or deep excessive pulse. Ingestion of contaminated food may cause nausea, vomiting, abdominal colic or vomiting alternating with diarrhea.

Analysis

The stomach decomposes food and stomach *qi* descends. An improper diet impairing the descending of stomach *qi* may cause stomachache, a foul breath and chest or diaphragm fullness. A thick greasy tongue coating and a slippery powerful pulse are signs of food retention (indigestion). The spleen transports and transforms water and food. An improper diet impairing the spleen may cause abdominal pain and diarrhea. Undigested food mixed with the ascending turbid *qi* may cause a thick greasy or yellow tongue coating. Ingestion of contaminated food may cause a sudden disorder of *qi* and blood, leading to vomiting alternating with diarrhea and abdominal colic.

Work–rest imbalance

Overview

This refers to conditions resulting from excessive physical/mental fatigue or physical inactivity.

Clinical manifestations

Overexertion may cause lassitude, reluctance to talk and reduced food ingestion. Physical inactivity may cause obesity, panting upon mild exertion, palpitations, weakness of the extremities and a soft weak pulse.

Analysis

Overexertion consumes *yuan*-primordial *qi* and results in lassitude and reluctance to talk. Physical inactivity may cause stagnation of *qi* and blood, leading to palpitations, shortness of breath and weakness of the extremities.

Sexual Indulgence

Overview

This refers to conditions of kidney essence consumption due to sexual indulgence, getting married at an early age or frequent childbirths.

Clinical manifestations

Dizziness, tinnitus, soreness and weakness of the low back and knee joints, bone-steaming tidal fever, palpitations, night sweats, spermatorrhea, dreaming of intercourse, scanty menstruation, amenorrhea, cold hands and feet, impotence, premature ejaculations, infertility, profuse thin clear leukorrhea and irregular menstruation.

Analysis

Sexual indulgence may consume kidney essence and result in insufficient supply to the brain marrow, thus leading to dizziness and tinnitus. Malnourishment of the skeleton may cause soreness and weakness of the low back and knee joints. Kidney yin deficiency may cause internal deficient fire, leading to bone-steaming tidal fiver. Deficient fire disturbing the heart–mind may cause palpitations. Fire expelling body fluids may cause night sweats. Fire disturbing the essence chamber may cause nocturnal emissions, dreaming of intercourse, scanty menstruation and amenorrhea. Kidney yang deficiency may cause cold hands and feet, impotence, premature ejaculations, infertility, profuse thin clear leukorrhea and irregular menstruation.

Trauma

Overview

This refers to injuries resulting from metallic knives, insects or animals and traumatic injuries.

Injury by metallic knives

Clinical manifestations

Local injury causes bleeding with redness, swelling and pain. Injury to the bones and tendons causes severe pain with restricted movement. Heavy bleeding may cause pallor, dizziness and a dark circle around the eyes. Toxic wind affecting the lesion may cause chills and fever, muscle twitching, trismus, a forced-smile facial look, opisthotonos and excessive salivation (this condition is known as tetanus).

Analysis

Metallic knives injuring the skin may cause bleeding with redness, swelling and pain. Severe damage to the collaterals (bones or tendons) may cause severe pain with restricted movement. Heavy bleeding may cause fainting. Wind toxins affecting the lesion may cause tetanus signs and symptoms.

Injury by insects or animals

This refers to injuries due to bites by poisonous insects, snakes, dogs, other animals or pets.

Clinical manifestations

Bites by poisonous insects may cause local redness, swelling, pain and rashes, coupled with numb painful extremities. In severe cases, headache and unconsciousness may also be present, followed by local pain, numbness, swelling, blisters, necrosis and ulceration. In rare cases, general poisoning symptoms may be present. These include dizziness, blurred vision, chest tightness, weakness of the extremities, trismus, difficult breathing and dilation of the pupils. Rabies may cause hydrophobia, photophobia and fear of noises, voices or telephones.

Analysis

Insect or animal bites may cause local redness, swelling and pain. Toxins affecting the meridians may cause numb painful extremities. Spreading of toxins over the body may cause headache and unconsciousness. Bites by poisonous snakes may cause numbness, pain, swelling, blisters, necrosis or ulceration of the affected skin. Spreading of snake venom may cause dizziness, blurred vision and trismus. Hydrophobia, photophobia and fear of noises, voices or telephones are typical signs of rabies.

Traumatic injuries

This refers to injuries due to falling, collision, contusion or squeezing.

Clinical manifestations

Local pain, swelling, lesions, bleeding and fracture; squeezing or falling may also cause hematemesis, blood in the urine or bloody stools; head trauma may cause dizziness, staring blankly or unconsciousness.

Analysis

Traumatic injuries may obstruct the circulation of meridian *qi* and blood, leading to local pain, swelling, lesion and bleeding. Squeezing or falling may damage the *zang–fu* organs, subsequently causing hematemesis, blood in the urine or bloody stools. Head trauma may disturb the mind, leading to dizziness, staring blankly or unconsciousness.

QUESTIONS

1. Describe the clinical manifestations of pestilence.
2. Describe the clinical manifestations of the seven emotions.
3. Describe the clinical manifestations of food injury, work–rest imbalance and sexual indulgence.

PATTERN IDENTIFICATION OF *QI*, BLOOD AND BODY FLUIDS

Pattern identification of *qi*, blood and body fluids aims to analyze complicated clinical manifestations and identify disorders of *qi*, blood and body fluids. This process is based of the theory of *qi*, blood and body fluids relating to the *zang–fu* organs.

Qi, blood and body fluids are closely associated with the *zang–fu* organs. They are the material foundation and also the products of normal functions of the *zang–fu* organs. Their production and transportation depends on the functions of the *zang–fu* organs. As a result, disorders of *qi*, blood and body fluids can interact with each other and affect the *zang–fu* organs.

Disorders of *qi*, blood and body fluids can be categorized into four types: *qi* disorder, blood, disorder, disorder of *qi* and blood, and disorder of body fluids.

Pattern Identification of *Qi* Disorders

The chapter "On Pain" in *the Basic Questions* (*Sù Wèn*, 素问) states that "almost all medical conditions start from *qi*." Both externally contracted and internally damaged conditions affect *qi* first, followed by blood, body fluids, *zang–fu* organs and meridians. There are four common patterns of *qi* disorders, namely *qi* deficiency, *qi* sinking, *qi* stagnation and abnormal *qi* activity.

Qi deficiency

Overview

This pattern refers to hypofunction of the *zang–fu* organs due to general or specific *qi* insufficiency. The main contributing factors include constitutional weakness due to chronic conditions, overexertion, aging and malnutrition.

Clinical manifestations

Lack of energy, reluctance to talk, mental fatigue, dizziness, blurred vision, spontaneous sweating, aggravated symptoms after physical exertion, a pale tongue with a white coating and a deficient weak pulse.

Analysis

Qi is the driving force of vital activities. *Qi* abundance guarantees normal functions of the *zang–fu* organs. *Qi* deficiency causes hypofunction of the *zang–fu* organs. Consequently, it is characterized by general hypofunction. Deficiency of *yuan*–primordial *qi* causes lack of energy, reluctance to talk and mental fatigue. *Qi* deficiency may impair the ascending of clean yang, resulting in dizziness and blurred vision. It may weaken the exterior, causing spontaneous sweating. Physical exertion may consume *qi* and therefore aggravate all symptoms. A pale tongue with a white coating and a deficient weak pulse are signs of *qi* failing to circulate blood.

Qi sinking

Overview

This pattern refers to failure of *qi* to ascend but instead sink. It often develops from *qi* deficiency, overexertion or injury to internal organs.

Clinical manifestations

Qi deficiency symptoms coupled with sinking symptoms: dizziness, blurred vision, lack of energy, lassitude, chronic diarrhea or dysentery, a falling sensation in the abdomen, presence of rectal or uterine prolapse, a pale tongue with a white coating and a weak pulse.

Analysis

This pattern is distinctively characterized by prolapse of internal organs. Since it is the further progression of *qi* deficiency, dizziness, blurred vision, lack of energy and lassitude also occur. Failure of spleen *qi* to ascend and subsequent sinking of clean yang may cause chronic diarrhea or dysentery. Failure of *qi* to ascend and maintain the normal anatomical positions of the internal organs may cause rectal or uterine prolapse. A pale tongue with a white coating and a weak pulse are signs of *qi* deficiency.

Qi stagnation

Overview

This pattern refers to obstructed flow of *qi* in specific tissue or *zang–fu* organs. The main contributing factors include emotional disturbance, pathogens entering the interior and yang–*qi* deficiency.

Clinical manifestations

Tightness, distension and wandering or paroxysmal pain.

Analysis

This pattern is distinctively characterized by tightness, distension and pain. Free flow of *qi* is essential for health. Stagnant flow of *qi* may cause tightness, distension or migratory pain in the *zang–fu* organs, meridians, muscles or joints. It is necessary to identify according to the locations and associated symptoms. For example, stomach *qi* stagnation due to food retention may cause gastric or abdominal distension, tightness and pain; liver *qi* stagnation may cause wandering pain in the hypochondriac region; *qi* stagnation affecting the heart and lungs may cause chest pain; and *qi* stagnation in meridians may cause muscle or joint pain.

Abnormal qi activity

Overview

This pattern refers to conditions due to abnormal *qi* activity, especially *qi* ascending of the lungs, stomach, liver and gallbladder.

Clinical manifestations

Ascending of lung *qi* may cause coughs and panting. Ascending of stomach *qi* may cause hiccups, belching, nausea and vomiting. Ascending of liver fire may cause headache, vertigo, syncope and vomiting of blood.

Analysis

Ascending of lung *qi* often results from external pathogens or internal turbid phlegm. External pathogens or internal turbid phlegm may impair the dispersing and descending of lung *qi*, resulting in coughs and panting. Cold fluid retention, turbid phlegm or food retention may impair the descending of stomach *qi*, resulting in hiccups, belching, nausea and vomiting. Anger may cause liver *qi* stagnation, which may over time transform into fire to ascend and result in headache, vertigo, syncope and vomiting of blood. There are four common patterns of blood disorder: blood deficiency, blood stasis, blood heat and blood cold.

Pattern Identification of Blood Disorders

Blood travels within the vessels to nurture the *zang–fu* organs and skin. Contraction of external pathogens or dysfunctions of the *zang–fu* organs may compromise the normal physiological functions of blood, leading to blood disorders.

Blood deficiency

Overview

This pattern refers to a general debilitating condition due to failure of blood to nourish the body. Numerous factors can contribute to blood deficiency. They include congenital deficiency, insufficient production of *qi* and blood due to weakness of the spleen and stomach, acute bleeding, chronic conditions, anxiety, blood stasis and intestinal parasites.

Clinical manifestations

A lusterless or sallow complexion, pale lips and nails, dizziness, blurred vision, palpitations, insomnia, numbness of the hands and feet, scanty menstruation in a pale color, a delayed period or amenorrhea, a pale tongue with a white coating and a thready weak pulse.

Analysis

This pattern is distinctively characterized by a pale complexion, pale lips and nails and general weakness. Failure of blood to nourish the skin may cause a pale complexion with pale lips and nails. Failure of blood to nourish the brain marrow and eyes may cause dizziness and blurred vision. Failure of blood to nourish the heart and heart–mind may cause palpitations and insomnia. Malnourishment of the meridians and muscles may cause numbness of the hands and feet. Insufficient blood within the vessels may cause a thready weak pulse. Also, insufficient blood may cause scanty menstruation in a pale color, a delayed period or amenorrhea.

Blood stasis

Overview

This pattern refers to conditions of unabsorbed blood outside the vessels and stagnant blood remaining within the meridians, tissues or *zang–fu* organs. The main contributing factors include cold retention, *qi* stagnation, *qi* deficiency and trauma.

Clinical manifestations

Stabbing pain in a fixed position, tenderness and aggravated pain at night; other signs and symptoms may include bluish-purple lumps, solid immobilized abdominal masses, recurrent bleeding in a dark-purple color, tarry stools, a dark complexion, rough scaly skin, dark-purple lips and nails, subcutaneous bruises, exposure of abdominal veins, varicose veins in the lower limbs, amenorrhea, a dark-purple tongue or a tongue with ecchymosis, and a thready hesitant pulse. The clinical manifestations of the blood stasis pattern can be generalized as pain, a purple color, stasis, clots and a hesitant pulse.

Analysis

This pattern is distinctively characterized by stabbing pain in a fixed position, tenderness, lumps, bleeding, dark-purple lips and nails and a hesitant pulse. Stagnant blood blocking the flow of *qi* may cause severe stabbing pain in a fixed position. Pressure may aggravate the blockage of *qi*, causing tenderness. The yin–*qi* becomes abundant at night; therefore the pain is especially aggravated at night. Persistent stagnant blood may form into bluish-purple lumps on the body surface or solid immobilized masses within the abdomen. It may also cause recurrent bleeding. It may impair the functions of *qi* and blood to nourish the body and skin, causing a dark complexion, rough scaly skin, and dark-purple lips and nails. Stagnant blood in other body parts may cause subcutaneous bruises, exposure of abdominal veins, varicose veins or amenorrhea. A dark-purple tongue and a thready hesitant pulse are signs of stagnant blood.

Blood heat

Overview

This pattern refers to conditions of exuberant fire–heat accelerating the circulation of blood. The main contributing factors include external contraction of fire–heat, excessive consumption of alcohol, overingestion of hot spicy food, anger and sexual indulgence.

Clinical manifestations

Hemoptysis, hematemesis, blood in the urine, nosebleed or gum bleeding, restlessness, a dry mouth with no desire to drink water, fever especially at night, a dark-red tongue and a rapid pulse; an earlier period with heavy menstruation may also be present. In summary, this pattern is character-ized by bleeding and heat signs.

Analysis

Exuberant fire–heat in the *zang–fu* organs may accelerate the circulation of blood, resulting in bleeding symptoms. Exuberant fire–heat damaging the lung, stomach and bladder collaterals may cause hemoptysis, hemate-mesis and blood in the urine, respectively. Blood–heat disturbing the mind may cause restlessness. Consumption of yin blood may cause a dry mouth, but without a desire to drink water, due to an absence of *qi* in the *qi* phase. Since blood is yin in nature, the fever becomes aggravated at night. Accelerated flow of blood may cause earlier periods with heavy menstruation. A dark-red tongue and a rapid pulse are signs of blood heat.

Blood cold

Overview

This pattern refers to conditions due to cold retention within the blood obstructing the *qi* activity and blood circulation. It can be caused by either contraction of a cold or internal yin exuberance due to yang deficiency.

Clinical manifestations

Pain on the hands, feet or abdomen with a preference for warmth, but intol-erance of cold, cold limbs in a bluish-purple color, a delayed period with dark-purple menstruation containing blood clots, a dark-purple tongue with a white coating and a deep slow hesitant pulse.

Analysis

This pattern is distinctively characterized by a dark-purple skin color and local pain with a preference for warmth. Cold is pathogenic yin in nature and may block the circulation of blood, leading to cold pain on the hands, feet and abdomen with a dark-purple skin color. Since normal blood circulation can be restored by warmth and aggravated by cold, the local pain can be alleviated by warmth. Cold attacking the uterus may cause lower abdominal pain and a delayed period with dark-purple menstruation containing blood clots. Failure of blood to ascend to nourish the tongue may cause a dark-purple tongue with a white coating. A deep slow hesitant pulse indicates cold retention or blood stasis.

QUESTIONS

1. Describe the patterns and distinctive differentiation points of *qi* disorders.
2. Describe the patterns and distinctive differentiation points of blood disorders.

Pattern Identification of *Qi* and Blood Disorders

In Chinese medicine, *qi* is the commander of blood, while blood is the mother of *qi*. *Qi* and blood are interdependent and can be mutually promoted. Physiologically, *qi* and blood work together to maintain equilibrium of the body. Pathologically, *qi* and blood can affect each other, either being impaired simultaneously or being the consequence of each other. There are five common patterns of *qi* and blood disorders: blood stasis due to *qi* stagnation, blood stasis due to *qi* deficiency, deficiency of *qi* and blood, *qi* failing to hold blood and *qi* collapse after blood loss.

Blood stasis due to qi stagnation

Overview

This pattern refers to conditions of blood stasis resulting from *qi* stagnation. The main contributing factors are emotional disturbance or contraction of external pathogens.

Clinical manifestations

Distension, tightness and wandering pain in the chest or hypochondriac regions, restlessness, irritability and masses in the hypochondrium coupled with stabbing pain and tenderness, amenorrhea, dysmenorrhea, dark-purple menstruation containing blood clots, a dark-purple tongue or a tongue with ecchymosis, and a hesitant pulse.

Analysis

This pattern is distinctively characterized by emotions, distension, tightness and stabbing pain on the chest and hypochondriac regions, and irregular menstruation. Since the liver maintains the free flow of *qi*, emotional disturbance or external pathogens attacking the liver meridian may cause liver *qi* stagnation and subsequent restlessness, irritability and distension, tightness and wandering pain in the chest or hypochondriac regions. Over time, *qi* stagnation may result in blood stasis and subsequent masses in the hypochondrium coupled with stabbing pain and tenderness. Since the liver stores blood, liver–blood stasis may cause amenorrhea or dysmenorrhea. A dark-purple tongue or a tongue with ecchymosis and a hesitant pulse are signs of internal stagnant blood.

Qi deficiency and blood stasis

Overview

This pattern refers to conditions due to concurrent *qi* deficiency and blood stasis. It is mainly caused by failure of *qi* to circulate blood.

Clinical manifestations

Lassitude, lack of energy, reluctance to talk, a pale or gray-dull complexion, stabbing pain in the chest or hypochondriac regions with tenderness and a fixed position, a pale-dark tongue or a tongue with ecchymosis, and a deep hesitant pulse.

Analysis

This pattern is distinctively characterized by concurrent *qi* deficiency and blood stasis symptoms. *Qi* deficiency symptoms include a pale complexion, lassitude, lack of energy and reluctance to talk. Blood stasis symptoms include stabbing pain with tenderness and a fixed position and a gray-dull complexion. Since *qi* deficiency and blood stasis are often associated with the heart and liver, the pain often occurs in the chest and hypochondriac regions. A pale tongue indicates deficiency, a deep pulse indicates an interior syndrome, a hesitant pulse indicates stasis and a tongue with ecchymosis indicates *qi* deficiency with blood stasis.

Deficiency of qi and blood

Overview

This pattern refers to conditions due to deficiency of both *qi* and blood. Chronic conditions or failure of blood to transform *qi* may contribute to it.

Clinical manifestations

A pale white or sallow complexion, dizziness, blurred vision, lack of energy, reluctance to talk, mental fatigue, spontaneous sweating, palpitations, insomnia, a pale tender tongue and a thready weak pulse.

Analysis

This pattern is distinctively characterized by concurrent *qi* deficiency and blood deficiency symptoms. *Qi* deficiency symptoms include lack of energy, reluctance to talk, mental fatigue, spontaneous sweating and a weak pulse. Blood deficiency symptoms include a sallow or pale white complexion, a pale tongue and a thready pulse. Failure of blood to nourish the heart may cause palpitations and insomnia. It is also necessary to identify the specific *zang–fu* organs related to deficiency of *qi* and blood prior to treatment.

Qi failing to hold blood

Overview

This pattern is also known as loss of blood due to *qi* deficiency, referring to a condition of concurrent *qi* deficiency and bleeding. The contributing factors include chronic conditions, overexertion, spleen deficiency and chronic bleeding.

Clinical manifestations

Hematemesis, blood in the urine, metrorrhagia and metrostaxis, subcutaneous bruises, shortness of breath, lassitude, a pale lusterless complexion, a pale tongue and a weak pulse.

Analysis

This pattern is distinctively characterized by bleeding and *qi* deficiency symptoms. Bleeding includes hematemesis, blood in the urine, subcutaneous bruises, and metrorrhagia and metrostaxis. *Qi* deficiency symptoms include shortness of breath and lassitude. Blood deficiency causes a pale lusterless complexion. A pale tongue and a thready weak pulse are signs of deficiency of *qi* and blood.

Qi collapse following bleeding

Overview

This pattern refers to *qi* collapse following heavy bleeding. It can be associated with the liver, stomach and lungs. Trauma, uterine bleeding or childbirth may also contribute to the pattern.

Clinical manifestations

A sudden pallor during bleeding, coupled with cold limbs, profuse sweating, a pale tongue and an extremely faint or hollow floating big scattering pulse; syncope may also be present.

Analysis

This pattern is distinctively characterized by sudden *qi* collapse during heavy bleeding. Since *qi* and blood are interdependent, heavy loss of blood may cause collapse of yang–*qi*, subsequently resulting in pallor and cold limbs. Failure of yang–*qi* to warm and consolidate the exterior may cause profuse sweating. The heart (mind) spirit scatters following *qi* collapse, leading to syncope. A pale tongue and an extremely faint or hollow floating big scattering pulse are signs of yang depletion and *qi* collapse following blood loss.

QUESTION

Describe the patterns and clinical manifestations of *qi* and blood disorders.

Pattern Identification of Body Fluid Disorders

Body fluids (or bodily fluids) are liquids inside the human body. They nourish the *zang–fu* organs, lubricate the joints and nurture the body skin. The production, distribution and discharge are mainly associated with the spleen (transportation and transformation), lungs (water path regulation) and kidneys (*qi* transformation).

Disorders of body fluids often manifest as either insufficient fluids or fluid retention. They can be attributed to multiple factors or dysfunctions of the *zang–fu* organs.

Insufficiency of fluids

Overview

This pattern refers to dryness symptoms due to failure of fluids to moisten the *zang–fu* organs or tissues. Insufficiency of fluids is attributed to either insufficient production or excessive consumption. Insufficient production can be caused by weakness of the spleen and stomach, inadequate drinking of water and *qi* deficiency. Excessive consumption may include dry heat damaging fluids, sweating, vomiting, diarrhea or loss of blood.

Clinical manifestations

Thirst, a dry throat, dry cracked lips, dry withered skin, dry stools, a dry red tongue and a thready rapid pulse.

Analysis

This pattern is distinctively characterized by dry skin, lips, tongue and throat, coupled with constipation, which are caused by insufficiency of fluids. A dry red tongue and a thready rapid pulse are signs of internal heat.

Water fluid retention

Water fluid retention mainly refers to phlegm fluid retention and edema resulting from abnormal water metabolism and distribution. The contributing factors include contraction of six external pathogens or emotional disturbance. Water fluid retention mainly manifests as four types: phlegm, fluid, water and dampness. Pattern identification of dampness has been discussed previously in the part under "Six External Pathogens." Edema, phlegm and fluid will therefore be discussed in the following:

Edema

Overview

Edema is an abnormal accumulation of fluid beneath the skin or in one or more cavities of the body. It can occur in the head, face, eyelids, four extremities, abdomen and even the entire body. It is important to identify yang edema from yin edema prior to treatment.

Subpatterns

Yang water

Yang water is excess in nature and often has an acute onset and a short duration. Causative factors include external contraction of wind or water-dampness retention.

Clinical manifestations

Edema begins with the eyelids and then spreads over the face or the entire body rapidly; scanty urine and thin shiny skin are present. Wind–cold may cause wind intolerance, chills, fever, no sweating, general pain, a thin white tongue coating and a floating tight pulse; wind–heat may cause a sore throat, a red tongue and a floating rapid pulse; wind–dampness may cause gradual general pitting edema, a general heavy sensation, gastric or abdominal discomfort, a poor appetite, nausea, vomiting, a white greasy tongue coating and a deep pulse.

Analysis

Yang edema is distinctively marked by *a sudden onset, rapid progression* and *edema starting from the eyelids (mainly spreading over the upper body)*. It is mainly caused by wind attacking the lung defense. Wind is pathogenic yang in nature and tends to attack the upper body first, causing edema from the eyelids, followed by the face. Impaired *qi* transformation of the urinary bladder may cause scanty urine. Wind is also liable to mix with other factors, like cold, heat or dampness, to attack the body, resulting in respective associated symptoms.

Yin water

Yin water is deficiency in nature and often has an insidious onset and a long duration. The causative factors include chronic conditions, antipathogenic *qi* deficiency, sexual indulgence and overexertion.

Clinical manifestations

Persistent pitting edema, especially below the low back, a bright pale complexion, mental fatigue, lassitude, gastric or abdominal distension, a poor appetite, loose stools, scanty urine, a pale tongue with a white slippery coating and a deep pulse; alternatively, aggravated edema, dysuria, cold pain in the low back and knee joints, cold limbs, cold intolerance, mental fatigue, a bright pale or gray-dull complexion, a pale swollen tongue with a white slippery coating and a deep slow weak pulse may also be present.

Analysis

Yin edema is distinctively marked by *an insidious onset, slow progression* and *pitting edema mainly involving the lower body*, coupled with *yang deficiency of the spleen and kidneys*. Since the spleen transports and transforms water dampness and the kidneys dominate water, chronic conditions or overexertion may cause yang–*qi* deficiency of the spleen and kidneys, leading to water–dampness retention in the lower *jiao*, which in turn leads to pitting edema mainly involving the lower limbs. Spleen yang deficiency causes gastric or abdominal distension, a poor appetite and loose stools. Since the spleen governs muscles, spleen deficiency with retention of water–dampness may cause a bright pale complexion, mental fatigue and lassitude. Since the lumbus houses the kidneys, kidney yang deficiency may cause cold pain in the low back and knee joints, cold limbs, cold intolerance and mental fatigue. A bright pale complexion indicates yang deficiency with water retention. A gray-dull complexion indicates kidney deficiency with water retention. A pale swollen tongue with a white slippery coating and a deep slow weak pulse are signs of internal yin cold due to yang deficiency of the spleen and kidneys.

Phlegm

Overview

Phlegm and fluid are mostly caused by dysfunctions of the *zang–fu* organs and subsequent water metabolic disorder. However, phlegm manifests more as water fluid retention in the *zang–fu* organs, meridians and tissues with a high concentration and appears more thick and sticky, while fluid appears more thin and clear. Six external pathogens and emotional disturbance may cause dysfunction of the *zang–fu* organs and further result in phlegm. It is believed by some scholars that phlegm is pathogenic yang in nature, whereas fluid is pathogenic yin in nature. Furthermore, phlegm results from heat, whereas fluid results from dampness. There are five types of phlegm: wind phlegm (ascribed to the liver), heat phlegm (ascribed to the heart), cold phlegm (ascribed to the kidneys), damp phlegm (ascribed to the spleen) and dry phlegm (ascribed to the lungs).

Subpatterns

Wind phlegm

Wind phlegm refers to exuberant phlegm with wind stirring. The contributing factors include hyperactive yang due to yin deficiency or internal phlegm due to overingestion of sweet and fatty food.

Clinical manifestations

Dizziness, blurred vision, fullness and tightness in the chest and hypochondriac regions, phlegm sounds in the throat, production of clear foamy sputum, sudden collapse, deviation of the mouth and eyes, a stiff tongue, numbness of the four extremities, hemiplegia, a red tongue with a greasy coating and a wiry thready slippery pulse.

Analysis

This pattern is distinctively marked by dizziness, chest and hypochondriac fullness, sudden collapse and phlegm sounds in the throat. Wind carrying phlegm to attack the mind may cause dizziness, blurred vision and phlegm sounds in the throat. Phlegm misting the mind may cause sudden collapse and a stiff tongue. Phlegm dampness flowing into meridians may cause numbness of the four extremities, hemiplegia, and deviation of the mouth and eyes. A red tongue with a greasy coating and a wiry thready slippery pulse are signs of internal wind stirring with phlegm dampness.

Heat phlegm

Heat phlegm is mostly caused by contraction of heat or exuberant yang–*qi* consuming fluids.

Clinical manifestations

Fever, restlessness, coughing with yellow thick sputum, loss of voice, constipation, dark-yellow urine, mania, a red tongue with a yellow greasy coating and a slippery rapid pulse.

Analysis

This pattern is distinctively marked by fever with restlessness, coughing with yellow thick sputum and a slippery rapid pulse. Internal disturbance of phlegm heat may cause mania. Exuberant heat may consume fluids, resulting in coughing with yellow thick sputum. Heat phlegm blocking *qi* activity may cause loss of voice. Phlegm heat in the stomach and intestine may cause constipation and dark-yellow urine. A red tongue with a yellow greasy coating and a slippery rapid pulse are signs of phlegm heat.

Cold phlegm

Cold phlegm refers to either concurrent cold and phlegm or exuberant phlegm coupled with cold symptoms. It is mostly caused by contraction of a cold or yin exuberance due to constitutional yang deficiency.

Clinical manifestations

Intolerance of cold, cold limbs, coughing with white thin sputum, a heavy sensation of the four extremities, stabbing pain of the bones and joints, and a deep slow pulse.

Analysis

This pattern is distinctively marked by coughing with white thin sputum and a deep slow pulse. Cold phlegm affecting yang–*qi* or constitutional yang deficiency may cause intolerance of cold, cold limbs and coughing with white thin sputum. Cold phlegm may impair the flow of meridian *qi*, leading to pain of the bones and joints, a heavy sensation of the four extremities and a deep slow pulse.

Damp phlegm

Damp phlegm (also known as phlegm dampness) is mostly caused by internal phlegm dampness due to spleen deficiency or water retention following contraction of external cold dampness.

Clinical manifestations

Chest discomfort, a poor appetite, nausea, vomiting, lassitude, drowsiness, production of profuse white sputum, a thick greasy tongue coating and a soft slippery pulse.

Analysis

This pattern is distinctively marked by production of profuse white sputum, nausea, vomiting, chest discomfort and a thick greasy tongue coating. Spleen deficiency with internal dampness may cause a poor appetite. Phlegm dampness obstructing the flow of *qi* may cause chest discomfort. Phlegm dampness impairing the descending of stomach *qi* may cause nausea and vomiting. Phlegm dampness blocking clean yang may cause lassitude and drowsiness. Failure of the spleen to transport and transform may cause profuse white sputum. A thick greasy tongue coating and a soft slippery pulse are signs of internal phlegm dampness.

Dry phlegm

Dry phlegm is mostly caused by either contraction of dryness or heat consuming the fluids.

Clinical manifestations

Coughing with scanty and extremely thick sticky sputum or blood-stained sputum, dry nose, mouth and throat, constipation and a thready slippery rapid pulse.

Analysis

This pattern is distinctively marked by scanty thick sticky sputum or blood-stained sputum. Dryness consuming fluids may cause coughing with thick sticky sputum. Dryness damaging the lung collaterals may cause blood-stained sputum. Dryness affecting the lungs and large intestine may cause dry nose, mouth and throat, and constipation. A thready slippery rapid pulse indicates phlegm heat damaging fluids.

Fluid retention

Overview

Fluid retention is sometimes termed "phlegm fluid" or "water fluid." Unlike phlegm, it is more thin and clear. It mostly results from water fluid retention due to yang deficiency or dysfunctions of the *zang–fu* organs. The contributing factors include an improper diet, overexertion or constitutional spleen yang deficiency coupled with contraction of cold–dampness. By the location of fluid retention, fluid retention can be categorized into four types: phlegm fluid retention, pleural fluid retention, subcutaneous fluid retention and thoracic fluid retention.

Subpatterns

Phlegm fluid retention

In a narrow sense, phlegm fluid retention refers to fluid retention in the stomach and intestines. The main contributing factors include contraction of cold–dampness, an improper diet and chronic conditions damaging spleen yang.

Clinical manifestations

Chest or hypochondriac fullness, a splashing sound in the stomach, vomiting of thin clear saliva, no thirst or thirst with no desire to drink water, dizziness, blurred vision, palpitations, shortness of breath, a white slippery tongue coating and a wiry slippery pulse.

Analysis

Water fluid retention in the stomach may cause a splashing sound. Ascending of the water retention may cause vomiting of thin clear saliva. Retention of water fluid in the middle *jiao* may cause no thirst or thirst with no desire to drink water. Water fluid retention obstructing clean yang may cause dizziness and blurred vision. Water retention affecting the heart and lungs may cause palpitations and shortness of breath. A white slippery tongue coating and a wiry slippery pulse are signs of water fluid retention.

Pleural fluid retention

This refers to water fluid retention in the chest and hypochondriac regions. It is mainly caused by contraction of external cold–dampness.

Clinical manifestations

Distending pain of the chest and hypochondrium (especially following coughing, rolling over or breathing), costal distension and fullness, shortness of breath, fast breathing and a deep wiry pulse.

Analysis

The chest and hypochondrium are pathways for *qi* ascending and descending, and water retention may cause distending pain of the chest and hypochondrium. Water fluid retention affecting the lungs may cause costal distension and fullness, shortness of breath, fast breathing and a deep wiry pulse.

Subcutaneous fluid retention

This refers to water retention in the muscles or four extremities. The main contributing factors include spleen deficiency, wind–cold binding the exterior and subsequent water–dampness retention.

Clinical manifestations

Pain of the extremities with a heavy sensation, edema in the limbs, dysuria, coughing with profuse white foamy sputum, a white slippery tongue coating and a wiry tight pulse; fever, chills and no sweating may also be present.

Analysis

Failure of lung and spleen *qi* to transport and distribute water may cause water retention in the muscles or four extremities, resulting in pain of the extremities with a heavy sensation or even edema in the limbs. Wind–cold binding the exterior may cause fever, chills and no sweating. Water retention affecting the lungs may cause coughing with profuse white foamy sputum. A white slippery tongue coating and a wiry tight pulse are signs of interior and exterior cold.

Thoracic fluid retention

This refers to water fluid retention in the chest and diaphragm. It is often caused by contraction of wind–cold or yang deficiency of the spleen and kidneys.

Clinical manifestations

Coughing, panting, chest fullness, shortness of breath, an inability to lie flat, facial puffiness, production of profuse white foamy sputum, a white greasy tongue coating and a wiry tight pulse.

Analysis

Water retention affecting the descending of lung *qi* may cause coughing and panting with an inability to lie flat. Failure of water fluid retention to be transported downward may cause facial puffiness. Water fluid retention with internal yin cold may cause production of profuse white foamy sputum. A white greasy tongue coating and a wiry tight pulse are signs of water fluid retention. Due to the hidden fluid and susceptibility to contraction of a cold, this pattern can be persistent and recurrent.

QUESTIONS

1. What are the two categories of disorders of the body fluids?
2. Describe the subpatterns and clinical manifestations of edema.
3. Describe the subpatterns and clinical manifestations of phlegm and fluid retention.

PATTERN IDENTIFICATION OF THE *ZANG–FU* ORGANS

Pattern identification of the *zang–fu* organs aims to summarize and analyze the clinical signs and symptoms and thus deduce the location (of the organs), nature and strength between antipathogenic *qi* and pathogenic factors. This process is based on the physiological functions and pathological features of the *zang–fu* organs. Since all vital activities and pathological changes are closely associated with the *zang–fu* organs, the holistic concept of Chinese medicine especially highlights the five *zang* organs. The occurrence and development of any medical conditions may eventually affect the *zang–fu* organs, resulting in their dysfunctions. As a result, this method plays a key role in the pattern identification system.

There are numerous pattern identification methods in Chinese medicine. Each has its own distinctive characteristics. However, the affected *zang–fu* organs have to be identified in the final conclusion prior to treatment. To do so, it is extremely important to understand the essential theories of Chinese medicine and be familiar with the physiological functions of the *zang–fu* organs as well as their connections.

Pattern identification of the *zang–fu* organs includes identification of the *zang* organs, *fu* organs and two or more organs. Pattern identification of the *zang* organs is particularly important. Owing to the internal–external connection between the *zang* and *fu* organs, pattern identification of the *fu* organs is covered by that of the *zang–fu* organs.

Pattern Identification of the Heart and Small Intestine

The heart is located within the chest. The heart meridian descends to connect with the small intestine. The two organs are internally–externally connected. The main physiological functions of the heart are to govern blood vessels, store the spirit–mind and dominate the life activity. The heart opens into the tongue. The physiological functions of the small intestine are to separate the clear from the turbid and to absorb the decomposed food.

The patterns of the heart can be classified into deficiency and excess. Deficient patterns are often caused by chronic conditions, constitutional deficiency and anxiety, while excessive patterns are often linked to cold retention, blood stasis, phlegm and fire disturbance.

Common signs and symptoms of the heart conditions include palpitations, chest pain, restlessness, insomnia, dream-disturbed sleep, poor memory and coma with delirium. The main pathology of the small intestine manifests as excessive heat in the small intestine.

Heart qi deficiency, heart yang deficiency and sudden collapse of heart yang

Overview

These three patterns manifest deficiency of heart yang (*qi*), hypofunction of the heart and sudden collapse of yang–*qi*. Over time, heart *qi* deficiency may develop into heart yang deficiency and sudden collapse of heart yang. The main contributing factors include constitutional deficiency, chronic conditions and age-related debilitation.

Clinical manifestations

Heart *qi* deficiency causes mild or severe palpitations, chest tightness and shortness of breath that can be aggravated by physical exertion, sweating, mental fatigue, a pale complexion, a pale tongue with a white coating and a deficient pulse.

Heart yang deficiency further causes cold intolerance, cold limbs, pallor, cardiac pain, a pale and swollen tongue with a white slippery coating and a faint or regularly/irregularly intermittent pulse.

A sudden collapse of heart yang may even cause profuse cold sweating, cold limbs, pallor, cyanosis, faint breathing, mental confusion or coma, a pale or dark-purple tongue and an extremely faint pulse.

Analysis

Failure of heart *qi* to circulate blood may cause mild or severe palpitations, chest tightness and shortness of breath. Physical exertion consumes *qi* and thus aggravates the symptoms. Since sweat is the liquid of the heart, heart *qi* deficiency causes sweating. Failure of *qi* and blood to ascend to nourish the face and tongue causes a pale complexion and a pale tongue with a white coating. Weakness of heart *qi* to circulate blood causes a deficient pulse.

Over time, heart *qi* deficiency may impair heart yang, leading to *qi* stagnation and subsequent cardiac pain. Failure of yang–*qi* to warm the body causes cold intolerance, cold limbs and pallor. Yang deficiency may produce internal cold, causing a pale swollen tongue and a white slippery tongue coating. Failure of heart yang to circulate blood causes a faint or regularly/irregularly intermittent pulse.

A sudden collapse of heart yang may cause scattering of *zang*-pectoral *qi*, further leading to faint breathing. Failure of yang–*qi* to consolidate the exterior causes cold profuse sweating. Failure of yang-*qi* to warm the body causes cold limbs. Failure of yang–*qi* to circulate blood to nourish the body causes pallor, cyanosis of the lips and an extremely faint pulse. Scattering of *qi* may disturb the heart–mind, resulting in mental confusion or even coma.

Differentiation

The distinctive points of heart *qi* deficiency include palpitations, shortness of breath, mental fatigue and general *qi* deficiency symptoms. In summary, heart *qi* deficiency involves heart-related symptoms plus *qi*-deficiency symptoms.

Heart yang deficiency develops from heart *qi* deficiency, involving heart-related symptoms plus yang deficiency symptoms. It is distinctively characterized by cold intolerance, cyanosis and stasis.

A sudden collapse of heart yang develops from heart *qi* deficiency and heart-yang deficiency, involving heart-related symptoms plus yang depletion symptoms. It is distinctively characterized by aggravated symptoms of heart *qi* deficiency and heart yang deficiency, coupled with mental confusion or unconsciousness.

Distinctive notes

Common heart-related symptoms of the three patterns are *mild or severe palpitations* and *chest tightness with shortness of breath.* Heart *qi* (yang) deficiency can cause worsened symptoms upon physical exertion. A sudden collapse of heart yang can cause life-threatening mental confusion, which requires immediate emergency measures.

Heart blood deficiency and heart yin deficiency

Overview

These two patterns manifest failure of heart yin and heart blood to nourish the heart. The main contributing factors include constitutional deficiency, loss of blood, chronic conditions consuming blood and internal fire transformed from emotion-induced *qi* stagnation.

Clinical manifestations

Common symptoms of the two patterns are *palpitations* and *insomnia or dream-disturbed sleep.*

Heart blood deficiency also causes dizziness, poor memory, pallor or a sallow complexion, pale lips and nails, and a thready weak pulse.

Heart yin deficiency also causes tidal fever, night sweats, feverish sensations on the palms, soles and chest, rosy cheeks, a dry throat, a red tongue with a scanty coating and a thready rapid pulse.

Analysis

Failure of heart yin and heart blood to nourish the heart causes mild or severe palpitations. Failure of yin and blood to nourish the heart–mind causes insomnia or dream-disturbed sleep. Failure of blood to nurture the brain causes dizziness and a poor memory. Failure of blood to ascend to nourish the face and tongue causes a pale or sallow complexion and pale lips and nails. Deficiency of heart blood causes a thready pulse. Yin deficiency may cause deficient heat, resulting in subsequent feverish sensations on the palms, soles and chest, tidal fever and night sweats. Ascending of deficient fire causes rosy cheeks. Failure of yin to ascend causes a dry throat. A red tongue with a scanty coating and a thready rapid pulse are typical signs of internal heat due to yin deficiency.

Differentiation

Other than *palpitations* and *insomnia or dream-disturbed sleep*, heart yin deficiency is distinctively characterized by a red tongue, a thready rapid pulse and/or night sweats; while heart blood deficiency is distinctively characterized by absence of redness (tongue and cheeks), heat or sweating but presence of a thready pulse, a pale tongue and a lusterless complexion.

Distinctive notes

It is easy to identify heart yin deficiency or heart blood deficiency by the heart-related symptoms plus either yin deficiency or blood deficiency symptoms. The heart-related symptoms include mild or severe palpitations, insomnia or dream-disturbed sleep and abnormal mental activities. Chest tightness, chest pain, night sweats, profuse sweating and tongue changes may also be present; however, these symptoms can also be caused by dysfunctions of other *zang–fu* organs. There is an exception, though: owing to the close association between blood and heart–spirit, presence of palpitations and insomnia without other manifestations is often diagnosed as heart blood deficiency.

In addition, heart blood deficiency coupled with restlessness, tidal fever and night sweats can be identified as deficiency of heart yin and blood.

Hyperactivity of heart fire

Overview

Hyperactivity of heart fire manifests an internal exuberance of heart fire. The main contributing factors include internal fire heat, six external pathogens, *qi* stagnation transforming into fire and overingestion of hot, spicy or fatty food.

Clinical manifestations

A red face, thirst with a desire to drink water, restlessness, insomnia, dark-yellow urine, dry stools, ulcerations, swelling and pain of the tongue, redness on the tip of the tongue and a rapid pulse; alternatively, hematemesis, bleeding from the nostrils, bloody urine, mania or skin sores may also be present.

Analysis

Ascending of exuberant fire causes a red face. Fire consuming fluids causes thirst with a desire to drink water. Internal exuberance of heart fire causes restlessness and insomnia. The heart opens into the tongue; ascending of fire heat along the meridian may cause redness on the tip of the tongue and subsequent ulcerations, swelling and pain. Dark-yellow urine, dry stools and a rapid pulse are typical signs of interior heat. Additionally, since the heart dominates blood and blood vessels, exuberant heart fire may accelerate the flow of blood, leading to hematemesis, bleeding from the nostrils or bloody urine. Heat disturbing the mind causes mania. Over time, internal toxic fire causes skin sores.

Differentiation

This pattern manifests as excessive fire and should be distinguished from heart yin deficiency which causes deficient fire. Combined fire and yin deficiency symptoms can be diagnosed as hyperactivity of fire due to (heart) yin deficiency.

Distinctive notes

The distinctive points of hyperactivity of heart fire include heart-related symptoms, especially involving the mental activities and tongue (redness, ulceration and pain), heat and excess.

Blockage of heart vessels

Overview

Blockage of heart vessels manifests obstructed circulation of heart blood. The main contributing factors include stasis, cold retention, phlegm, and *qi* stagnation due to aging or chronic conditions.

Clinical manifestations

Mild or severe palpitations, chest tightness with intermittent chest pain radiating to the shoulder, back and arms. Stasis causes a stabbing chest pain, a dark-purple tongue or a tongue with ecchymosis or petechiae, severe chest tightness, a white greasy tongue coating and a deep slippery pulse. Phlegm causes an oppressive chest pain, obesity, a general heavy sensation, a white greasy tongue coating and a deep slippery pulse. Cold retention causes a sudden intense chest pain that can be alleviated by warmth, cold intolerance, cold limbs, a pale tongue with a white coating and a deep slow or deep tight pulse. *Qi* stagnation causes a distending chest pain that is associated with emotions, a light red or dark-red tongue and a wiry pulse.

Analysis

Failure of heart yang (*qi*) to circulate blood to nourish the heart causes mild or severe palpitations and subsequent blood stasis and phlegm retention. This may further cause chest pain that can radiate to the shoulder, back and arms along the meridian.

Clinically, blockage of heart vessels can be caused by one factor (of phlegm, stasis, *qi* stagnation and cold retention) alone or in combination.

Differentiation

This pattern is distinctively characterized by chest tightness and pain. In modern medicine, it can be seen in patients with coronary artery disease, angina or myocardial infarction. The chest tightness and pain can be caused by trauma, pulmonary or pleural conditions, or mental stress. In addition, this pattern is more commonly seen in elderly males, accompanied by *qi* deficiency, yang deficiency, yin deficiency, blood deficiency, excessive cold or phlegm.

Distinctive notes

The distinctive points of this pattern include intermittent recurrent chest tightness and pain. Laboratory findings can help confirm the diagnosis and predict prognosis.

Phlegm misting the heart–mind

Overview

Phlegm misting the heart–mind manifests turbid phlegm disturbing the heart–mind. The main contributing factors include internal dampness transforming into phlegm and emotional disturbance.

Clinical manifestations

Gastric fullness, nausea, phlegm sounds in the throat, mental confusion or unconsciousness, slurred speech, a white greasy tongue coating and a slippery pulse; alternatively, mental depression, apathy, dementia expression, muttering to oneself and abnormal behaviors may also be present. In some cases, a sudden collapse, unconsciousness, phlegm sounds in the throat, salivation, uncontrollable jerking movements of the arms and legs, and a staring spell can be present.

Analysis

This pattern is often seen in a critical stage of depression, epilepsy or other chronic conditions, such as stroke.

Depression causes dementia expression and abnormal behaviors. It often results from emotional disturbance and subsequent liver *qi* stagnation. Epilepsy causes a sudden collapse with uncontrollable jerking movements of the arms and legs. It is often congenital or linked to a sudden fright. Since the liver dominates tendons and opens into the eyes, internal stirring of liver wind may cause a staring spell. Ascending of liver *qi* causes phlegm sounds in the throat.

External or internal turbid dampness may obstruct the ascending of clean yang and descending of stomach *qi*, resulting in gastric fullness and nausea. Over time, the turbid dampness may transform into phlegm to disturb the mind, leading to mental confusion, slurred speech or even loss of consciousness. A white greasy tongue coating and a slippery pulse are typical signs of internal phlegm turbidity.

Differentiation

This pattern should be distinguished from hyperactivity of heart fire. Both may cause abnormal mental activities. However, hyperactivity of heart fire mainly causes excessive heat symptoms, while phlegm misting the heart–mind mainly causes phlegm symptoms, including phlegm sounds in the throat, a white greasy tongue coating, gastric fullness, nausea and salivation.

If coupled with fire heat symptoms, the new pattern can be diagnosed as phlegm fire disturbing the mind.

Distinctive notes

The distinctive points of this pattern include abnormal mental activities (due to phlegm disturbing the mind), gastric discomfort and nausea (due to ascending of phlegm turbidity) and recurrent attacks.

Phlegm fire disturbing the mind

Overview

Phlegm fire disturbing the mind manifests phlegm fire affecting the heart–mind. The main contributing factors include internal phlegm fire transformed from *qi* stagnation and heat phlegm disturbing the mind following an external contraction of heat.

Clinical manifestations

Red face and eyes, fever, restlessness, manic delirium, yellow sticky sputum, a red tongue with a yellow greasy coating and a slippery rapid pulse; alternatively, insomnia, restlessness, dizziness, blurred vision, profuse sputum and chest tightness may be present. In some cases, illogical speech, crying or laughing with no apparent reason and manic behaviors may be present.

Analysis

Qi stagnation transforming into fire may consume fluid and form phlegm, which then ascend to disturb the mind, leading to red face and eyes, fever and restlessness. Exuberant heat also causes yellow sticky sputum. Phlegm fire disturbing the heart–mind causes mental confusion and subsequent manic delirium. Internal exuberance of phlegm fire causes a red tongue with a yellow greasy coating and a slippery rapid pulse.

Differentiation

This pattern should be distinguished from hyperactivity of heart fire and phlegm misting the heart–mind. Hyperactivity of heart fire is marked by restlessness, insomnia and dark-yellow urine. Phlegm misting the heart–mind is marked by dementia expression, mental confusion and a white greasy tongue coating. This pattern is marked by mania, mental confusion and phlegm sounds in the throat.

Distinctive notes

The distinctive points of this pattern include excessive phlegm, exuberant heat and mental confusion.

Excessive heat in the small intestine

Overview

Excessive heat in the small intestine manifests exuberant interior heat in the small intestine. It is mainly caused by downward transmission of heart fire to the small intestine.

Clinical manifestations

Restlessness, thirst, mouth or tongue ulcerations, painful urination with a burning sensation in the urethra, bloody urine, a red tongue with a yellow coating and a rapid pulse.

Analysis

Internal heart fire can disturb the mind and cause restlessness. Fire consuming fluids causes thirst. Ascending of heart fire causes mouth or tongue ulcerations. Since the heart is internally–externally connected with the small intestine, heart fire can be transmitted down to the small intestine, leading to painful urination with a burning sensation. Exuberant heat damaging yang collaterals causes bloody urine. A red tongue with a yellow coating and a rapid pulse are typical signs of heat.

Differentiation

This pattern, also known as downward transmission of heart fire to the small intestine, should be distinguished from damp–heat in the urinary bladder. Common symptoms of the two include dark-yellow urine with a burning sensation in the urethra. However, this pattern also causes symptoms due to hyperactivity of heart fire, while damp–heat in the urinary bladder mainly causes low back pain and lower abdominal distension.

Distinctive notes

The distinctive points of this pattern include symptoms of hyperactivity of heart fire, scanty painful urination with a burning sensation and an absence of low back pain.

Summary

The patterns and diagnosis points for the heart and small intestine:

Patterns	Distinctive Diagnosis Points
Heart *qi* deficiency	Palpitations, shortness of breath, mental fatigue and general hypofunction
Heart yang deficiency	Heart *qi* deficiency + deficiency cold symptoms
Sudden collapse of heart yang	Heart yang deficiency + yang depletion symptoms
Heart yin deficiency	Palpitations etc. + yin deficiency symptoms
Heart blood deficiency	Palpitations etc. + blood deficiency symptoms
Hyperactivity of heart fire	Heart-related symptoms + heat + excess syndrome
Blockage of the heart vessels	Chest tightness + recurrent attacks + lab tests
Phlegm misting the mind	Abnormal mental activities + ascending turbid phlegm
Phlegm fire disturbing the mind	Phlegm + heat + mental confusion
Excessive heat in the small intestine	Hyperactive heart fire + scanty painful urination + an absence of low back pain

---

QUESTIONS

1. How do you understand pattern identification of the *zang–fu* organs and its significance?
2. List the main pathologies and common symptoms of the heart.
3. Distinguish heart *qi* deficiency from heart yang deficiency and sudden collapse of heart yang, and distinguish heart blood deficiency from heart yin deficiency.
4. List the causative factors and clinical manifestations of blockage of the heart vessels.

Pattern Identification of the Lungs and Large Intestine

The lungs reside in the chest. They govern *qi* and dominate respiration. They also govern dispersing and descending, and regulate the waterway. Externally the lungs connect with the skin and body hair, and they are internally–externally connected with the large intestine. They open into the nose. The physiological function of the large intestine is to govern transmission and discharge wastes.

The main pathologies of the lungs manifest either as a dysfunction of the lungs in governing *qi* dispersing and descending as well as *wei*, or as an abnormality of the lungs in regulating the water metabolism. The patterns of the lungs can be classified into deficiency and excess. Deficient patterns include lung *qi* deficiency and lung yin deficiency. Excessive patterns are often caused by contraction of six external pathogens and phlegm dampness obstructing the lungs. The patterns of the large intestine include damp–heat retention, insufficiency of liquid and yang–*qi* deficiency.

Common signs and symptoms of the lung conditions include cough, panting or fast breathing, chest tightness or pain and hemoptysis.

Lung qi deficiency

Overview

Lung *qi* deficiency manifests weakness of lung *qi* and hypofunction of the lungs. The main contributing factors include chronic cough consuming lung *qi*, lung deficiency due to chronic conditions and insufficient *qi* production.

Clinical manifestations

Weak coughing, panting and shortness of breath that can be aggravated by physical exertion, profuse thin clear sputum, a low voice with reluctance to talk, a pale complexion or pallor and mental fatigue; alternatively, wind intolerance, spontaneous sweating, and susceptibility to the common cold may be present. The tongue is pale with a white coating. The pulse is deficient.

Analysis

Deficiency of lung *qi* causes weak coughing, panting and shortness of breath that can be aggravated by physical exertion. Failure of lung *qi* to regulate the waterway causes water retention and subsequent clear thin profuse phlegm. Weakness of lung *qi* causes a low voice with reluctance to talk. A pale complexion or pallor, mental fatigue, a pale tongue with a white coating and a deficient pulse are typical signs of *qi* deficiency. Failure of lung *qi* to defend the exterior causes spontaneous sweating, wind intolerance and resultant susceptibility to the common cold.

Differentiation

This pattern should be distinguished from heart *qi* deficiency. Heart *qi* deficiency also causes shortness of breath, lack of energy and sweating; however, it causes mild or severe palpitations and an abnormal pulse as well.

In regard to coughing and susceptibility to the common cold, this pattern should be distinguished from wind–cold binding the lungs, which involves a short duration and an absence of deficient symptoms.

Distinctive notes

The distinctive points of this pattern are weak coughing and panting, shortness of breath (followed by phlegm and spontaneous sweating) and general hypofunction of the body. However, it is necessary to rule out other conditions that may affect the lungs.

Lung yin deficiency

Overview

Lung yin deficiency manifests internal deficient heat due to insufficiency of lung yin. The main contributing factors include chronic coughing damaging yin, tuberculosis or dry heat damaging yin.

Clinical manifestations

Unproductive coughs or coughing with scanty sticky sputum, weight loss, feverish sensations on the palms, soles and chest, night sweats, rosy cheeks, a dry mouth and throat, a dry red tongue and a thready rapid pulse; coughing up blood and hoarseness may also be present.

Analysis

Since the lungs like moistening but dislike dryness, lung yin deficiency may produce internal deficient heat to consume fluids and form phlegm, thus resulting in unproductive coughs or coughing with scanty sticky sputum. Failure of lung yin to nourish the muscles causes weight loss. Failure of lung yin (fluids) to ascend causes a dry mouth and throat. Exuberant internal deficient heat causes feverish sensations on the palms, soles and chest. Ascending of deficient fire causes rosy cheeks. Deficient heat disturbing the yin fluids causes night sweats. Deficient heat damaging lung collaterals causes coughing up of blood. Failure of lung yin to moisten the throat causes a hoarse voice. A dry red tongue and a thready rapid pulse are typical signs of internal heat due to yin deficiency.

Differentiation

This pattern should be distinguished from dry heat attacking the lungs. Dry heat attacking the lungs is often acute and is more commonly seen in autumn. It is marked by damage to fluids, such as dry nose and throat and unproductive coughs. However, it does not give yin damage signs, such as weight loss, rosy cheeks, tidal fever, night sweats, a red tongue and a thready pulse.

Distinctive notes

The distinctive points of this pattern include an unproductive cough or coughing with scanty sputum, a recurrent extended duration and yin deficiency symptoms, including weight loss, night sweats, a smaller tongue body and a thready pulse. For concurrent deficient heat, a red tongue, rosy cheeks, feverish sensations on the palms, soles and chest, a low-grade fever and a rapid pulse may also be present.

Wind–cold binding the lungs

Overview

Wind–cold binding the lungs manifests external wind–cold affecting lung *qi*.

Clinical manifestations

Coughing with white thin sputum, slight cold intolerance, a mild fever, an absence of sweating, a stuffy or runny nose, a white tongue coating and a floating tight pulse.

Analysis

External wind–cold obstructing lung *qi* causes coughing. Cold is yin in nature, causing white thin sputum. The lung opens into the nose; lung *qi* obstruction causes a stuffy or runny nose. Wind–cold binding *wei* causes slight cold intolerance, a mild fever and an absence of sweating. A white tongue coating and a floating tight pulse are typical signs of wind–cold attacking the exterior.

Differentiation

This pattern should be distinguished from a wind–cold exterior syndrome and cold attacking the lungs. A wind–cold exterior syndrome also results from an external contraction; however, this pattern is especially marked by lung-related symptoms. Cold attacking the lungs mainly causes coughing with profuse sputum, but with no obvious signs of an exterior syndrome.

Distinctive notes

The distinctive points of this pattern include a wind–cold exterior syndrome, lung-related symptoms and unproductive coughs or coughing with scanty sticky sputum (due to binding of lung *qi*).

Cold attacking the lungs

Overview

Cold attacking the lungs manifests cold retention in the lungs.

Clinical manifestations

Coughing with white thin clear sputum, panting, cold limbs, a pale tongue with a white coating and a slow pulse.

Analysis

Cold retention in the lungs blocks yang *qi* and causes ascending of lung *qi*, leading to coughing with white thin clear sputum and panting. Failure of lung *qi* to warm the body causes cold limbs. Cold retention impairs the circulation of *qi* and blood, resulting in a pale tongue with a white coating and a slow pulse.

Differentiation

This pattern should be distinguished from wind–cold binding the lungs. See the previous pattern for reference.

Distinctive notes

The distinctive points of this pattern include an excessive cold syndrome, such as cold limbs, a pale tongue with a white coating, a slow pulse and white thin clear sputum, and lung-related symptoms, such as coughing and panting.

Phlegm dampness obstructing the lungs

Overview

Phlegm dampness obstructing the lungs manifests accumulated phlegm dampness impairing the lung system. The main contributing factors include spleen *qi* deficiency, chronic coughing or contraction of cold–dampness.

Clinical manifestations

Coughing with profuse white sticky sputum, chest tightness, a pale tongue with a white greasy coating and a slippery pulse; panting with phlegm sounds in the throat may also be present.

Analysis

External pathogens attacking the lungs may impair the dispersing and descending of lung *qi*, causing water retention and subsequent phlegm dampness. Failure of spleen *qi* to transport and transform causes internal phlegm and further affects the lungs. Chronic coughing may also impair the lungs' function in regulating water passage, leading to water retention. All these factors contribute to coughing with profuse white sticky sputum. Phlegm dampness may also obstruct flow of lung *qi*, resulting in chest tightness or even panting with phlegm sounds in the throat. A pale tongue with a white greasy coating and a slippery pulse are typical signs of internal phlegm dampness.

Differentiation

This pattern is marked by a chronic duration and profuse sputum. It is worth noting that a critical condition of phlegm dampness may affect the heart as well, leading to concurrent symptoms of heart *qi* deficiency, heart yang deficiency or even sudden collapse of heart yang.

Distinctive notes

The distinctive points of this pattern include a recurrent extended duration of coughing (unlike an acute attack of external pathogens attacking the lungs), phlegm dampness symptoms (profuse white sticky sputum, phlegm sounds, a greasy tongue coating and a slippery or wiry pulse) and lung-related symptoms (coughing, panting and chest tightness).

Wind–heat attacking the lungs

Overview

Wind–heat attacking the lungs manifests external wind–heat impairing *wei*.

Clinical manifestations

Coughing with yellow thick sputum, fever, slight intolerance of wind–cold, a dry mouth with a sore throat, redness on the tip of the tongue with a thin yellow coating and a floating rapid pulse.

Analysis

Wind–heat may impair the dispersing and descending of lung *qi*, causing coughing. Heat is yang in nature and tends to consume fluids, leading to yellow thick sputum. Wind–heat attacking *wei* causes fever and slight intolerance of wind–cold. Wind–heat consuming fluids may cause a dry mouth with a sore throat. Redness on the tip of the tongue with a thin yellow coating indicates heat in the upper *jiao*. A floating rapid pulse is a typical sign of wind–heat attacking the lungs.

Differentiation

This pattern should be distinguished from dryness attacking the lungs and heat accumulating in the lungs. As mentioned in the pattern of lung yin deficiency, dry heat attacking the lungs is often acute and is more commonly seen in autumn. Heat accumulating in the lungs manifests interior heat in the lungs. In addition, both wind–heat attacking the lungs and dry heat attacking the lungs have a short duration and can cause concurrent symptoms of an exterior syndrome.

Distinctive notes

The distinctive points of this pattern include a wind–heat exterior syndrome and lung-related symptoms.

Heat accumulating in the lungs

Overview

Heat accumulating in the lungs manifests internal retention of heat in the lungs. The main contributing factors include contraction of warmth–heat or wind–heat or wind–cold transforming into heat after attacking the lungs.

Clinical manifestations

Coughing with yellow thick sputum, panting, fast breathing, a strong fever, thirst, restlessness, nasal flaring, a red tongue with a yellow coating and a rapid pulse; alternatively, chest pain, coughing up smelly sputum containing mucus or blood, constipation and scanty dark-yellow urine may also be present.

Analysis

Buildup of heat in the lungs can impair the dispersing and descending of lung *qi*, causing coughing, panting and fast breathing. Accumulated heat can consume fluid and thus form phlegm, causing yellow thick sputum. Exuberant interior heat causes a strong fever and thirst. Heat disturbing the mind may cause restlessness. Phlegm heat impairing the airway may cause nasal flaring (indicative of a critical condition). Over time, heat may damage lung collaterals, leading to *qi* stagnation, blood stasis and subsequent chest pain and coughing up of smelly sputum containing mucus and blood. Interior heat consuming fluids may cause constipation or scanty dark-yellow urine.

Differentiation

See the previous pattern for reference.

Distinctive notes

The distinctive points of this pattern include an excessive interior heat syndrome (from yellow sputum, fever to coughing up purulent blood and a strong or tidal fever) and lung-related symptoms, such as, coughing, panting, sputum, nasal flaring, and chest pain.

Dryness attacking the lungs

Overview

Dryness attacking the lungs manifests pathogenic dryness attacking the lung *wei*, particularly in autumn.

Clinical manifestations

Unproductive coughs or coughing with scanty sticky sputum (which may contain blood and is difficult to expectorate), chest pain, dry skin, lips and nose, fever, slight intolerance of wind–cold, a red tongue with a white or yellow coating and a rapid pulse.

Analysis

Dryness attacking the lungs may cause unproductive coughs or coughing with scanty sticky sputum. Dryness may damage the fluid, causing dry skin, lips and nose. Over time, coughing may damage the lung collaterals, leading to chest pain and coughing up of blood. Dryness attacking *wei* may cause fever and slight intolerance of wind–cold. The severity of fever and chills varies in an exterior syndrome. A warm-dryness exterior syndrome is similar to a wind–heat exterior syndrome. Dryness damaging fluids may cause a red tongue with a white coating and a floating rapid pulse, while dry heat attacking the lungs may cause a yellow tongue coating and a thready rapid pulse.

Differentiation

See the previous patterns for reference.

Distinctive notes

The distinctive points of this pattern include an acute onset in autumn, symptoms due to damage to fluids (such as unproductive coughs, sticky sputum and dry lips and nose) and lung-related symptoms (such as coughing with sputum).

In addition, cool-dryness may also give concurrent cold signs, while warm-dryness may also give heat signs.

Damp–heat in the large intestine

Overview

Damp–heat n the large intestine manifests damp–heat impairing the functions of the large intestine. The main contributing factors include external contraction of damp–heat and an improper diet.

Clinical manifestations

Abdominal pain, passing of stools containing blood or white mucus, tenesmus or emergent diarrhea mixed with smelly yellow feces, a red tongue with a yellow greasy coating and a slippery rapid or soft rapid pulse; a sense of incomplete emptying after diarrhea, a burning sensation of the anus, scanty dark-yellow urine, fever and thirst may also be present.

Analysis

Damp–heat may obstruct the *qi* activity of the large intestine, leading to abdominal pain and tenesmus. Over time, damp–heat may damage the collaterals, resulting in blood or mucus in the stools. Downward flow of damp–heat may cause emergent diarrhea mixed with yellow smelly feces. Dampness may obstruct the *qi* activity of the large intestine, causing a sense of incomplete emptying after diarrhea. Heat accumulating in the intestine may cause a burning sensation of the anus and scanty dark-yellow urine. Exuberant heat damaging fluids may cause thirst, fever and smelly sticky feces. A red tongue with a yellow greasy coating is a typical sign of damp–heat. More dampness than heat may cause a soft rapid pulse, while more heat than dampness may cause a slippery rapid pulse.

Differentiation

Diarrhea can be caused by either deficiency or excess patterns. Excess patterns are more related to the large intestine, while deficiency patterns are more related to the spleen. There are two excess patterns for diarrhea: damp–heat in the large intestine and food injury, which is often associated with a history of binge eating. Deficiency patterns include yang–*qi* deficiency of the large intestine, spleen deficiency and deficiency of the spleen and kidneys (diarrhea before dawn).

Distinctive notes

The distinctive points of this pattern include large-intestine-related symptoms (such as abdominal pain and diarrhea), an excess syndrome with a short duration and damp–heat symptoms (such as a yellow greasy tongue coating, and smelly or watery feces mixed with blood or mucus).

Insufficiency of liquid in the large intestine

Overview

Insufficiency of liquid in the large intestine manifests failure of body fluids to moisten and nourish the large intestine. The main contributing factors include chronic febrile conditions damaging yin, constitutional yin deficiency and loss of yin blood after childbirth.

Clinical manifestations

Difficult passing of dry stools, one bowel movement in several days, a dry mouth and throat, a dry tongue with a dry yellow coating and a thready hesitant pulse; alternatively, a foul breath and dizziness may also be present.

Analysis

Failure of fluids to moisten the large intestine may cause difficult passing of dry stools and one bowel movement in several days. Failure of fluids to ascend may cause a dry mouth and throat. Ascending of turbid *qi* may cause a foul breath and dizziness. Dry heat consuming yin fluids may cause a dry tongue with a dry yellow coating and a thready hesitant pulse.

Differentiation

This pattern is marked by dry stools with insufficient fluids. It should be distinguished from constipation due to *qi* deficiency (marked by *qi* deficiency symptoms), blood deficiency (often seen after childbirth or loss of blood), stomach yin deficiency (marked by retching, belching, an increased appetite and a dark red tongue with a peeled coating) and yang deficiency (often seen in the elderly and marked by strain during bowel movements).

Distinctive notes

The distinctive points of this pattern include difficult passing of dry stools and a dry mouth and throat. It is often seen at the later stages of yin fluid consumption.

Chronic diarrhea due to deficiency of the large intestine

Overview

Chronic diarrhea due to deficiency of the large intestine manifests yang–qi deficiency of the large intestine. Persistent diarrhea or dysentery can contribute to this condition.

Clinical manifestations

Severe diarrhea, fecal incontinence or even a prolapsed rectum, dull abdominal pain with a preference for pressure and warmth, a pale tongue with a white slippery coating, and a deep weak pulse.

Analysis

Chronic diarrhea or dysentery may damage yang–qi of the large intestine, further causing severe diarrhea, fecal incontinence or a prolapsed rectum. Yang deficiency may produce internal cold and qi stagnation, further resulting in a dull abdominal pain with a preference for pressure and warmth. A pale tongue with a white slippery coating and a deep weak pulse are typical signs of yang deficiency.

Differentiation

See the pattern of damp–heat in the large intestine for reference.

Distinctive notes

The distinctive points of this pattern include chronic diarrhea (not acute), absence of excess symptoms (such as a foul breath, a yellow greasy tongue coating, a severe abdominal pain and smelly feces) and presence of fecal incontinence or frequent diarrhea.

Summary

The patterns and diagnosis points for the lungs and large intestine:

Patterns	Distinctive diagnosis points
Lung *qi* deficiency	Weak coughing, shortness of breath and general hypofunction
Lung yin deficiency	Common lung-related symptoms + yin deficiency symptoms
Wind–cold binding the lungs	Wind–cold exterior syndrome + lung-related symptoms
Cold attacking the lungs	Excess cold syndrome + lung-related symptoms
Phlegm dampness obstructing the lungs	Recurrent chronic coughing with panting + phlegm dampness symptoms + lung-related symptoms
Wind–heat attacking the lungs	Wind–heat exterior syndrome + lung-related symptoms
Heat accumulating in the lungs	Excess interior heat syndrome + lung-related symptoms
Damp–heat in the large intestine	Large-intestine-related symptoms + excess syndrome + damp–heat symptoms
Insufficiency of liquid in the large intestine	Difficult passing of dry stools + a dry mouth and throat + the later stages of yin fluid damage
Chronic diarrhea due to deficiency of the large intestine	Chronic diarrhea + absence of excess syndrome + fecal incontinence or frequent diarrhea

QUESTIONS

1. How do you distinguish lung yin deficiency from dryness attacking the lungs?
2. Compare the clinical manifestations due to wind–cold binding the lungs and cold attacking the lungs.
3. How do you distinguish wind–heat attacking the lungs from heat accumulating in the lungs and dryness attacking the lungs?
4. List the clinical manifestations and distinctive diagnosis points of the three large intestine patterns.

Pattern Identification of the Spleen and Stomach

The spleen and stomach both reside in the middle *jiao* (energizer). The spleen governs the transportation and transformation of water, food and the body fluids. The stomach receives and decomposes food. Spleen *qi* ascends, while stomach *qi* descends. The spleen and stomach are therefore known as the acquired base and source of *qi* and blood production. They are internally–externally connected through meridians. The spleen also controls blood with vessels and governs the muscles of the four limbs. It opens into the mouth and its luster shows in the lips.

The patterns of the spleen and stomach can be classified into cold, heat, deficiency and excess. Common signs and symptoms of the spleen conditions include abdominal pain, bloating, diarrhea, edema, lack of energy and fatigue. Common symptoms of the stomach include stomachache, a poor appetite, vomiting, belching and hiccups.

Spleen qi deficiency

Overview

Spleen *qi* deficiency manifests failure of spleen *qi* to transport and transform. The main contributing factors include an improper diet, overexertion and chronic conditions consuming spleen *qi*.

Clinical manifestations

A poor appetite, gastric or abdominal fullness and distension (especially after eating food), loose stools, mental fatigue, lack of *qi*, reluctance to talk, pallor or a sallow complexion, a pale tongue with a white coating and a moderate weak pulse; edema or weight loss may also be present.

Analysis

Failure of spleen *qi* to transport and transform may cause a poor appetite and gastric or abdominal fullness and distension, especially after eating food. Water retention due to spleen *qi* deficiency may cause loose stools. Failure of the spleen to nourish muscles and the four limbs causes fatigue. Spleen *qi* deficiency causes lack of *qi* and reluctance to talk. Water–dampness due to spleen deficiency causes pallor and edema. Insufficient production of *qi* and blood causes weight loss and a sallow complexion. A pale tongue with a white coating and a floating weak pulse are typical signs of spleen *qi* deficiency.

Differentiation

Symptoms due to spleen *qi* deficiency vary greatly. However, it can be identified by *qi* deficiency symptoms coupled with exclusion of other organs, such as the heart and kidneys. Also, this pattern should be distinguished from dampness syndromes, which will be discussed later.

Distinctive notes

The distinctive points of this pattern include *qi* deficiency symptoms and hypofunction of the stomach, such as a poor appetite, bloating (especially after eating food), diarrhea, weight loss, a lusterless complexion or facial puffiness. In addition, dampness and phlegm need to be excluded, such as a swollen tongue with a greasy tongue coating and obesity.

Spleen yang deficiency

Overview

Spleen yang deficiency manifests failure of spleen yang to warm and transport. It often develops from spleen *qi* deficiency. The main contributing factors include overingestion of cold or raw food, overuse of cool or cold-property medications and kidney yang deficiency.

Clinical manifestations

Bloating, a poor appetite, dull abdominal pain with a preference for warmth and pressure, cold intolerance, cold limbs, thin loose stools, a pale swollen tongue with a white slippery coating and a deep, slow or weak pulse. A general heavy sensation, edema in the limbs, dysuria or profuse white thin clear leukorrhea may also be present.

Analysis

Failure of spleen yang to transport and transform may cause bloating and a poor appetite. Yang deficiency may produce internal cold retention and *qi* stagnation, causing abdominal pain with a preference for warmth and pressure. Yang deficiency may cause water–dampness retention and subsequent thin loose stools. Failure of spleen yang to warm the body may cause cold intolerance and cold limbs. Internal water–dampness may impair the *qi* transformation of the urinary bladder, leading to dysuria. Water–dampness in the body may cause a general heavy sensation. Downward flow of water–dampness may cause profuse white thin clear leukorrhea. A pale and swollen tongue with a white slippery coating and a deep slow weak pulse are typical signs of internal cold–dampness due to yang–*qi* deficiency.

Differentiation

This pattern can be identified by spleen *qi* deficiency symptoms coupled with cold intolerance or cold limbs. However, spleen yang deficiency can cause other accompanying symptoms, such as diarrhea, edema or white thin clear leukorrhea.

Distinctive notes

The distinctive points of this pattern include a chronic duration, spleen-related symptoms (such as appetite, digestion and muscle) and yang deficiency symptoms. Also, excessive dampness needs to be excluded.

Spleen *qi* sinking

Overview

Spleen *qi* sinking manifests loosened tendons or muscles and prolapsed internal organs due to spleen *qi* deficiency. The main contributing factors include an improper diet, overexertion and chronic conditions affecting the spleen.

Clinical manifestations

A falling sensation of the epigastrium or abdomen (particularly after eating food), frequent urges for bowel movements with a falling sensation of the anus, persistent diarrhea or dysentery, rectal prolapse, uterine prolapse, turbid urine, dizziness, blurred vision, a general heavy sensation, fatigue, a low voice, reluctance to talk, a pale tongue with a white coating and a weak pulse.

Analysis

Failure of spleen *qi* to transport and transform may cause inadequate supply to internal organs and subsequent prolapse, such as uterine prolapse or stomach prolapse. Stomach prolapse causes a falling sensation of the stomach, especially after eating food. Sinking of spleen *qi* causes frequent urges for bowel movements with a falling sensation of the anus, persistent diarrhea or dysentery. Failure of the spleen to distribute nutrients may affect the urinary bladder, leading to turbid urine. Failure of spleen yang to ascend may cause dizziness and blurred vision. Spleen *qi* deficiency causes a general heavy sensation, fatigue, a low voice and reluctance to talk. A pale tongue with a white coating and a weak pulse are typical signs of spleen *qi* weakness.

Differentiation

See the pattern of spleen *qi* deficiency for reference.

Distinctive notes

The distinctive points of this pattern include spleen *qi* deficiency, sinking of organs (such as stomach prolapse, rectal prolapse or uterine prolapse), sinking of *qi* (such as dizziness and blurred vision) and sinking of nutrients (such as turbid urine). Sinking of organs is most distinctive for identification.

It is worth noting that some symptoms can also be seen in kidney deficiency. This will be discussed later, in pattern identification of the kidneys and urinary bladder.

The spleen failing to control blood within the vessels

Overview

The spleen failing to control blood within the vessels manifests bleeding conditions due to spleen deficiency. The main contributing factors are chronic conditions and overexertion.

Clinical manifestations

Bloody stools, bloody urine, subcutaneous bruises, bleeding gums, heavy menstruation, uterine bleeding, a pale tongue with a white coating and a thready weak pulse; dizziness, mental fatigue, lassitude, reluctance to talk, a poor appetite, loose stools and a lusterless complexion may also be present.

Analysis

Failure of the spleen to control blood within the vessels may cause bloody stools, bloody urine, subcutaneous bruises and bleeding gums. This may further result in weakness of the *chong* and *ren* meridians, leading to heavy menstruation or uterine bleeding. Insufficient production of *qi* and blood may cause dizziness, mental fatigue, lassitude, reluctance to talk and a lusterless complexion. Spleen deficiency may also cause internal turbid dampness, resulting in a poor appetite and loose stools. A pale tongue with a white coating and a thready weak pulse are typical signs of deficiency.

Differentiation

This pattern should be distinguished from other patterns that may cause bleeding. Other than trauma, pathogenic heat and stagnant blood may also contribute to bleeding. Pathogenic heat often causes bright red blood, while stagnant blood causes dark blood and often involves a long duration. The spleen failing to control blood in the vessels often causes pale-colored blood coupled with spleen deficiency symptoms.

Distinctive notes

This pattern can be considered a severe pattern of spleen *qi* deficiency. It can be identified on the basis of spleen *qi* deficiency with bleeding.

Cold–dampness obstructing the spleen

Overview

Cold–dampness obstructing the spleen manifests internal cold–dampness affecting spleen yang. The main contributing factors include an improper diet (overingestion of cold food) and internal exuberance of dampness.

Clinical manifestations

Gastric or abdominal distension, oppression and pain, nausea, vomiting, a poor appetite, tastelessness, no thirst, loose stools, a heavy sensation of the head and body, a dark-yellow complexion, a pale swollen tongue with a white greasy slippery coating and a soft moderate pulse. Dark-gray yellow face and eyes, edema in the limbs, scanty urine and profuse leukorrhea may also be present.

Analysis

Internal cold–dampness obstructing spleen yang may cause gastric or abdominal distension, oppression and pain with a poor appetite. Failure of stomach *qi* to descend may cause nausea and vomiting. Cold–dampness (yin in nature) retention causes tastelessness and no thirst. Downward flow of dampness causes loose stools. Dampness has the property of heaviness and stickiness, causing a heavy sensation of the head and body. It may impair the circulation of *qi* and blood, leading to a lusterless complexion. Failure of spleen yang to disperse may cause overflow of bile, leading to dark-gray yellow face and eyes. Cold–dampness may cause the failure of yang–*qi* to transform water dampness, resulting in edema in the limbs. Cold–dampness may also impair the *qi* transformation of the urinary bladder, leading to scanty urine. Internal exuberance of cold–dampness causes a pale and swollen tongue with a white greasy or white slippery coating and a soft moderate pulse.

Differentiation

This pattern should be distinguished from spleen yang deficiency. Both patterns can cause failure of the spleen to transport and transform, cold signs, and dampness symptoms. However, cold–dampness obstructing the spleen is an excess pattern with a short duration and often causes a white greasy or white slippery coating and a soft moderate pulse, while spleen yang deficiency is a deficiency pattern with a long duration and often causes a white slippery tongue coating and a slow deep pulse.

Distinctive notes

The distinctive points of this pattern include a short duration, an absence of spleen *qi* deficiency symptoms and obvious cold–dampness symptoms.

Damp–heat accumulating in the spleen

Overview

Damp–heat accumulating in the spleen manifests internal damp–heat affecting the middle *jiao*. The main contributing factors include over-ingestion of sweet fatty food, excessive consumption of alcohol and external contraction of damp–heat.

Clinical manifestations

Gastric or abdominal discomfort, nausea, vomiting, a poor appetite, dark-yellow urine, loose stools, a heavy sensation in the limbs, bright or orange yellow face, eyes and skin, skin itching, persistent unresolved fever, a red tongue with a yellow greasy coating and a soft rapid pulse.

Analysis

Damp–heat may impair the transportation and transformation of the spleen and affect the descending of stomach *qi*, thus resulting in gastric or abdominal discomfort, nausea, vomiting and a poor appetite. Dampness has the property of heaviness and stickiness, causing a heavy sensation of the head and body. Downward flow of damp–heat may cause loose stools and scanty dark-yellow urine. Damp–heat scorching the liver and gallbladder may cause overflow of bile, resulting in yellow face and eyes in a bright orange color and skin itching. Hidden damp–heat may cause persistent unresolved fever. A red tongue with a yellow greasy coating and a soft rapid pulse are typical signs of internal damp–heat.

Differentiation

This pattern should be distinguished from dampness obstructing the spleen and stomach, external contraction of damp–heat, and damp–heat in the liver and gallbladder. It is different from cold obstructing the spleen and stomach in "heat" symptoms. External contraction of damp–heat is often seen in summer or autumn with a short duration and obvious exterior syndrome manifestations, such as fever, chills and general pain. Damp–heat in the liver and gallbladder causes distending pain and discomfort in the hypochondriac regions.

Distinctive notes

The distinctive points of this pattern are jaundice, fever and diarrhea, either alone or in combination. In addition, damp–heat symptoms (such as a yellow greasy tongue coating) and spleen stomach symptoms (such as a poor appetite and gastric or abdominal fullness and distension) are present.

Stomach yin deficiency

Overview

Stomach yin deficiency manifests a condition of internal deficient heat due to insufficiency of stomach yin. The main contributing factors include chronic stomach conditions, yin fluid consumption at the later stages of febrile conditions, overingestion of hot spicy food and emotional disturbance transforming into fire.

Clinical manifestations

A dull gastric pain, an increased appetite, gastric discomfort, retching, belching, a dry mouth and throat, constipation, scanty dark-yellow urine, a dry red tongue and a thready rapid pulse.

Analysis

Stomach yin deficiency may cause internal deficient heat to affect the descending of stomach *qi*, thus resulting in a dull gastric pain, an increased appetite and gastric discomfort. Deficient heat may disturb the stomach, resulting in ascending of stomach *qi* and subsequent retching and hiccups. Failure of stomach yin to moisten the throat causes a dry mouth and throat. Failure of stomach yin to moisten the large intestine causes constipation. A dry red tongue and a thready rapid pulse are typical signs of internal heat due to yin deficiency.

Differentiation

This pattern should be distinguished from stomach fire. Stomach fire is an excess pattern and causes a foul breath, a yellow tongue coating and a rough tongue. However, stomach fire may gradually result in stomach yin deficiency with hyperactivity of fire.

Distinctive notes

The distinctive points of this pattern include yin deficiency symptoms with abnormal digestion. In the case of presence of spleen *qi* deficiency symptoms, the pattern can be identified as spleen yin deficiency.

Food retention

Overview

Food retention manifests indigestion of food in the stomach. The main contributing factors include an improper diet and constitutional deficiency of the spleen and stomach.

Clinical manifestations

Gastric distension and pain, loss of appetite, belching, acid reflux, vomiting (the gastric distension and pain can be relieved after vomiting or flatus), a thick greasy tongue coating and a slippery pulse. Smelly loose stools may also be present.

Analysis

Food retention may impair the descending of stomach *qi* and result in gastric distension and pain. Retention of undigested food causes loss of appetite. Failure of stomach *qi* to descend and ascending of turbid *qi* may cause belching, acid reflux and vomiting. Vomiting can temporarily downregulate stomach *qi* and thus alleviate the gastric distension and pain. Downward flow of undigested food may cause flatus and smelly loose stools. Ascending of turbid stomach *qi* causes a thick greasy tongue coating. A slippery pulse is indicative of an excess syndrome.

Differentiation

This pattern should be distinguished from spleen deficiency. Spleen deficiency is a deficiency pattern and is characterized by deficiency symptoms. A history of food injury is not necessary for spleen deficiency.

Distinctive notes

This pattern can be identified by a history of food injury and exclusion of spleen *qi* deficiency and stomach fire.

Stomach cold

Overview

Stomach cold results from overingestion of cold food. It manifests a condition of yin cold retention in the stomach.

Clinical manifestations

Mild or spasmodic gastric pain that can be aggravated by cold and relieved by warmth, tastelessness, no thirst, a pale tongue with a white slippery coating and a deep or wiry pulse. Alternatively, mental fatigue, cold intolerance, cold limbs, preference for warmth (the gastric pain can be alleviated after eating food) and watery vomiting may also be present.

Analysis

Stomach cold can be classified into cold attacking the stomach and deficiency and cold of stomach *qi*. Cold has the property of contraction and can cause *qi* stagnation, resulting in gastric pain. Cold is yin in nature and can therefore aggravate pain. Yin pathogens do not consume fluids, causing tastelessness and no thirst. Over time, yang–*qi* can be damaged, followed by a transformation into a deficiency pattern. Binding of spleen *qi* causes mental fatigue. Failure of yang–*qi* to warm the body causes cold intolerance, cold limbs and preference for warmth. Eating food can activate yang–*qi* and therefore alleviate pain. Failure of stomach *qi* to warm and transform nutrients, as well as ascending of stomach *qi* may cause watery vomiting. A pale tongue with a white slippery pulse is a typical sign of internal yin cold with water retention. A deep pulse is indicative of cold. Water retention causes a wiry pulse.

Differentiation

This pattern should be distinguished from the spleen conditions. Stomach cold mainly causes stomachache, while spleen cold mainly causes diarrhea. In addition, deficiency is much more common in the spleen conditions than in the stomach conditions.

Distinctive notes

Cold attacking the stomach and deficiency and cold in the stomach can be identified by the duration. The former is acute, while the latter is chronic and lingering, involving mild symptoms with deficiency symptoms, such as a cold sensation of the stomach with a preference for warmth and a lusterless complexion.

Stomach heat

Overview

Stomach heat manifests exuberance of stomach fire. The main contributing factors include heat attacking the stomach, liver *qi* stagnation transforming into fire and overingestion of hot spicy fatty food.

Clinical manifestations

Gastric pain with a burning sensation, acid reflux, fast hunger even with an increased appetite, thirst with a desire to drink cold water, swelling, pain, ulcers or even bleeding gums, a foul breath, constipation, dark-yellow urine, a red tongue with a yellow coating and a slippery rapid pulse.

Analysis

Internal exuberance of stomach fire may impair the stomach collaterals, causing gastric pain with a burning sensation. Fire transformed from liver *qi* stagnation may affect the stomach, leading to ascending of stomach fire and subsequent gastric discomfort and acid reflux. Hyperactive stomach fire causes an increased appetite but fast hunger. Heat consuming fluids may cause thirst with a desire to drink cold water. Since the stomach meridian passes through the gums, ascending of stomach fire may cause swelling, pain, ulceration and even bleeding gums. Ascending of turbid stomach *qi* causes a foul breath. Heat consuming fluids in the intestines causes constipation and scanty dark-yellow urine. A red tongue with a yellow coating and a slippery rapid pulse are typical signs of exuberant heat.

Differentiation

This pattern should be distinguished from damp–heat due to spleen deficiency. Generally, the stomach can be identified by gastric pain, vomiting and acid reflux, while the spleen can be identified by abdominal distension and diarrhea.

Distinctive notes

This pattern can be concluded by a heat syndrome plus stomach pain or ascending of stomach *qi*. However, it is worth noting that mouth or gum ulcerations can also be known as ascending of stomach fire; and acid reflux can also be known as liver fire affecting the stomach.

Summary

The patterns and diagnosis points for the spleen and stomach:

Patterns	Distinctive Diagnosis Points
Spleen *qi* deficiency	*Qi* deficiency symptoms + spleen-related symptoms
Spleen yang deficiency	Spleen-related symptoms + yang deficiency symptoms + exclusion of excessive dampness
Spleen *qi* sinking	Spleen *qi* deficiency + sinking symptoms
Spleen failing to control blood in the vessels	Spleen *qi* deficiency + bleeding
Cold–dampness obstructing the spleen	A short duration + absence of spleen *qi* deficiency + obvious cold–dampness symptoms
Damp–heat accumulating in the spleen	Jaundice (yellow face, eyes and skin) + fever or diarrhea
Stomach yin deficiency	Yin deficiency symptoms + abnormal digestion
Food retention	A history of food injury + exclusion of spleen *qi* deficiency and stomach fire
Stomach cold	Be clear about cold attacking the stomach and deficiency and cold of stomach *qi*
Stomach heat	Heat syndrome + stomachache or ascending of stomach *qi*

QUESTIONS

1. Describe the clinical manifestations of cold–dampness obstructing the spleen and spleen yang deficiency. How do you distinguish these two patterns?
2. Describe the clinical manifestations and pathogenesis of the spleen failing to control blood in the vessels and spleen *qi* sinking.
3. List the main pathologies of the stomach.
4. Describe the clinical manifestations and diagnosis points of stomach yin deficiency and food retention.
5. Distinguish between excessive stomach cold and deficient stomach cold.

Pattern Identification of the Liver and Gallbladder

The liver resides in the right-side hypochondriac area, and the gallbladder is attached to the liver. They are internally–externally connected through meridians. The liver maintains free flow of *qi*, i.e. it regulates *qi* activity, emotions, bile secretion and discharge, digestion and absorption of the spleen and stomach, as well as the transportation and distribution of *qi*, blood and body fluids. In addition, it helps to regulate ovulation, menstruation and semen. Another main function of the liver is to store blood and regulate the blood volume. The liver opens into the eyes, its tissue shows in tendons and its luster manifests in nails.

The physiological functions of the gallbladder are to store and discharge bile and help to digest food. The gallbladder is also associated with emotions. Its functions are regulated and controlled by the liver. A normal function of the liver in maintaining the free flow of *qi* can guarantee normal bile storage and discharge, thus maintaining normal physiological functions of the body.

The main pathologies of the liver manifest either as a dysfunction of the liver in maintaining free flow of *qi* or as a disorder of the liver in storing the blood. Common signs and symptoms of the liver conditions include a distending or wandering pain in the chest or hypochondriac area, restlessness, irritability, dizziness, headache with a sense of distension, tremor of the limbs, convulsions of the hands and feet, blurred vision, irregular menstruation and distending pain of the testes. The patterns of the liver conditions can be classified into cold, heat, deficiency and excess.

The main pathologies of the gallbladder manifest as either an abnormal function of the gallbladder in storing and discharging the bile or emotional disturbance. Common signs and symptoms of the gallbladder conditions include a bitter taste, a tendency to panic, insomnia and jaundice.

Liver qi stagnation

Overview

Liver *qi* stagnation manifests an abnormal function of the liver in maintaining the free flow of *qi*. The main contributing factors include mental irritation, depression and chronic conditions of other organs. This pattern is characterized by *qi* stagnation, along with varying symptoms in different body parts where the *qi* stagnation stays.

Clinical manifestations

Depression, restlessness, irritability, frequent sighing, distension, tightness or wandering pain in the chest or hypochondriac regions, a foreign body sensation in the throat (also known as plum stone *qi* or globus hystericus), an enlarged thyroid, abdominal masses, breast distension or masses, irregular menstruation, dysmenorrhea, amenorrhea and a wiry pulse.

Analysis

The liver is closely associated with emotions. Mental irritation or emotional disturbance may cause liver *qi* stagnation, resulting in depression, restlessness, irritability and frequent sighing. Since the liver meridian passes through the hypochondriac regions and lower (lateral) abdomen, liver *qi* stagnation may cause distension, tightness or wandering pain in the chest or hypochondriac regions. Over time, *qi* stagnation may produce phlegm to ascend with *qi*, leading to a foreign body sensation, an enlarged thyroid or abdominal masses. *Qi* stagnation may also cause blood stasis, affecting the *chong* and *ren* meridians and thus resulting in breast distension and masses, irregular menstruation, dysmenorrhea or amenorrhea. A wiry pulse is indicative of a liver condition.

Persistent liver *qi* stagnation may transform into fire, developing ascending of liver fire. Liver *qi* stagnation may also affect the spleen, developing liver *qi* affecting the spleen. Additionally, it may further result in blood stasis.

Differentiation

This pattern should be distinguished from ascending of liver fire. Liver *qi* stagnation is marked by *qi* depression, *qi* stagnation and emotional fluctuations, while ascending of liver fire is mainly marked by fire–heat symptoms.

Distinctive notes

The distinctive points of this pattern are mental irritation, emotional depression and dysfunction of the liver in maintaining the free flow of *qi*. The severity of this pattern is closely linked to emotions.

Ascending of liver fire

Overview

Ascending of liver fire manifests the fire transformed from liver *qi* stagnation ascending along the pathway of the liver meridian. The main contributing factors include persistent liver *qi* stagnation, overingestion of hot warm food and internal buildup of damp–heat.

Clinical manifestations

Dizziness, headache with a sense of distension, tinnitus, a red face, redness, swelling and pain of the eyes, restlessness, irritability, insomnia or dream-disturbed sleep, a dry mouth with a bitter taste, constipation, scanty dark-yellow urine, a red tongue with a yellow coating and a wiry rapid pulse; alternatively, a burning pain in the hypochondriac regions, hematemesis, heavy menstruation or an earlier menstrual period may also be present.

Analysis

Ascending liver fire may disturb the head, leading to dizziness and headache with a sense of distension. Since the liver opens into the eyes, ascending of liver fire along the meridian may cause redness, swelling and pain of the eyes. Since the gallbladder is attached to the liver and the gallbladder meridian enters the ears, liver fire may affect the gallbladder and result in tinnitus. Internal disturbance of liver fire may cause restlessness, irritability, insomnia or dream-disturbed sleep. Liver fire affecting the liver collaterals may cause a burning pain in the hypochondriac regions. Fire–heat consuming fluids may cause a dry mouth with a bitter taste, constipation and scanty dark-yellow urine. Liver fire may accelerate the flow of blood, further resulting in hematemesis, heavy menstruation and an earlier menstrual period. A red tongue with a yellow coating and a wiry rapid pulse are typical signs of an excess liver syndrome.

Ascending of liver fire develops from liver *qi* stagnation. Left uncontrolled, this pattern may further result in hyperactivity of liver yang transforming into wind.

Differentiation

This pattern should be distinguished from hyperactivity of liver yang. Both patterns show a red face and eyes, restlessness and irritability; however, hyperactivity of liver yang also causes soreness and weakness of the low back and knee joints due to liver yin deficiency.

Distinctive notes

The distinctive point of this pattern is a history of liver *qi* stagnation coupled with obvious symptoms caused by internal heat transforming into fire.

Liver blood deficiency

Overview

Liver blood deficiency manifests failure of the liver in regulating blood and subsequent malnourishment of the relevant *zang–fu* organs. The main contributing factors include insufficient production of blood, loss of blood and chronic conditions consuming liver blood. It generally involves liver-related symptoms of a systemic blood deficiency.

Clinical manifestations

Vertigo, tinnitus, dry eyes, blurred vision, poor vision or night blindness, a pale lusterless or sallow complexion, numbness or tremor of the hands and feet, muscle spasm or twitching, dry nails, scanty menstruation in a pale color, amenorrhea, pale lips, a pale tongue with a thin coating and a thready pulse.

Analysis

Failure of liver blood to nourish the mind may cause vertigo and tinnitus. Since the liver opens into the eyes, liver blood deficiency causes dry eyes, blurred vision, poor vision or night blindness. Failure of liver blood to ascend and nourish the head and face may cause a pale lusterless or sallow complexion, and a pale tongue and lips. Since the tissue of the liver shows in tendons and its luster manifests in nails, liver blood deficiency causes numbness or tremor of the hands and feet, muscle spasm or twitching, dry nails and a thready pulse. Failure of liver blood to nourish the *chong* and *ren* may cause scanty menstruation in a pale color or amenorrhea. Left untreated, liver blood deficiency may further develop into blood deficiency generating wind.

Differentiation

This pattern should be distinguished from heart blood deficiency. Both patterns have blood deficiency symptoms; however, they can be identified by heart- or liver-related symptoms. Additionally, this pattern needs to be distinguished from liver yin deficiency. Liver blood deficiency is mainly marked by blood deficiency, while liver yin deficiency is mainly marked by deficient heat.

Distinctive notes

The distinctive points of this pattern include blood deficiency symptoms and liver-related symptoms.

Liver yin deficiency

Overview

Liver yin deficiency manifests deficient heat due to insufficiency of liver yin fluids. The main contributing factors include liver *qi* stagnation transforming into fire and damage to yin fluids at the later stages of liver conditions or febrile diseases.

Clinical manifestations

Vertigo, tinnitus, dry painful eyes, pain in the hypochondriac regions, hot flushes, feverish sensations on the palms, soles and chest, tidal fever, night sweats, a dry mouth, twitching of the hands and feet, a dry red tongue and a wiry thready rapid pulse.

Analysis

Failure of liver yin to nourish the head and eyes may cause vertigo and tinnitus. Since the liver opens into the eyes, liver yin deficiency causes dry painful eyes. Failure of liver yin to nourish the liver meridian may cause pain in the hypochondriac regions. Yin deficiency may produce internal heat and result in hot flushes, feverish sensations on the palms, soles and chest, tidal fever, night sweats, a dry mouth, a dry red tongue and a wiry thready pulse. Failure of liver yin to nourish tendons or muscles may cause twitching of the hands and feet.

It is worth noting that liver yin deficiency may affect the kidneys, leading to yin deficiency of the liver and kidneys and subsequent hyperactivity of liver yang.

Differentiation

This pattern should be distinguished from ascending of liver fire. Both patterns have heat symptoms; however, this pattern manifests deficient heat in the liver, while ascending of liver fire manifests excessive heat in the liver.

Distinctive notes

The distinctive points of this pattern include general yin deficiency symptoms and liver-related symptoms.

Hyperactivity of liver yang

Overview

Hyperactivity of liver yang manifests failure of liver yin to control liver yang. It is characterized by liver yin deficiency and hyperactivity of liver yang. The main contributing factors include liver *qi* transforming into fire to consume liver yin and yin deficiency of the liver and kidneys.

Clinical manifestations

Vertigo, tinnitus, headache with a sense of distension, a top-heavy feeling, red face and eyes, restlessness, irritability, insomnia or dream-disturbed sleep, soreness and weakness of the low back and knee joints, feverish sensations on the palms, soles and chest, hot flushes, a red tongue and a wiry powerful or wiry thready rapid pulse.

Analysis

Hyperactive yang due to yin deficiency of the liver and kidneys may cause vertigo, tinnitus, headache with a sense of distension, a top-heavy feeling and red face and eyes. Liver *qi* stagnation transforming into fire may cause restlessness, irritability, insomnia or dream-disturbed sleep. Failure of liver yin to nourish tendons or muscles may cause soreness and weakness of the low back and knee joints. Internal deficient heat due to yin deficiency causes feverish sensations on the palms, soles and chest, hot flushes, a red tongue and a wiry powerful or wiry thready rapid pulse.

Differentiation

This pattern should be distinguished from ascending of liver fire and liver yin deficiency. See the previous patterns for reference.

Distinctive notes

The distinctive points of this pattern include manifestations due to yin deficiency of the liver and kidneys and symptoms due to hyperactivity of liver yang.

Internal stirring of liver wind

Overview

Internal stirring of liver wind manifests a set of clinical symptoms including vertigo, tremor and convulsions. It is mainly caused by failure of yin fluids and essence blood of the liver and kidneys to nourish tendons and constrain yang. Clinically, this pattern can be subcategorized into liver yang transforming into wind, extreme heat generating wind, yin deficiency stirring wind and blood deficiency generating wind.

Liver yang transforming into wind

Overview

This develops from hyperactivity of liver yang. It is mainly caused by failure of yin fluid deficiency of the liver and kidneys to constrain yang.

Clinical manifestations

Vertigo, headache, a top-heavy feeling, unstable walking, a red tongue with a thin or greasy coating and a wiry powerful pulse; alternatively, neck rigidity, tremor of the limbs, numbness of the hands and feet, slurred speech, a deviated tongue, sudden collapse, unconsciousness, deviated mouth and eyes, hemiplegia, tongue stiffness and phlegm sounds in the throat may also be present.

Analysis

This pattern often follows hyperactivity of liver yang. Hyperactive liver yang disturbing the mind may cause vertigo, headache, a top-heavy feeling and unstable walking. Ascending of liver wind carrying disordered *qi* and blood may cause neck rigidity, tremor of the limbs and numbness of the hands and feet. Ascending of liver wind carrying turbid phlegm may cause slurred speech with a deviated tongue. Liver wind mixed with turbid phlegm may disturb the mind, leading to sudden collapse, unconsciousness, tongue stiffness and phlegm sounds in the throat. Wind phlegm obstructing the meridians may cause deviation of the mouth and eyes and hemiplegia. A red tongue and a wiry powerful pulse are typical signs of hyperactivity yang transforming into wind.

With pre-existing hyperactivity of liver yang, presence of aggravated headache and dizziness, tremor of the hands and feet and numbness of the limbs can be identified as liver yang transforming into wind. These symptoms are warning signs of a stroke. Stroke-related symptoms, including sudden collapse, unconsciousness, tongue stiffness, hemiplegia and phlegm sounds in the throat, can be life-threatening.

Differentiation

This pattern should be distinguished from hyperactivity of liver yang. Both patterns have vertigo and headache; however, this pattern is more severe than hyperactivity of liver yang, coupled with the presence of tremor or numbness of the limbs. In severe cases of this pattern, sudden collapse and hemiplegia may also occur.

Distinctive notes

The distinctive notes of this pattern include a history of hyperactivity of liver yang and presence of wind stirring or abnormal mental activities.

Extreme heat generating wind

Overview

Extreme heat generating wind manifests stirring of liver wind due to exuberant heat consuming yin fluid. It is often caused by a high-grade fever.

Clinical manifestations

A high-grade fever, delirium, manic restlessness, uncontrollable jerking movements of the arms and legs, neck rigidity, opisthotonos, trismus, a staring spell, coma, a red tongue with a yellow coating and a wiry rapid pulse.

Analysis

Exuberant heat causes a high-grade fever. Heat disturbing the mind may cause manic restlessness. Heat consuming body fluids may cause malnourishment of the tendons and muscles, leading to tremor of the hands and feet, neck rigidity, opisthotonos, trismus and a staring spell. Heat misting the mind may cause coma and delirium. A red tongue with a yellow coating and a wiry rapid pulse are typical signs of exuberant heat.

Differentiation

This pattern should be distinguished from liver yang transforming into wind. Both patterns have wind stirring symptoms; however, this pattern is marked by a high-grade fever with wind, while liver yang transforming into wind is linked to a history of liver yin deficiency and hyperactivity of liver yang.

Distinctive notes

This pattern is distinctively marked by high fever and wind stirring.

Yin deficiency stirring wind

Overview

Yin deficiency stirring wind manifests failure of yin fluid to nourish tendons and muscles. It is often caused by severe deficiency of yin fluid and is commonly seen in the later stages of externally contracted conditions or internally damaged miscellaneous diseases.

Clinical manifestations

Twitching of the hands, feet and muscles, tidal fever in the afternoon, feverish sensations on the palms, soles and chest, night sweats, a dry mouth and throat, weight loss, a red tongue with a scanty coating and a wiry rapid pulse.

Analysis

Severe consumption of yin fluid in the later stages of febrile or miscellaneous diseases may cause twitching of the hands, feet and muscles. Yin deficiency may produce internal heat, causing tidal fever in the afternoon, feverish sensations on the palms, soles and chest, a dry mouth and throat, weight loss, a red tongue with a scanty coating and a wiry rapid pulse.

Differentiation

This pattern should be distinguished from liver yang transforming into wind and extreme heat generating wind. All three patterns have wind stirring symptoms; however, liver yang transforming into wind is marked by hyperactive yang due to yin deficiency, extreme heat generating wind is marked by high fever with wind stirring, and yin deficiency stirring wind is marked by yin deficiency symptoms with twitching of the hands and feet.

Distinctive notes

This pattern involves yin deficiency and wind stirring.

Blood deficiency generating wind

Overview

Blood deficiency generating wind manifests failure of blood to nourish the tendons and muscles. It is often caused by heavy bleeding or chronic conditions.

Clinical manifestations

Twitching of the hands, feet and muscles, numbness with impaired movement of the limbs, vertigo, tinnitus, dry eyes with blurred vision, a lusterless or sallow complexion, dry nails, a pale tongue and a wiry thready or thready pulse.

Analysis

Since the liver stores blood and opens into the eyes, its tissue shows in the tendons and its luster manifests in the nails, liver blood deficiency may cause twitching of the hands, feet and muscles, numbness with impaired movement of the limbs and dry nails. Failure of liver blood to ascend to nourish the brain may cause vertigo, tinnitus, dry eyes with blurred vision and a lusterless or sallow complexion. A pale tongue and a wiry thready or thready pulse are typical signs of liver blood deficiency.

Differentiation

This pattern should be distinguished from yin deficiency stirring wind. Both patterns have wind stirring symptoms; however, yin deficiency stirring wind is marked by tidal fever and night sweats, while blood deficiency generating wind is marked by a lusterless complexion and a pale tongue.

Distinctive notes

The distinctive points of this pattern include deficient wind stirring and blood deficiency symptoms.

Cold retention in the liver meridian

Overview

Cold retention in the liver meridian manifests *qi* stagnation and blood stasis within the liver meridian. It is often caused by contraction of cold.

Clinical manifestations

Lower (lateral) abdominal pain with a cold sensation; the pain may radiate to the testes or scrotum, coupled with a falling sensation and tenderness; the pain may also radiate to the thigh, the pain can be aggravated by cold and relieved by warmth; a pale tongue with a white or dark coating and a deep wiry pulse. Cold intolerance, cold limbs and pallor may also be present.

Analysis

Since the liver meridian passes around the genitalia and lower abdomen, cold retention in the liver meridian may cause cold pain in the lower abdomen, testes and scrotum with a falling sensation or a pain radiating to the thigh. Cold has the property of contraction and can affect the circulation of *qi* and blood, leading to tenderness and pain that can be aggravated by cold and alleviated by warmth. Cold can obstruct yang–*qi* and thus cause cold intolerance, cold limbs, pallor and a pale tongue with a white coating. A deep wiry pulse is indicative of a liver condition.

Differentiation

This pattern should be distinguished from cold hernia, also known as the small intestine herniated into the scrotum. Cold hernia is marked by pain alone without cold symptoms.

Distinctive notes

This pattern is distinctively marked by pain in the lower abdomen and testes with a falling sensation as well as cold symptoms (such as cold limbs, and the pain can be aggravated by cold).

Damp–heat in the liver and gallbladder

Overview

Damp–heat in the liver and gallbladder manifests internal accumulation of damp–heat in the liver and gallbladder. The main contributing factors include external contraction of damp–heat, internal damp–heat due to spleen deficiency and overingestion of sweet, fatty food.

Clinical manifestations

Burning or distending pain in the hypochondriac regions, masses in the hypochondrium region with tenderness upon palpation, yellow eyes, yellow urine and yellow body skin (bright-orange-like yellow), fever, a bitter taste, a poor appetite, nausea, vomiting, bloating, constipation or diarrhea, a red tongue with a yellow greasy coating and a wiry rapid or wiry slippery pulse.

Analysis

Internal buildup of damp–heat may affect *qi* activities, causing burning or distending pain in hypochondriac regions or masses with tenderness upon palpation. Damp–heat may impair the function of the liver in maintaining the free flow of *qi*, leading to overflow of bile and subsequently a bitter taste, yellow eyes and yellow urine. A bright-orange-like yellow indicates yang jaundice. Internal damp–heat may affect the descending of stomach *qi*, leading to nausea, vomiting, bloating and constipation or diarrhea. A red tongue with a yellow greasy coating and a wiry rapid or wiry slippery pulse are typical signs of damp–heat in the liver and gallbladder.

Differentiation

This pattern should be distinguished from damp–heat in the spleen and stomach. Both patterns have internal damp–heat; however, other than jaundice, damp–heat in the spleen and stomach causes a poor appetite, nausea, vomiting, gastric fullness and a greasy tongue coating, while damp–heat in the liver and gallbladder mainly causes jaundice and pain in the hypochondriac regions.

Distinctive notes

This pattern is distinctively marked by damp–heat symptoms, jaundice and pain in the hypochondriac regions.

Gallbladder *qi* stagnation with phlegm retention

Overview

Gallbladder *qi* stagnation with phlegm retention manifests internal phlegm heat due to dysfunction of the liver and gallbladder in maintaining the free flow of *qi*. It is mainly caused by emotional disturbance and resultant phlegm dampness.

Clinical manifestations

Panic, insomnia, restlessness, timidity, a bitter taste, nausea, chest tightness, distension in the hypochondriac regions, dizziness, blurred vision, tinnitus, a yellow greasy tongue coating and a wiry slippery pulse.

Analysis

Qi stagnation may produce phlegm, dampness and heat to affect gallbladder *qi*, leading to panic, insomnia, restlessness and timidity. Phlegm heat may cause a bitter taste, nausea, chest tightness and distension in the hypo-chondriac regions. Ascending of phlegm heat may cause dizziness, blurred vision and tinnitus. A yellow greasy tongue coating and a wiry slippery pulse are typical signs of internal phlegm heat.

Differentiation

This pattern should be distinguished from phlegm fire disturbing the heart, which is marked by restlessness, abnormal mental activities, incoherent speech and mania.

Distinctive notes

This pattern is distinctively marked by panic, insomnia and timidity, coupled with chest tightness, nausea and a yellow greasy tongue coating.

Summary

The patterns of the liver and gallbladder conditions:

Patterns	Distinctive Diagnosis Points
Liver *qi* stagnation	*Qi* depression, *qi* stagnation and emotional fluctuations
Ascending of liver fire	A history of liver *qi* stagnation + heat symptoms
Liver yin deficiency	Yin deficiency symptoms + liver-related symptoms
Hyperactivity of liver yang	Yin deficiency symptoms + hyperactive yang symptoms
Liver yang transforming into wind	A history of hyperactivity of liver yang + wind stirring or abnormal mental activities
Extreme heat generating wind	High-grade fever + wind stirring
Yin deficiency generating wind	Yin deficiency symptoms + wind stirring
Blood deficiency generating wind	Blood deficiency symptoms + wind stirring
Cold retention in the liver meridian	Pain with a falling sensation in the lower abdomen and testes + cold intolerance, cold limbs and cold-aggravated pain
Damp–heat in the liver and gallbladder	Damp–heat symptoms + jaundice or pain in the hypochondriac regions
Gallbladder stagnation with phlegm retention	Panic, insomnia, timidity + phlegm heat symptoms (such as chest tightness, nausea and a yellow greasy tongue coating)

QUESTIONS

1. Describe the clinical manifestations of liver *qi* stagnation, ascending of liver fire, liver blood deficiency, liver yin deficiency and hyperactivity of liver yang.
2. Analyze the etiology and pathogenesis of the above five patterns.
3. How can you distinguish liver *qi* stagnation from ascending of liver fire, liver yin deficiency, hyperactivity of liver yang and internal stirring of liver wind? Try to analyze the interactions between their etiology and pathogenesis.
4. Describe the clinical manifestations of cold retention in the liver meridian, damp–heat in the liver and gallbladder, and gallbladder stagnation with phlegm retention.

Pattern Identification of the Kidneys and Urinary Bladder

The kidneys reside in the lumbar region — one on the left and the other on the right. The urinary bladder is located at the center of the lower abdomen. They kidneys are internally–externally connected with the urinary bladder through meridians. They store essence, govern reproduction, controls bone and produce marrow to supplement the brain. As a result, the kidneys are also known as the congenital base. They also govern water and absorb *qi*. They open into the ears, their tissue shows in the bone and luster manifests in the hair.

The physiological function of the urinary bladder is to store and discharge urine. A normal function of the urinary bladder depends on the *qi* transformation of the kidneys.

The main pathologies of the kidneys manifest abnormal functions of the kidneys, often causing deficiency patterns. Common signs and symptoms of the kidney conditions include soreness and weakness of the low back and knee joints, tinnitus, deafness, prematurely graying hair, loosened teeth, impotence, nocturnal emissions, sterility due to a low sperm count, scanty menstruation or amenorrhea, edema, and abnormal urination and bowel movements.

The main pathologies of the urinary bladder mainly manifest as abnormal micturition, such as dysuria, frequent urgent painful urination, enuresis and urinary incontinence.

Kidney yang deficiency

Overview

Kidney yang deficiency manifests a condition due to yang–*qi* deficiency of the kidneys. The main contributing factors include constitutional yang deficiency, sex indulgence, aging, chronic conditions, contraction of external pathogens and conditions of other organs.

Clinical manifestations

Soreness, weakness or pain of the low back and knee joints, cold intolerance, cold limbs, dizziness, a low spirit, a bright pale or dark complexion, impotence, sterility, diarrhea mixed with undigested food, diarrhea before dawn, a pale tongue with a white coating and a deep thready weak pulse.

Analysis

Since the lumbus houses the kidneys and the kidneys dominate bones, failure of kidney yang to warm and nourish the lumbus and bones may cause soreness, weakness or pain of the low back and knee joints. Failure of yang–*qi* to warm the body may cause cold intolerance and cold limbs. Failure of clean yang to ascend may cause dizziness and a low spirit. Failure of yang–*qi* to circulate blood may cause a bright pale or dark complexion. Kidney yang deficiency may cause fire declining of the vital gate, resulting in impotence and sterility. Kidney yang deficiency may further cause spleen yang deficiency and subsequent diarrhea mixed with undigested food or diarrhea before dawn. A pale tongue with a white coating and a deep thready weak pulse are typical signs of kidney yang deficiency.

Differentiation

This pattern should be distinguished from a general yang deficiency syndrome. General yang deficiency is marked by deficiency and cold of the body, while kidney yang deficiency also includes kidney-related symptoms.

Distinctive notes

This pattern is distinctively marked by hypofunction of the kidneys and deficiency cold symptoms.

Kidney yin deficiency

Overview

Kidney yin deficiency manifests a condition due to insufficiency of kidney yin fluid. The main contributing factors include chronic conditions, febrile diseases, congenital deficiency, sex indulgence, loss of blood or fluids, and overingestion of dry and warm-property food or medications.

Clinical manifestations

Soreness, weakness or pain of the low back and knee joints, vertigo, tinnitus, insomnia or dream-disturbed sleep, weight loss, tidal fever, night sweats, feverish sensations on the palms, soles and chest, a dry mouth and throat, nocturnal emissions, premature ejaculations, scanty menstruation, amenorrhea or uterine bleeding, a red tongue with a scanty coating and a thready rapid pulse.

Analysis

Failure of kidney yin to nourish the lumbus and bones may cause soreness, weakness or pain of the low back and knee joints. Failure of kidney yin to fill up the brain marrow may cause vertigo and tinnitus. Failure of kidney water to constrain heart fire may cause insomnia or dream-disturbed sleep. Kidney yin deficiency may cause internal heat, resulting in weight loss, tidal fever, night sweats, feverish sensations on the palms, soles and chest, a dry mouth and throat, a red tongue with a scanty coating and a thready rapid pulse. Internal deficient heat due to kidney yin deficiency may cause nocturnal emissions and premature ejaculations. Kidney yin deficiency may affect essence blood, leading to scanty menstruation or amenorrhea. Internal deficient fire may also accelerate the flow of blood, resulting in uterine bleeding.

Differentiation

This pattern should be distinguished from a general yin deficiency syndrome. General yin deficiency syndrome is marked by yin deficiency with internal heat, while this pattern also includes the kidney-related symptoms.

Distinctive notes

This pattern is distinctively marked by kidney deficiency symptoms and clinical manifestations due to internal deficient heat.

Insufficiency of kidney essence

Overview

Insufficiency of kidney essence manifests delayed growth and development due to deficiency of kidney essence. The main contributing factors include congenital maldevelopment, constitutional weakness, hypofunction of the spleen and stomach, sexual indulgence and severe chronic conditions.

Clinical manifestations

Delayed growth and development, delayed closure of the fontanelle, short stature, mental retardation, skeletal flaccidity, slow movements, sterility, scanty menstruation or amenorrhea, premature aging, loss of hair with loosened teeth, tinnitus, deafness, soreness and weakness of the low back and knee joints, a dull spirit, a poor memory, a small tongue and a thready weak pulse.

Analysis

Since the kidneys store essence and dominate growth and reproduction, failure of kidney essence may cause delayed growth in children, delayed closure of the fontanelle and short stature. Failure of kidney essence to supplement the brain marrow may cause mental retardation, skeletal flaccidity, slow movements, a dull spirit and a poor memory. Deficiency of kidney essence may also cause sterility and scanty menstruation or amenorrhea. Since the kidneys open into the ears and their tissue shows in bone, kidney essence deficiency may cause loss of hair (hair is known as the extension of blood, and blood and essence share the same source), loosened teeth, tinnitus, deafness, and soreness and weakness of the low back and knee joints. Premature aging, a small tongue and a thready weak pulse are typical signs of deficiency.

Differentiation

This pattern should be distinguished from kidney yang deficiency and kidney yin deficiency. All three patterns have kidney deficiency. Both kidney yang deficiency and kidney yin deficiency have obvious cold and heat symptoms. However, this pattern has no visible cold or heat symptoms.

Distinctive notes

This pattern is distinctively characterized by severe delayed growth and development or severe reproductive hypofunction.

Weakness of kidney qi

Overview

Weakness of kidney *qi* manifests a condition due to infirmness of kidney *qi*. The main contributing factors include congenital deficiency, sex indulgence, aging and chronic conditions.

Clinical manifestations

Clear profuse urine, frequent urination, urine dribbling, urinary incontinence, enuresis, increased urination at night, spermatorrhea, premature ejaculations, thin clear leukorrhea, susceptibility to miscarriage, mental fatigue, lassitude, soreness and weakness of the low back and knee joints, hearing impairment, pallor, a pale tongue with a white coating and a thready weak deep pulse.

Analysis

Failure of kidney *qi* to constrain the urinary bladder may cause clear profuse urine, frequent urination, urine dribbling, urinary incontinence, enuresis, and increased urination at night. Failure of kidney *qi* to constrain the essence chamber may cause spermatorrhea, premature ejaculations, thin clear leukorrhea and susceptibility to miscarriage. Kidney *qi* deficiency may also cause hypofunction of the other organs and meridians, leading to mental fatigue, lassitude, soreness and weakness of the low back and knee joints, hearing impairment, pallor, a pale tongue with a white coating and a thready weak deep pulse.

Differentiation

Abnormal urination in this pattern should be distinguished from damp–heat in the urinary bladder. Damp–heat in the urinary bladder is characterized by frequent urgent painful urination, scanty dark-yellow urine, a yellow greasy tongue coating and a rapid pulse. This pattern has no damp–heat symptoms. Also, it has no obvious cold or heat symptoms, unlike kidney yang deficiency and kidney yin deficiency.

Distinctive notes

This pattern is distinctively marked by an uncontrollable urinary bladder, insecurity of the essence chamber or *dai* meridian and kidney *qi* deficiency.

The kidneys failing to receive qi

Overview

The kidneys failing to receive *qi* manifests a condition due to kidney-*qi* deficiency. It is often caused by chronic lung conditions.

Clinical manifestations

Panting and shortness of breath that can be aggravated by physical exertion, an inability to lie flat, breathing with an open mouth and raised shoulders, more exhalation than inhalation, a low voice, soreness and weakness of the low back and knee joints; in severe cases, chest tightness, cold limbs, a bluish complexion, cold sweats and a deficient floating rootless pulse may also be present. Alternatively, a red face, restlessness, a dry mouth and throat, a red tongue and a thready rapid pulse may be present.

Analysis

The lungs govern respiration and the kidneys dominate the receiving of *qi*. Lung *qi* deficiency may cause panting and shortness of breath that can be aggravated by physical exertion. Kidney *qi* deficiency causes an inability to lie flat, breathing with an open mouth and raised shoulders, more exhalation than inhalation and a low voice, as well as soreness and weakness of the low back and knee joints. The kidneys failing to receive *qi* may affect chest yang, resulting in chest tightness, cold limbs, pallor and cold sweats. A deficient floating rootless pulse is a critical sign of yang–*qi* failure. Those with a yin deficiency constitution may have internal deficient fire–heat and thus present with a red face, restlessness, a dry mouth and throat, a red tongue and a thready rapid pulse.

Differentiation

Panting with shortness of breath in this pattern should be distinguished from lung *qi* deficiency. Lung *qi* deficiency alone often causes weak coughing and lack of *qi* without more exhalation than inhalation. Also, this pattern should be distinguished from kidney yang deficiency and kidney yin deficiency, in that they do not involve lung-related symptoms.

Distinctive notes

This pattern is distinctively marked by more exhalation than inhalation (due to the kidneys failing to receive *qi*) and panting with shortness of breath (due to lung *qi* deficiency).

Damp–heat in the urinary bladder

Overview

Damp–heat in the urinary bladder manifests a condition of pathogenic damp-heat accumulating in the urinary bladder. The main contributing factors include external contraction of damp–heat, an improper diet, and internal damp–heat due to spleen deficiency.

Clinical manifestations

Frequent urgent painful urination, scanty dark-yellow urine, urine dribbling, lower abdominal distension, a red tongue with a yellow greasy coating and a rapid pulse; fever, low back pain, bloody urine, urine containing stones and turbid urine may also be present.

Analysis

Damp–heat in the urinary bladder may impair its *qi* transformation, leading to frequent urgent painful urination, urine dribbling and lower abdominal distension. Exuberant heat causes scanty dark-yellow urine. More dampness causes turbid urine. Damp–heat damaging the collaterals may cause bloody urine. Over time, buildup of damp–heat may cause urine containing stones. Accumulated damp–heat may affect the kidneys, resulting in low back pain. A red tongue with a yellow greasy coating and a rapid pulse are typical signs of internal accumulation of damp–heat.

Differentiation

This pattern should be distinguished from an uncontrollable urinary bladder, which is mainly characterized by frequent and dribbling urination but with no urgency and pain during urination.

Distinctive notes

The distinctive points of this pattern include irritation signs of the urinary bladder (frequent urgent painful urination) and internal accumulation of damp–heat.

Summary

The patterns of the kidneys and urinary bladder:

Patterns	Distinctive diagnosis points
Kidney yang deficiency	Yang deficiency + kidney-related symptoms
Kidney yin deficiency	Yin deficiency + kidney-related symptoms
Kidney essence insufficiency	Severe delayed growth and development + reproductive hypofunction
Weakness of kidney *qi*	Uncontrollable urinary bladder + insecurity of the essence chamber or uncontrollable *dai* meridian
Kidneys failing to receive *qi*	Lung *qi* deficiency + more exhalation than inhalation
Damp–heat in the urinary bladder	Irritation signs of the bladder + internal buildup of damp–heat

---

QUESTIONS

1. List the similarities and differences of signs and symptoms due to kidney yang deficiency, kidney yin deficiency, kidney essence insufficiency, weakness of kidney *qi* and the kidneys failing to receive *qi*.
2. Describe the clinical manifestations caused by damp–heat in the urinary bladder.

Pattern Identification of Two or More *Zang–Fu* Organs

Since the human body is an integral whole, the *zang–fu* organs are physiologically interconnected and pathologically interactive. Pathologies of one organ may, under certain circumstances, affect another organ. Pathological transmissions often develop between organs having special connections, such as internal–external connection via meridians, mutual generation/restriction and overaction/counteraction. Common patterns involving two or more *zang–fu* organs are as follows:

Disharmony between the heart and kidneys

Overview

Disharmony between the heart and kidneys manifests a condition due to incoordination between the heart and kidneys. The main contributing factors include external pathogens, chronic conditions, sexual indulgence and emotional disturbance.

Clinical manifestations

Restlessness, insomnia, palpitations, vertigo, tinnitus, a poor memory, feverish sensations on the palms, soles and chest, a dry mouth and throat, soreness and weakness of the low back and knee joints, nocturnal emissions, leukorrhea, a red tongue and a thready rapid pulse.

Analysis

Failure of kidney yin to control heart fire may cause restlessness, insomnia, palpitations and a poor memory. Failure of kidney water to supplement the brain may cause vertigo, tinnitus, and soreness and weakness of the low back and knee joints. Kidney yin deficiency may produce internal deficient and subsequent feverish sensations on the palms, soles and chest, a dry mouth and throat, a red tongue and a thready rapid pulse. Deficient fire may further disturb the essence chamber, leading to nocturnal emissions and leukorrhea.

Differentiation

This pattern should be distinguished from hyperactivity of heart fire, which is characterized by restlessness and insomnia alone without kidney yin deficiency symptoms.

Distinctive notes

This pattern is distinctively marked by hyperactivity of heart fire and deficiency of kidney yin.

Deficiency of the heart and spleen

Overview

Deficiency of the heart and spleen manifests a condition due to deficiency of spleen *qi* and heart blood. The main contributing factors include an improper diet, overexertion, anxiety and chronic conditions or chronic bleeding.

Clinical manifestations

Mild or severe palpitations, insomnia, dream-disturbed sleep, a lusterless complexion, a poor appetite, bloating, diarrhea, dizziness, a poor memory, mental fatigue, scanty menstruation in a pale color, a pale tongue and a thready weak pulse.

Analysis

Failure of heart blood to nourish the heart may cause mild or severe palpitations. Failure of heart blood to nourish the heart–mind may cause insomnia or dream-disturbed sleep. Failure of *qi* and blood to ascend to nourish the brain may cause dizziness and a poor memory. Spleen *qi* deficiency causes a lusterless complexion, a poor appetite, bloating, diarrhea and mental fatigue. Deficiency of *qi* and blood may cause scanty or dribbling menstruation in a pale color, a pale tongue and a thready weak pulse. The spleen is the source of *qi* and blood generation. The heart dominates blood and blood vessels, and the spleen controls blood in the vessels. Spleen *qi* deficiency may cause insufficient generation of blood. Failure of spleen *qi* to control blood in vessels may cause loss of blood. Likewise, blood deficiency may worsen *qi* deficiency.

Differentiation

This pattern should be distinguished from deficiency of *qi* and blood, which is characterized by general *qi* and blood deficiency.

Distinctive notes

This pattern is distinctively marked by symptoms due to heart blood deficiency and spleen *qi* deficiency, coupled with general *qi* and blood deficiency.

Blood deficiency of the heart and liver

Overview

Blood deficiency of the heart and liver manifests a hypofunction of the heart and liver due to blood deficiency. The main contributing factors include chronic conditions, loss of blood and conditions of other *zang–fu* organs.

Clinical manifestations

Mild or severe palpitations, insomnia, dream-disturbed sleep, a poor memory, dizziness, tinnitus, a lusterless complexion, dry eyes, blurred vision, dry nails, numbness of the limbs, amenorrhea or scanty menstruation in a pale color, a pale tongue and a thready weak pulse.

Analysis

Failure of heart blood to nourish the heart and heart–mind may cause mild or severe palpitations, insomnia and dream-disturbed sleep. Failure of heart and liver blood to ascend to nourish the brain may cause a poor memory, dizziness, tinnitus and a lusterless complexion. Since the liver opens into the eyes, dominates tendons and its luster manifests in the nails, liver blood deficiency may cause dry eyes, blurred vision, dry nails, and numbness of the limbs. Insufficient blood in the liver may also cause amenorrhea or scanty menstruation in a pale color. A pale tongue and a thready weak pulse are typical signs of blood deficiency.

Differentiation

This pattern should be distinguished from either heart blood deficiency or liver blood deficiency alone.

Distinctive notes

This pattern is distinctively marked by blood deficiency symptoms and symptoms involving both the heart and liver.

Yang deficiency of the heart and kidneys

Overview

Yang deficiency of the heart and kidneys manifests internal cold retention due to yang–*qi* deficiency of the heart and kidneys. The main contributing factors include external contraction of cold, constitutional yang deficiency, chronic conditions and overexertion.

Clinical manifestations

Mild or severe palpitations, mental fatigue, lassitude, cold intolerance, cold limbs, dysuria, facial puffiness or edema in the lower limbs, pale-gray or bluish lips and nails, a pale-purple tongue with a white slippery coating and a deep thready pulse.

Analysis

The heart dominates the heart–mind and mental activities. Failure of heart yang to warm and nourish the heart may cause mild or severe palpitations, mental fatigue, and lassitude. Kidney yang deficiency causes cold intolerance and cold limbs. Kidney yang deficiency may impair the *qi* transformation of the urinary bladder, resulting in dysuria. Yang–*qi* deficiency may cause water retention and subsequent facial puffiness and edema in the lower limbs. Failure of heart and kidney yang to circulate *qi* and blood may cause blood stasis, leading to pale-gray or bluish lips and nails and a pale-purple tongue. A white slippery tongue coating and a deep thready pulse are typical signs of internal exuberance of yin cold due to yang deficiency.

Differentiation

This pattern should be distinguished from either heart yang deficiency or kidney yang deficiency alone.

Distinctive notes

This pattern is distinctively marked by yang deficiency (with internal yin cold) symptoms and symptoms involving both the heart and kidneys.

Qi deficiency of the heart and lungs

Overview

Qi deficiency of the heart and lungs manifests a hypofunction of the heart and lungs due to *qi* deficiency. The main contributing factors include chronic lung conditions, aging and anxiety.

Clinical manifestations

Mild or severe palpitations, coughing, panting and shortness of breath that can be aggravated by physical exertion, mental fatigue, a bright pale complexion, spontaneous sweating, a low voice, chest tightness, production of clear thin sputum, a pale tongue with a white coating and a deep weak or regularly/irregularly intermittent pulse.

Analysis

Failure of heart *qi* to nourish the heart may cause mild or severe palpitations. Lung *qi* deficiency causes coughing, panting and shortness of breath that can be aggravated by physical exertion. *Qi* deficiency of the heart and lungs causes mental fatigue, a bright pale complexion, spontaneous sweating and a low voice. Failure of lung *qi* to distribute fluids may cause thin clear sputum. A pale tongue with a white coating and a deep weak or regularly/irregularly intermittent pulse are typical signs of impaired circulation of *qi* and blood.

Differentiation

This pattern should be distinguished from either heart *qi* deficiency or lung *qi* deficiency alone. Heart *qi* deficiency is marked by mild or severe palpitations, while lung *qi* deficiency is marked by weak coughing or panting.

Distinctive notes

This pattern is distinctively marked by general *qi* deficiency and symptoms involving both the heart and lungs.

Qi deficiency of the lungs and spleen

Overview

Qi deficiency of the lungs and spleen manifests a hypofunction of the lungs and spleen due to *qi* deficiency. The main contributing factors include chronic lung conditions, overexertion and other chronic conditions.

Clinical manifestations

Persistent coughing and panting, shortness of breath, fatigue, production of profuse white thin sputum, a poor appetite, bloating, diarrhea, a low voice with reluctance to talk, a bright pale complexion, facial puffiness, edema on the feet, a pale tongue with a white coating and a thready weak pulse.

Analysis

The spleen is known as the source of phlegm, while the lungs are the container of phlegm. Failure of spleen *qi* to transport and transform may cause a poor appetite, bloating and diarrhea. Spleen deficiency may produce internal phlegm dampness, resulting in profuse white thin sputum. The phlegm dampness may, in turn, affect the lungs, resulting in persistent coughing and panting. *Qi* deficiency of the lungs and spleen may cause shortness of breath, fatigue, a low voice with reluctance to talk and a bright pale complexion. It may also cause water retention and subsequent facial puffiness or edema on the feet. A pale tongue with a white coating and a thready weak pulse are typical signs of *qi* deficiency.

Differentiation

This pattern should be distinguished from either lung *qi* deficiency or spleen *qi* deficiency alone. Lung *qi* deficiency is marked by persistent coughing, panting, shortness of breath and fatigue, while spleen *qi* deficiency is marked by a poor appetite, bloating and diarrhea.

Distinctive notes

This pattern is distinctively marked by general *qi* deficiency and symptoms involving both the lungs and spleen.

Yang deficiency of the spleen and kidneys

Overview

Yang deficiency of the spleen and kidneys manifests a condition due to yang–*qi* weakness of the spleen and kidneys. The main contributing factors include external contraction of cold, chronic conditions, chronic diarrhea and deficiency of other organs.

Clinical manifestations

Diarrhea mixed with undigested food, fecal incontinence, diarrhea before dawn, cold intolerance, cold limbs, lower abdominal pain with a cold sensation, soreness and weakness of the low back and knee joints, dysuria, a bright pale complexion, facial puffiness or edema in the limbs, a pale swollen tongue with a white slippery coating and a deep thready pulse.

Analysis

Failure of spleen and kidney yang (*qi*) to warm, transform and hold may cause diarrhea mixed with undigested food, fecal incontinence and diarrhea before dawn. Yang–*qi* deficiency may produce internal yin cold, resulting in cold intolerance, cold limbs, lower abdominal pain with a cold sensation and a bright pale complexion. Failure of kidney yang to perform *qi* transformation of the urinary bladder may cause soreness and weakness of the low back and knee joints, and dysuria. Yang–*qi* deficiency may also cause water retention and subsequent facial puffiness or edema in the limbs. A pale swollen tongue with a white slippery coating and a deep thready pulse are typical signs of yang deficiency with internal cold.

Differentiation

This pattern should be distinguished from either spleen yang deficiency or kidney yang deficiency alone. Also, it needs to be distinguished from water retention due to yang deficiency, which is mainly characterized by edema.

Distinctive notes

This pattern is distinctively characterized by yang deficiency of both the spleen and the kidneys, coupled with internal exuberance of yin cold.

Yin deficiency of the lungs and kidneys

Overview

Yin deficiency of the lungs and kidneys manifests a condition of insufficient liquids in the lungs and kidneys. The main contributing factors include external contraction of pathogens (later transforming into heat), chronic lung conditions and sexual indulgence.

Clinical manifestations

Unproductive coughs or coughing with scanty sputum containing blood, a dry mouth and throat, weight loss, soreness and weakness of the low back and knee joints, bone-steaming tidal fever, rosy cheeks, night sweats, nocturnal emissions, irregular menstruation, a red tongue with a scanty coating and a thready rapid pulse.

Analysis

Lung yin deficiency may cause internal heat to impair the descending of lung *qi*, resulting in unproductive coughs or coughing with scanty sputum. Deficient heat damaging the lung collaterals may cause blood in the sputum. Internal deficient heat causes a dry mouth and throat. Failure of the lungs and kidneys yin to nourish muscles and tendons may cause weight loss and soreness and weakness of the low back and knee joints. Internal deficient heat may also cause bone-steaming tidal fever. Ascending of deficient fire may cause rosy cheeks and night sweats. Deficient fire disturbing the essence chamber may cause nocturnal emissions. Deficient fire affecting the *chong* and *ren* meridians may cause irregular menstruation. A red tongue with a scanty coating and a thready rapid pulse are typical signs of internal heat due to yin deficiency.

Differentiation

This pattern should be distinguished from either lung yin deficiency or kidney yin deficiency alone.

Distinctive notes

This pattern is distinctively marked by general yin deficiency and symptoms involving both the lungs and the kidneys.

Yin deficiency of the liver and kidneys

Overview

Yin deficiency of the liver and kidneys manifests a condition due to insufficient liquids in the liver and kidneys. The main contributing factors include chronic conditions, sexual indulgence and emotional disturbance.

Clinical manifestations

Soreness and weakness of the low back and knee joints, dry eyes, blurred vision, tinnitus, a poor memory, pain in the hypochondriac regions, feverish sensations on the palms, soles and chest, rosy cheeks, night sweats, a dry mouth and throat, insomnia or dream-disturbed sleep, nocturnal emissions, scanty menstruation or uterine bleeding, a red tongue with a scanty coating and a thready rapid pulse.

Analysis

Failure of liver and kidney yin to nourish tendons and muscles may cause soreness and weakness of the low back and knee joints. The liver opens into the eyes, so liver yin deficiency causes dry eyes and blurred vision. The kidneys open into the ears, so kidney yin deficiency causes tinnitus. Failure of liver and kidney yin to supplement the brain may cause a poor memory. The liver meridian passes through the hypochondriac regions, so failure of liver yin to nourish the meridians may also cause pain in the hypochondriac regions. Internal deficient heat due to yin deficiency of the liver and kidneys may cause feverish sensations on the palms, soles and chest, rosy cheeks, night sweats, and a dry mouth and throat. Deficient heat disturbing the mind may cause insomnia or dream-disturbed sleep. Deficient fire disturbing the essence chamber may cause nocturnal emissions. Deficient fire affecting the *chong* and *ren* meridians may cause scanty menstruation or uterine bleeding. A red tongue with a scanty coating and a thready rapid pulse are typical signs of internal heat due to yin deficiency.

Differentiation

This pattern should be distinguished from either liver yin deficiency or kidney yin deficiency alone. Also, it needs to be distinguished from yin deficiency of the lungs and kidneys.

Distinctive notes

This pattern is distinctively characterized by internal heat due to yin deficiency and deficient fire, as well as symptoms involving both the liver and the kidneys.

Disharmony between the liver and the spleen

Overview

Disharmony between the liver and the spleen manifests a condition due to failure of the spleen to transport and transform and failure of the liver to maintain the free flow of *qi*. The main contributing factors include liver *qi* stagnation, an improper diet and overexertion.

Clinical manifestations

Distension, fullness or wandering pain in the chest and hypochondriac regions, frequent sighing, emotional depression or restlessness, irritability, a poor appetite, bloating, diarrhea, paroxysmal abdominal pain and diarrhea, a white or greasy tongue coating and a wiry pulse.

Analysis

Liver *qi* stagnation may cause distension, fullness or wandering pain in the chest and hypochondriac regions. Failure of the liver to maintain the free flow of *qi* may cause frequent sighing, depression or restlessness and irritability. Failure of the spleen to transport and transform may cause a poor appetite, bloating, diarrhea and paroxysmal abdominal pain and diarrhea (often related to emotions). A white or greasy tongue coating is indicative of dampness in the middle *jiao*. A wiry pulse is indicative of a liver condition.

Differentiation

This pattern should be distinguished from either liver *qi* stagnation or spleen deficiency with dampness retention alone.

Distinctive notes

This pattern is distinctively characterized by symptoms due to liver *qi* stagnation and manifestations due to spleen deficiency.

Disharmony between the liver and the stomach

Overview

Disharmony between the liver and the stomach manifests a condition due to failure of the liver to maintain the free flow of *qi* and failure of stomach *qi* to descend. The main contributing factors include liver *qi* stagnation and cold attacking the liver and stomach.

Clinical manifestations

Liver *qi* affecting the stomach may cause distension, tightness and pain in the stomach and hypochondriac regions, belching, acid reflux, hiccups, vomiting, restlessness, irritability, a red tongue with a thin yellow coating and a wiry pulse.

Cold attacking the liver and stomach may cause parietal headache, vomiting of saliva, cold limbs, cold intolerance, a pale tongue with a white coating and a deep wiry pulse.

Analysis

Liver *qi* stagnation may transform into fire and affect the stomach, leading to distension, tightness and pain in the stomach and hypochondriac regions. Failure of the stomach *qi* to descend may cause belching, acid reflux, hiccups and vomiting. Liver fire causes restlessness, irritability, a red tongue with a thin yellow coating and a wiry pulse. After attacking the liver and stomach, pathogenic cold may ascend along the pathway of the liver meridian, causing parietal headache. Pathogenic cold may impair the descending of stomach *qi* and result in vomiting of saliva. Cold may damage yang and result in cold limbs and cold intolerance. A pale tongue with a white coating and a deep wiry pulse are typical signs of yin cold.

Differentiation

Liver *qi* attacking the stomach in this pattern should be distinguished from damp–heat in the spleen and stomach alone. Both can have gastric distension and pain, belching, acid reflux, hiccups and vomiting; however, damp–heat in the spleen and stomach may not produce symptoms involving liver *qi* stagnation affecting the stomach. Also, cold attacking the liver and stomach needs to be distinguished from cold attacking the stomach. Both can have gastric pain and vomiting; however, cold attacking the stomach may not produce symptoms involving liver cold and *qi* stagnation.

Distinctive notes

This pattern is distinctively characterized by clinical manifestations involving both the liver and the stomach. It is necessary to distinguish cold from heat.

Liver fire attacking the lungs

Overview

Liver fire attacking the lungs manifests a condition due to liver fire affecting the descending of lung *qi*. The main contributing factors include liver *qi* stagnation, heat in the liver meridian affecting the lungs and chronic conditions.

Clinical manifestations

Paroxysmal coughing with difficult-to-expectorate sputum, distending pain in the chest and hypochondriac regions, frequent sighing, restlessness, irritability, dizziness, red eyes, a bitter taste, breast distension, irregular menstruation, a red tongue with a yellow coating and a wiry pulse.

Analysis

Liver *qi* stagnation may impair the descending of lung *qi*, causing paroxysmal coughing with difficult-to-expectorate sputum. Unresolved liver *qi* stagnation may cause distending pain in the chest and hypochondriac regions, frequent sighing, restlessness and irritability. Ascending of liver fire may cause dizziness, red eyes and a bitter taste. Persistent liver *qi* stagnation may further cause breast distension and irregular menstruation.

A red tongue with a yellow coating and a wiry pulse are typical signs of liver *qi* stagnation transforming into fire.

Differentiation

This pattern should be distinguished from dryness attacking the lungs, which is characterized by unproductive coughs or coughing with scanty sputum and a dry throat and lips; however, it may not cause symptoms involving liver *qi* transforming into fire.

Distinctive notes

This pattern is distinctively characterized by paroxysmal coughing with difficult-to-expectorate sputum (due to failure of lung *qi* to descend) and symptoms due to liver *qi* stagnation transforming into fire.

QUESTIONS

1. Describe the clinical manifestations of disharmony between the heart and the kidneys, as well as its distinctive diagnosis points.
2. List the similarities and differences of clinical manifestations between deficiency of the heart and spleen and blood deficiency of the heart and liver.
3. Describe the clinical manifestations of yang deficiency of the heart and spleen, as well as its distinctive diagnosis points.
4. List the similarities and differences of clinical manifestations between *qi* deficiency of the heart and lungs and *qi* deficiency of the lungs and spleen.
5. Describe the clinical manifestations of yang deficiency of the spleen and kidneys, as well as its distinctive diagnosis points.
6. List the similarities and differences of clinical manifestations between yin deficiency of the lungs and kidneys and yin deficiency of the liver and kidneys.
7. How do you distinguish disharmony between the liver and the spleen and disharmony between the liver and the stomach?
8. Describe the clinical manifestations of liver fire attacking the lungs. How do you distinguish it from dryness attacking the lungs?

Review

The patterns of the liver conditions (except for internal stirring of liver wind)

Patterns	Clinical Manifestations	Pathogenesis
Liver *qi* stagnation	Depression, restlessness, irritability, frequent sighing, distension, tightness or wandering pain in the chest and hypochondriac regions, globus hystericus, breast distension and irregular menstruation. The pulse is wiry	Dysfunction of the liver in maintaining the free flow of *qi*
Ascending of liver fire	Dizziness, distending headache, tinnitus, a red face, redness, swelling and pain of the eyes, restlessness, irritability, insomnia, a dry mouth with a bitter taste, constipation and dark-yellow urine. The tongue is red with a yellow coating. The pulse is wiry and rapid	Liver *qi* stagnation transforming into fire
Liver blood deficiency	Vertigo, tinnitus, dry eyes, blurred vision, poor eyesight, night blindness, a pale lusterless complexion, numbness of the hands and feet, and dry nails. The tongue is pale, with a thin coating. The pulse is thready	Liver blood failing to nourish
Liver yin deficiency	Vertigo, tinnitus, dry painful eyes, pain in the hypochondriac regions, hot flushes, feverish sensations on the palms, soles and chest, tidal fever, night sweats and a dry mouth. The tongue is dry and red. The pulse is wiry, thready and rapid	Liver yin failing to nourish
Hyperactivity of liver yang	Vertigo, tinnitus, distending headache, a top-heavy feeling, red face and eyes, restlessness, irritability, insomnia, soreness and weakness of the low back and knee joints. The tongue is red. The pulse is wiry and powerful or wiry, thready and rapid	Hyperactive yang due to yin deficiency of the liver and kidneys

(Continued)

(*Continued*)

Patterns	Clinical Manifestations	Pathogenesis
Cold retention in the liver meridian	Cold pain in the lower (lateral) abdomen and testes (may radiate to the thighs) with a falling sensation, tenderness, cold intolerance, cold limbs and pallor. The tongue is pale, with a white coating. The pulse is deep and wiry	Cold retention causing meridian *qi* stagnation
Damp–heat in the liver and gallbladder	Burning and distending pain in the hypochondriac regions with palpable masses, tenderness, yellow eyes, urine and skin (bright orange color), fever, a bitter taste and a poor appetite. The tongue is red with a yellow greasy coating. The pulse is wiry and rapid or wiry and slippery	Dysfunction of the liver and gallbladder due to internal damp–heat
Gallbladder stagnation with phlegm	Panic, insomnia, restlessness, timidity, a bitter taste, nausea, chest tightness, distension in the hypochondriac regions, dizziness and blurred vision. The tongue coating is yellow and greasy. The pulse is wiry and slippery	Gallbladder *qi* stagnation with phlegm heat

The subpatterns of internal stirring of liver wind

Subpatterns	Clinical Manifestations	Pathogenesis
Liver yang transforming into wind	Vertigo, headache, a top-heavy feeling, neck rigidity, tremor of the limbs, numbness of the hands and feet, slurred speech, deviated tongue and hemiplegia. The tongue is red with a thin or greasy coating. The pulse is wiry	Hyperactive liver yang transforming into wind
Extreme heat transforming into wind	High-grade fever, delirium, manic restlessness, convulsions of the hands and feet, neck rigidity, opisthotonos, trismus and even coma. The tongue is red, with a yellow coating. The pulse is wiry and rapid	Exuberant heat with malnourishment of tendons and muscles

(*Continued*)

(Continued)

Subpatterns	Clinical Manifestations	Pathogenesis
Yin deficiency generating wind	Twitching of the hands, feet and muscles, tidal fever in the afternoon, feverish sensations on the palms, soles and chest, night sweats, a dry mouth and throat, and weight loss. The tongue is red, with a scanty coating. The pulse is wiry and rapid	Failure of yin fluids to nourish the tendons and muscles
Blood deficiency generating wind	Twitching of the hands, feet and muscles, numbness of the limbs, impaired movement, dry eyes, blurred vision, a lusterless complexion and dry nails. The tongue is pale. The pulse is wiry and thready, or thready	Failure of blood to nourish the tendons and muscles

The patterns of the kidney conditions

Patterns	Clinical Manifestations	Pathogenesis
Kidney yang deficiency	Soreness, weakness or pain of the low back and knee joints, cold intolerance, cold limbs, vertigo, a low spirit, a bright pale or dark complexion, impotence, sterility and diarrhea. The tongue is pale, with a white coating. The pulse is deep, thready and weak	Failure of kidney yang to warm the body
Kidney yin deficiency	Soreness, weakness or pain of the low back and knee joints, vertigo, tinnitus, insomnia, weight loss, tidal fever, night sweats, feverish sensations on the palms, soles and chest, a dry mouth and throat, nocturnal emissions and premature ejaculations. The tongue is red with a scanty coating. The pulse is thready and rapid	Internal deficient heat due to yin deficiency

(Continued)

(Continued)

Patterns	Clinical Manifestations	Pathogenesis
Kidney essence insufficiency	Delayed growth and development, delayed closure of the fontanelle, short stature, mental retardation, sterility, amenorrhea and premature aging. The tongue is small and thin. The pulse is thready and weak	Insufficiency of kidney essence to support growth and development
Kidney *qi* weakness	Profuse thin clear urine, urine dribbling, urinary incontinence, increased urination at night, spermatorrhea, premature ejaculations, clear leukorrhea or tendency of miscarriage. The tongue is pale. The pulse is thready and deep	Kidney *qi* failing to hold urine
The kidneys failing to receive *qi*	Panting and shortness of breath (especially after exertion), breathing with an open mouth and raised shoulders, more exhalation than inhalation, soreness and weakness of the low back and knee joints, chest tightness, cold limbs, a bluish complexion and cold sweats. The pulse is deficient and rootless	Deficiency and failure of kidney *qi*
Damp–heat in the urinary bladder	Frequent urgent painful urination, scanty dark-yellow urine, urine dribbling, lower abdominal distension, bloody urine, urine mixed with stones and turbid urine. The tongue is red with a yellow greasy coating. The pulse is rapid	Downward flow of damp–heat affecting the bladder

The patterns of two or more zang–fu organs

Patterns	Clinical Manifestations	Pathogenesis
Disharmony between the heart and the kidneys	Restlessness, insomnia, palpitations, vertigo, tinnitus, a poor memory, feverish sensations on the palms, soles and chest, a dry mouth and throat, soreness and weakness of the low back and knee joints, nocturnal emissions and leukorrhea. The tongue is red. The pulse is thready and rapid	Kidney yin deficiency with hyperactivity of heart fire
Deficiency of the heart and spleen	Mild or severe palpitations, insomnia, dream-disturbed sleep, a lusterless complexion, a poor appetite, bloating, diarrhea, dizziness, a poor memory, mental fatigue and scanty menstruation. The tongue is pale. The pulse is thready and weak	Deficiency of spleen *qi* and heart blood
Blood deficiency of the heart and liver	Mild or severe palpitations, insomnia, dream-disturbed sleep, a lusterless complexion, dizziness, tinnitus, dry eyes, blurred vision, dry nails and numbness of the limbs. The tongue is pale. The pulse is thready and weak	Blood failing to nourish the heart and liver
Yang deficiency of the heart and spleen	Mild or severe palpitations, cold intolerance, cold limbs, mental fatigue, dysuria, edema in the limbs and pale-gray lips and nails. The tongue is pale, with a white slippery coating. The pulse is deep and thready	Yang of the heart and spleen failing to warm
Qi deficiency of the heart and lungs	Mild or severe palpitations, coughing, panting, shortness of breath (especially after exertion), mental fatigue, a bright pale complexion, spontaneous sweating, a low voice, chest tightness and clear thin sputum. The tongue is pale with a white coating. The pulse is deep and weak	Heart *qi* deficiency with lung *qi* weakness

(Continued)

(Continued)

Patterns	Clinical Manifestations	Pathogenesis
Qi deficiency of the lungs and spleen	Persistent coughing, panting, shortness of breath, fatigue, white thin profuse sputum, a poor appetite, bloating, loose stools, a low voice with reluctance to talk, a bright pale complexion, facial puffiness and edema on the feet. The tongue is pale with a white coating. The pulse is thready and weak	Spleen and lung *qi* deficiency
Yang deficiency of the spleen and kidneys	Diarrhea mixed with undigested food, fecal incontinence, diarrhea before dawn, cold intolerance, cold limbs, cold pain in the lower abdomen, soreness and weakness of the low back and knee joints, dysuria, a bright pale complexion and edema. The tongue is pale. The pulse is deep and thready	Internal cold due to yang deficiency of the spleen and kidneys
Yin deficiency of the lungs and kidneys	Unproductive coughs or coughing with scanty sputum, a dry mouth and throat, weight loss, soreness and weakness of the low back and knee joints, tidal fever, night sweats, nocturnal emissions and irregular menstruation. The tongue is red with a scanty coating. The pulse is thready and rapid	Internal deficient fire due to lung and kidney yin deficiency
Yin deficiency of the liver and kidneys	Soreness and weakness of the low back and knee joints, dry eyes, blurred vision, tinnitus, a poor memory, feverish sensations on the palms, soles and chest, night sweats, a dry mouth, insomnia, nocturnal emissions and scanty menstruation. The tongue is red with a scanty coating. The pulse is thready and rapid	Internal deficient fire due to liver and kidney yin deficiency
Disharmony between the liver and the spleen	Fullness, distension and wandering pain in the chest or hypochondriac regions, frequent sighing, depression, restlessness, irritability, a poor appetite, bloating, loose stools and paroxysmal abdominal pain and diarrhea. The tongue coating is white or greasy. The pulse is wiry	Liver *qi* affecting the transportation and transformation of the spleen

(Continued)

(*Continued*)

Patterns	Clinical Manifestations	Pathogenesis
Disharmony between the liver and the stomach	Gastric distension, tightness and pain in the stomach and hypochondriac regions, belching, acid reflux, hiccups, vomiting, restlessness and irritability. The tongue is red with a thin yellow coating. The pulse is wiry. Parietal headache, vomiting of saliva, cold intolerance and cold limbs may also be present	Liver *qi* affecting the descending of stomach *qi*
Liver fire attacking the lungs	Paroxysmal coughing with difficult-to-expectorate sputum, distending pain in the chest and hypochondriac regions, frequent sighing, restlessness, irritability, dizziness, red eyes, a bitter taste, breast distension and irregular menstruation. The tongue is red with a yellow coating. The pulse is wiry	Liver fire affecting the dispersing and descending of lung *qi*

PATTERN IDENTIFICATION OF MERIDIANS

Meridians are pathways through which *qi* and blood circulate. They connect the interior with the exterior and the upper body with the lower body. The tissues and *zang–fu* organs are connected through meridians. Meridians play an extremely important role in coordinating the holistic vital activities involving the *zang–fu* organs, four extremities, bones, sense organs, orifices, muscles, tendons and skin. Pathologically, they can also be the pathways for disease transmission. For example, external pathogens may attack the exterior and enter the *zang–fu* organs via meridians, and pathological changes in one organ may spread to another through meridians as well.

Pattern identification of meridians is based on the meridians as well as the related *zang–fu* organs. It aims to identify the location, etiology, pathogenesis and nature of the conditions and thus provide treatment plans.

This section covers two parts: patterns of the twelve regular meridians and patterns of the eight extra meridians. Since pattern identification of meridians is not as important as that of the *zang–fu* organs, "Differentiation" and "Distinctive notes" will not be presented.

Pattern Identification of the Twelve Regular Meridians

Pattern of the (hand–taiyin) lung meridian

Overview

This pattern manifests conditions along the pathway of the lung meridian as well as lung-related problems.

Clinical manifestations

Fever, chills, sweating, pain in the shoulder and back with a cold sensation, pain in the supraclavicular fossa, lung distension, coughing, panting, chest fullness and distention, restlessness, scanty but frequent urination, shortness of breath and feverish sensations on the palms and soles.

Analysis

Since the lungs dominate the skin and skin hair, wind–cold may obstruct *wei* yang (*qi*), causing fever and chills. Wind has the property of opening the striae or pores, resulting in sweating. Cold may impair the (lung) meridian *qi* flow, leading to cold pain in the shoulder and back as well as pain in the supraclavicular fossa. Failure of lung *qi* to disperse and descend may cause lung distension, coughing and panting. Lung *qi* blockage may cause chest distension and fullness, and restlessness. Failure of the lungs to regulate water passage may cause scanty frequent urination. Lung *qi* deficiency causes shortness of breath. Lung yin deficiency causes feverish sensations on the palms and soles.

Pattern of the (hand–yangming) large intestine meridian

Overview

This pattern manifests conditions along the pathway of the large intestine meridian as well as large-intestine-related problems.

Clinical manifestations

Toothache, a sore throat, nosebleed, runny nose, swelling of the neck, a dry mouth, pain on the anterior aspect of the shoulder and anterior border of the extensor aspect of the upper limbs, numbness, pain and impaired flexion and extension of the thumbs and index fingers, abdominal pain, bowel sounds and diarrhea or constipation.

Analysis

Since, from the shoulder, a branch of the large intestine meridian travels upward over the muscle at the side of the neck, passing through the lower gums, and terminates beside the opposite nostril, impaired flow of meridian *qi* may cause toothache, a sore throat, nosebleed, a runny nose, swelling of the neck and a dry mouth. Since the large intestine meridian begins at the outside corner of the index fingernail, and runs along the edge of the finger, between the two tendons of the thumb, reaching the anterior side of the shoulder along the anterior border of the lateral aspect of the arm, impaired flow of meridian *qi* may cause pain on the anterior aspect of the shoulder and the anterior border of the extensor aspect of the upper limbs, numbness, and pain and impaired flexion and extension of the thumb and index fingers. Downward flow of damp–heat to the large intestine may cause abdominal pain and bowel sounds. Dysfunction of the large intestine may cause diarrhea. Heat consuming the liquid of the large intestine may cause constipation.

Pattern of the (foot–yangming) stomach meridian

Overview

This pattern manifests conditions along the pathway of the large intestine meridian as well as large-intestine-related problems.

Clinical manifestations

Fever, especially on the front part of the body, a swollen sore throat, nosebleed, toothache, deviated mouth and eyes, pain in the chest, abdomen and along the lateral aspects of the lower limbs, pain on the dorsum of the feet, numbness and impaired movement of the middle toes, gastric pain, vomiting, fast hunger even with an increased appetite, abdominal distension and fullness, edema, panic and mania.

Analysis

Since the stomach meridian travels on the front part of the body, exuberant *qi* may cause fever especially on that part of the body. The stomach meridian starts beside the nose, then passes into the upper gums and around the mouth. From the jaw it descends along the throat to the collarbone and passes through the diaphragm. The superficial path continues down over the abdomen to the pubic area, then continues down the anterior thigh, passing just to the outside of the kneecap, and terminates at the middle toe. Ascending of stomach fire along the pathway of the meridian may cause a swollen sore throat, nosebleed and toothache. Wind attacking the meridian may cause deviated mouth and eyes. External pathogens affecting the flow of meridian *qi* may cause pain on the chest, abdomen or along the lateral aspect of the lower limbs, pain on the dorsum of the feet, and numbness and impaired movement of the middle toes. External pathogens attacking the stomach may cause gastric pain. Adverse ascending of stomach *qi* may cause vomiting. Exuberant stomach heat may cause a fast hunger even with an increased appetite. Since the stomach is internally–externally connected with the spleen, the spleen failing to transport and transform may cause water retention and subsequent abdominal fullness and distension and edema. Stomach heat disturbing the heart may cause panic and mania.

Pattern of the (foot–taiyin) spleen meridian

Overview

This pattern manifests conditions along the pathway of the spleen meridian as well as spleen-related problems.

Clinical manifestations

Stiffness and pain of the tongue, vomiting after eating food, gastric pain, bloating, frequent belching, a heavy sensation, fatigue, impaired movement, swelling, pain and a cold sensation along the medial aspect of the thigh, numbness and impaired movement of the great toes, physical inactivity, a poor appetite, restlessness, loose stools or diarrhea, edema and jaundice.

Analysis

Since the spleen meridian reaches the root of the tongue, impaired circulation of meridian *qi* may cause stiffness and pain of the tongue. Spleen conditions may affect the descending of stomach *qi*, thus causing vomiting. Obstructed flow of *qi* may cause gastric pain. Failure of the spleen to transport and transform may cause bloating and frequent belching. Dampness obstructing the spleen may cause a heavy sensation, fatigue and physical inactivity. Since the spleen meridians starts from the great toe and runs upward along the medial aspect of the thigh, impaired circulation of meridian *qi* may cause swelling, pain and a cold sensation along the medial aspect of the thigh, and numbness and impaired movement of the great toes. As the spleen is internally–externally connected with the stomach, failure of the spleen to transport and transform may impair the descending of stomach *qi*, leading to a poor appetite and restlessness. Spleen deficiency may cause water retention and affect the conduction of the large intestine, leading to loose stools or diarrhea. Water retention may also cause edema. Spleen deficiency can also affect the liver and gallbladder, leading to overflow of bile and subsequent jaundice.

Pattern of the (hand–shaoyin) heart meridian

Overview

This pattern manifests conditions along the pathway of the heart meridian as well as heart-related problems.

Clinical manifestations

A dry throat, thirst with a desire to drink water, pain in the axillary or along the medial aspect of the arm, warmth and pain of the palms, cardiac pain, palpitations, insomnia and abnormal mental activities.

Analysis

Since a branch of the heart meridian travels along the throat, heat in the heart meridian may cause a dry throat. Heat consuming yin fluids may cause thirst with a desire to drink water. The heart meridian comes out of the axillary fossa, so impaired flow of meridian *qi* may cause pain in the axillary. Impaired flow of meridian *qi* may also cause pain along the pathway, i.e. the medial aspect of the arms and palms. An impediment to the heart vessels may cause cardiac pain. Malnourishment of the heart–mind may cause palpitations and insomnia, as well as abnormal mental activities.

Pattern of the (hand–taiyang) small intestine meridian

Overview

This pattern manifests conditions along the pathway of the small intestine meridian as well as small-intestine-related problems.

Clinical manifestations

Deafness, yellow eyes, swelling of the cheeks, a swollen sore throat, a stiff neck, pain in the shoulder and medial brachial muscle, distending pain of the lower abdomen, frequent urination and diarrhea or constipation.

Analysis

Since a branch of the small intestine meridian travels along the cheek and outer canthus of the eyes and then enters the ears, impaired flow of meridian *qi* may cause deafness, yellow eyes, swollen cheeks, a swollen sore throat and a stiff neck. The small intestine starts from the outside corner of the small fingernail, runs along the posterior border of the lateral aspect of the forearm and reaches the shoulder; impaired flow of meridian *qi* may therefore cause pain in the shoulder and medial brachial muscle. *Qi* stagnation of the small intestine may cause distending pain of the lower abdomen. Failure of the small intestine to separate clear from turbid may cause frequent urination and diarrhea or constipation.

Pattern of the (foot–taiyang) bladder meridian

Overview

This pattern manifests conditions along the pathway of the urinary bladder meridian as well as bladder-related problems.

Clinical manifestations

Chills, fever, nasal congestion, nosebleed, headache, pain of the eyes, pain along the neck, low back, buttocks and along the posterior aspect of the lower limbs, numbness of the small toes, lower abdominal distension and fullness, dysuria and enuresis.

Analysis

Since the bladder meridian governs the exterior of the entire body, pathogenic factors attacking the meridian may cause chills, fever, nasal congestion and nosebleed. The bladder meridian reaches the vertex to connect with the brain; pathogenic *qi* along the pathway of the meridian may therefore cause headache. Since the bladder meridian starts from the inner canthus, one branch travels along the back to the lumbus, passes through the popliteal fossa, then continues downward to the external malleolus and terminates at the small toes. Impaired flow of meridian *qi* may cause pain in the eyes, neck, low back, buttocks and the posterior aspect of the lower limbs and numbness of the small toes. Impaired *qi* transformation of the urinary bladder may cause fullness and distension of the lower abdomen, dysuria and enuresis.

Pattern of the (foot–shaoyin) kidney meridian

Overview

This pattern manifests conditions along the pathway of the kidney meridian as well as kidney-related problems.

Clinical manifestations

Pain on the posterior border of the medial aspect of the thigh, warmth and pain in the soles, a dry tongue, a swollen sore throat, restlessness, cardiac pain, hemoptysis, panting, a dark complexion, panic, enuresis, nocturnal emissions and irregular menstruation.

Analysis

Since the kidney meridian starts from the small toe, crosses the soles, comes out of the ankle bone to the heel, rises along the medial aspect of the thigh and then internally ascends in line with the lumbar spine, where it enters the kidneys, impaired flow of meridian *qi* may cause pain on the posterior border of the medial aspect of the thigh, and warmth and pain on the soles. Since the kidney meridian also travels along the throat to the root of the tongue and one branch comes out of the lung to connect with the heart, disorder of the meridian may cause a dry tongue, a swollen sore throat, restlessness and cardiac pain. Kidney yin (essence) insufficiency may cause internal deficient fire, leading to hemoptysis. As the kidneys are known as the root of *qi*, kidney deficiency may cause panting. Kidney deficiency may also affect the circulation of *qi* and blood, leading to a dark complexion. The emotion of the kidneys manifests as fear, and kidney *qi* deficiency may cause panic. Failure of the kidneys to constrain the urinary bladder may cause enuresis. Insecurity of kidney *qi* may cause enuresis. Kidney deficiency may also affect the *chong* and *ren* meridians, leading to irregular menstruation.

Pattern of the (hand–jueyin) pericardium meridian

Overview

This pattern manifests conditions along the pathway of the pericardium meridian as well as pericardium-related problems.

Clinical manifestations

A warm sensation on the palms, spasm of the arms and elbows, swelling of the axilla (armpit), chest fullness, cardia pain, palpitations, a red face, restlessness and mania.

Analysis

The pericardium meridian starts from the chest, leaves the pericardium and travels upward to the axilla, then runs along the midline of the medial aspect of the upper limbs to the palms; disorder of this meridian may therefore causes a warm sensation on the palms, spasm of the arms and elbows, swelling of the axilla (armpit) and chest fullness. A problem of the pericardium may obstruct the heart vessels, leading to cardiac pain and palpitations. The luster of the heart shows in the face, and heat in the pericardium may cause a red face. Since the heart dominates the mind (spirit), a disordered pericardium may cause restlessness and mania.

Pattern of the (hand–shaoyang) sanjiao meridian

Overview

This pattern manifests conditions along the pathway of the *sanjiao* meridian as well as *sanjiao*-related problems.

Clinical manifestations

Deafness, pain behind the ears, a swollen sore throat, pain on the outer canthus, swollen painful cheeks, pain in the shoulder and arm and along the lateral aspect of the elbow, impaired movement of the small and index fingers, bloating, edema, enuresis and dysuria.

Analysis

Since a branch of the *sanjiao* meridian comes out of the collarbone region, ascends the side of the neck and around the back of the ear, and continues to the front of the ear and crosses to the outer canthus, impaired flow of meridian *qi* may cause deafness, pain behind the ears, a swollen sore throat, pain on the outer canthus and swollen painful cheeks. Since the *sanjiao* meridian starts from the ring finger, passes between the knuckles of the ring and small fingers to the wrist, then ascends between the two bones of the forearm (radius and ulna), through the tip of the elbow, and ascends to the shoulder, disorder of the meridian may cause pain in the shoulder and arm and along the lateral aspect of the elbow, and impaired movement of the small and index fingers. Since *sanjiao* regulates *qi* and water passage, *qi* stagnation of *sanjiao* may cause bloating. Impaired *qi* transformation may cause water retention, leading to edema. Impaired *qi* transformation of the urinary bladder may cause enuresis and dysuria.

Pattern of the (foot–shaoyang) gallbladder meridian

Overview

This pattern manifests conditions along the pathway of the gallbladder meridian as well as gallbladder-related problems.

Clinical manifestations

Headache, forehead pain, blurred vision, pain of the outer canthus, swollen painful collarbone, swollen painful armpit, pain in the chest, thigh and along the lateral aspect of the lower limbs, impaired movement of the small and fourth toes, a bitter taste, jaundice, pain in the hypochondriac regions, frequent sighing, malaria, anger, panic, timidity and insomnia.

Analysis

Since the gallbladder meridian starts from the outer canthus and reaches the forehead, disorder of this meridian may cause headache, forehead pain, blurred vision and pain of the outer canthus. A branch of the gallbladder meridian curves behind the ear, reaches the top of the shoulder and crosses the lateral side of the ribcage, then continues downward to the thigh and reaches the region between the fourth and fifth toes; disorder of this meridian may cause swollen painful collarbone, swollen painful armpit, pain on the chest, thighs and along the lateral aspect of the lower limbs, and impaired movement of the small and fourth toes. Since the gallbladder stores and discharges bile, overflow of bile causes a bitter taste and jaundice. Gallbladder *qi* stagnation causes pain in the hypochondriac regions and frequent sighing. Since *shaoyang* disorder manifests as alternating chills and fever, malaria is also covered. Gallbladder *qi* stagnation transforming into fire may cause anger. Since the gallbladder governs decision-making, dysfunctions of the gallbladder may cause panic, timidity and insomnia.

Pattern of the (foot–jueyin) liver meridian

Overview

This pattern manifests conditions along the pathway of the liver meridian as well as liver-related problems.

Clinical manifestations

Low back pain with an inability to bend or look up, fullness and distension of the chest and hypochondriac regions, lower (lateral) abdominal pain, hernia, parietal headache, a dry throat, vertigo, a bitter taste and emotional depression or irritability.

Analysis

Since the branch and divergent collaterals of the liver meridian pass through the lumbar region, impaired flow of meridian *qi* may cause low back pain with an inability to bend or look up. Since the liver meridian winds around the external genitalia, reaches the lower abdomen and spreads over the hypochondriac regions, impaired flow of meridian *qi* may cause fullness and distension of the chest and hypochondriac regions, lower (lateral) abdominal pain and hernia. Since the liver meridian ascends to the eye system along the throat, emerges from the forehead and reaches the vertex of the head, impaired flow of meridian *qi* may cause a dry throat and vertigo. Since the liver maintains the free flow of *qi*, liver *qi* stagnation transforming into fire may cause a bitter taste and emotional depression or irritability.

QUESTIONS

1. Describe the clinical manifestations of the lung, large intestine and stomach meridians. List the related *zang–fu* organs of these meridians.
2. Describe the clinical manifestations of the spleen, heart and small intestine meridians. List the related *zang–fu* organs of these meridians.
3. Describe the clinical manifestations of the bladder, kidney and pericardium meridians. List the related *zang–fu* organs of these meridians.
4. Describe the clinical manifestations of the *sanjiao*, gallbladder and liver meridians. List the related *zang–fu* organs of these meridians.

Pattern Identification of the Eight Extra Meridians

The eight extra meridians include the *du* meridian, *ren* meridian, *chong* meridian, *dai* meridian, *yinwei* meridian, *yangwei* meridian, *yinqiao* meridian and *yangqiao* meridian. They are termed "extra" meridians because they are different from the twelve regular meridians in the pathways and relationships to the *zang–fu* organs.

The eight extra meridians are important components of the meridian system. They facilitate the interactions between meridians and regulate the *qi* and blood of the twelve regular meridians. The surplus *qi* and blood of the twelve regular meridians can be stored in the eight extra meridians, while the *qi* and blood of the eight extra meridians can supplement the *qi* and blood of the twelve regular meridians when necessary.

The eight extra meridians are especially associated with the liver, kidneys, uterus, brain and marrow. Among these, the uterus, brain and marrow are directly linked to those meridians. Clinical conditions due to functional disorders of the *chong*, *ren*, *du* and *dai* meridians can be commonly seen in clinical practice.

Pattern of the du meridian

Overview

This pattern manifests conditions along the pathway of the *du* meridian as well as problems of related organs.

Clinical manifestations

Pathogenic factors attacking the *du* meridian may cause opisthotonos, stiffness of the neck and back, trismus, headache, convulsions of the four extremities, coma, fever, a white or yellow tongue coating and a wiry or rapid pulse.

Deficiency of the *du* meridian may cause dizziness, a heavy sensation of the head, vertigo, a poor memory, tinnitus, deafness, lumbar soreness and weakness, rickets, a pale tongue and a thready weak pulse.

Yang deficiency of the *du* meridian may cause cold intolerance on the back and spine, impotence, low sperm counts, nocturnal emissions, a falling sensation of the lower abdomen with infertility, lumbar soreness, a pale tongue and a deficient weak pulse.

Analysis

Since the *du* meridian starts from the perineum, travels within the spine, ascends to enter the brain and reaches the vertex along the forehead, pathogenic factors attacking the meridian may cause opisthotonos, stiffness of the neck and back, trismus, headache, convulsions of the four extremities, coma, fever, a white or yellow tongue coating and wiry or rapid pulse.

Since the *du* meridian enters the brain and meets with the liver meridian at the vertex of the head, it is closely associated with the liver and kidneys, and failure of the meridian to supplement the brain may cause dizziness, a heavy sensation of the head, vertigo and a poor memory. Because the ears are connected with the brain, brain marrow insufficiency may cause tinnitus and deafness. Since the *du* meridian ascends inside the spine, malnourishment of this meridian may cause lumbar soreness and weakness, and rickets. A pale tongue and a thready weak pulse are signs of deficiency.

The *du* meridian is known as the "sea of yang meridians"; yang–*qi* deficiency in it may cause cold intolerance on the back and spine, impotence, low sperm counts, nocturnal emissions, a falling sensation of the lower abdomen with infertility and lumbar soreness. A pale tongue and a deficient weak pulse are also signs of deficiency.

Pattern of the ren meridian

Overview

This pattern manifests conditions along the pathway of the *ren* meridian as well as problems of related organs.

Clinical manifestations

Obstructed *qi* flow of the *ren* meridian may cause amenorrhea, infertility, white leukorrhea, lower abdominal masses with fullness, distension and migratory pain, distending pain of the testes and hernia.

Deficiency of the *ren* meridian may cause increased fetal movement, a falling sensation of the lower abdomen, vaginal bleeding, possible miscarriage, a delayed period, amenorrhea, dribbling menstruation, dizziness, blurred vision, lumbar soreness and weakness of the low back and knee joints, a pale tongue and a thready weak pulse.

Analysis

The *ren* meridian, known as the "sea of yin meridians," starts from the uterus, travels along the front of the body along the anterior midline and acts to regulate the *qi* and blood of the yin meridians. Blocked *qi* flow of the *ren* meridian may cause amenorrhea. Failure of *qi* and blood to nourish the uterus may cause infertility and white leukorrhea.

Qi stagnation may cause lower abdominal masses with fullness, distension and migratory pain. Blockage of the *ren* meridian may cause *qi* stagnation in the liver meridian, causing a distending pain of the testes and hernia.

The *ren* meridian regulates menstruation, promotes reproduction and secures pregnancy; deficiency of the *ren* meridian may cause increased fetal movement, a falling sensation of the lower abdomen, vaginal bleeding and possible miscarriage. Failure of the *ren* meridian to regulate menstruation may cause a delayed period, amenorrhea or dribbling menstruation. Deficiency of the *ren* meridian may also cause deficiency of *qi* and blood, leading to dizziness, blurred vision, lumbar soreness and weakness of the low back and knee joints, a pale tongue and a thready weak pulse.

Pattern of the chong meridian

Overview

This pattern manifests conditions along the pathway of the *chong* meridian as well as problems of related organs.

Clinical manifestations

Adverse *qi* ascending of the *chong* meridian may cause a sudden *qi* ascending from the lower abdomen, nausea, vomiting, coughing, hematemesis, abdominal cramp, gushing pain in the epigastric region and severe morning sickness due to pregnancy.

Deficiency of the *chong* meridian may cause scanty menstruation in a pale color, amenorrhea, infertility, delayed menarche, premature menopause, lower abdominal pain, dizziness, blurred vision, palpitations, insomnia, maldevelopment of the male reproductive organs, thin beard or pubic hair, sterility, a pale tongue and a thready weak pulse.

Qi stagnation in the *chong* meridian may cause unsmooth menstruation, scanty menstruation, a delayed period, breast pain or distension, insufficient lactation and migratory lower abdominal masses.

Analysis

Since the *chong* meridian regulates the *qi* and blood of the twelve regular meridians, disordered *qi* activity of the meridian may cause a sudden *qi* ascending from the lower abdomen, nausea, vomiting, coughing and hematemesis.

The *chong* meridian originates from the uterus; so adverse *qi* flow may cause abdominal cramp, gushing pain in the epigastric region and severe morning sickness due to pregnancy.

The *chong* meridian, known as the "sea of blood," promotes reproduction and regulates menstruation; deficiency of the meridian with insufficiency of blood may cause scanty menstruation in a pale color, amenorrhea, infertility, delayed menarche, premature menopause and lower abdominal pain.

Failure of blood to nourish the *chong* meridian may cause dizziness, blurred vision, palpitations and insomnia.

Insufficiency of blood causes maldevelopment of the male reproductive organs, thin beard or pubic hair, sterility, a pale tongue and a thready weak pulse.

Obstructed *qi* flow of the *chong* meridian may cause unsmooth menstruation, scanty menstruation, a delayed period, breast pain or distension, insufficient lactation and migratory lower abdominal masses.

Pattern of the dai meridian

Overview

This pattern manifests conditions along the pathway of the *dai* meridian as well as problems of related organs.

Clinical manifestations

Lingering white leukorrhea, uterine prolapse, miscarriage, abdominal distension and fullness, pain around the umbilicus, low back and spine, lumbar soreness and weakness, a pale tongue with a white coating and a weak pulse.

Analysis

Since the *dai* meridian encircles the lumbar region, binds all longitudinal meridians, regulates meridian *qi*, secures the fetus and dominates leukorrhea, deficiency of the meridian may cause lingering white leukorrhea, uterine prolapse and miscarriage.

Qi stagnation of the *dai* meridian may cause abdominal distension and fullness.

Malnourishment of the *dai* meridian may cause pain around the umbilicus, low back and spine, lumbar soreness and weakness, a pale tongue with a white coating and a weak pulse.

Pattern of the yinwei and yangwei meridians

Overview

This pattern manifests conditions along the pathway of the *yinwei* and *yangwei* meridian as well as problems of related organs.

Clinical manifestations

Dull cardiac or chest pain, restlessness, emotional depression, mental fatigue, pain in the hypochondriac regions, low back pain, flaccidity of the limbs and persistent irregular fever.

Analysis

Since the *yinwei* and *yangwei* meridians connect all meridians and regulate *qi* and blood, deficiency of the *yinwei* meridian and subsequent malnourishment of the heart may cause dull cardiac or chest pain and restlessness.

Deficiency of the *yangwei* meridian and subsequent malnourishment of yang meridians may cause persistent irregular fever.

Deficiency of both the *yinwei* and *yangwei* meridians may cause emotional depression, mental fatigue, pain in the hypochondriac regions, low back pain and flaccidity of the limbs.

Pattern of the yinqiao and yangqiao meridians

Overview

This pattern manifests conditions along the pathway of the *yinqiao* and *yangqiao* meridians as well as problems of related organs.

Clinical manifestations

Muscle wasting, paralysis or weakness of the legs, unstable walking, weakness of the feet, drowsiness or insomnia, prolapse of the eyelids, abnormal closing and opening of the eyes, a pale tongue with a white coating and a deficient pulse.

Analysis

Since the *yinqiao* and *yangqiao* meridians travel in the lower limbs to maintain the normal physiological activities of those limbs, deficiency of *qi* and blood in these two meridians may cause muscle wasting, paralysis or weakness of the legs, unstable walking and weakness of the feet.

Since the *yinqiao* and *yangqiao* meridians ascend to the inner canthus, yin–yang disorder of these two meridians may cause either drowsiness or insomnia. Deficiency and malnourishment of the two meridians may cause abnormal closing and opening of the eyes.

A pale tongue with a white coating and a deficient pulse are signs of deficiency and weakness.

QUESTIONS

1. Describe the clinical manifestations of the *du, ren, chong* and *dai* meridians.
2. Describe the clinical manifestations of the *yinwei, yangwei, yinqiao* and *yangqiao* meridians.

PATTERN IDENTIFICATION OF THE SIX MERIDIANS

Pattern identification of the six meridians is a method to differentiate externally contracted febrile diseases developed by Zhang Zhong-jing (150–219 A.D.), a distinguished physician in the Eastern Han Dynasty (25–220 A.D.).

Externally contracted febrile diseases may cause varying clinical manifestations. Pattern identification of the six meridians aims to generalize these manifestations — taking yin and yang as the general principle — into six patterns: *taiyang* disease, *yangming* disease, *shaoyang* disease, *taiyin* disease, *shaoyin* disease and *jueyin* disease. These six patterns can tell about the pathological changes involving the *zang–fu* organs, meridians, *qi*, blood, *ying* and *wei*.

Based on the strength between antipathogenic *qi* and pathogenic factors, the nature of the pathogens and progression of the disease, pattern identification of the six meridians aims to analyze, compare, summarize and induce the disease location, nature and pathogenesis, thus providing the basis for treatment plans. Clinically, this method applies not only to externally contracted febrile conditions but also to internally damaged miscellaneous conditions.

Pattern Identification of *Taiyang* Disease

A *taiyang* disease develops at the early stage of externally contracted febrile conditions due to wind–cold attacking the exterior. It is mainly characterized by a floating pulse, headache, neck stiffness and chills. By the nature of the pathogens and individualized constitutions, *taiyang* diseases can be categorized into two types: wind invasion and cold invasion.

Wind invasion

Overview

This pattern manifests a condition following wind–cold (particularly wind) attacking the body surface.

Clinical manifestations

Fever, chills, intolerance of wind, sweating and a floating moderate pulse; alternatively, headache, a general pain, low back pain, a stuffy runny nose and a thin white tongue coating may also be present.

Analysis

The struggle between wind–cold and *wei* may cause fever. Wind–cold binding *wei* may cause chills or intolerance of wind. Wind opens the striae and pores, leading to sweating. A floating pulse is indicative of an exterior syndrome. The pulse is also moderate (relative to tightness). A rapid pulse may also be present in the case of fever. Since cold has the property of contracting, impaired free flow of *qi* may cause headache, a general ache and low back pain. Wind–cold affecting the lungs (the lungs open into the nose) may cause a stuffy or runny nose. A thin white tongue coating is indicative of contraction of wind–cold.

Differentiation

This pattern should be distinguished from an exterior heat syndrome. Both patterns can have fever, chills and a floating pulse; however, an exterior syndrome only causes mild intolerance of cold, a short duration, thirst, a red swollen painful throat and redness on the tip of the tongue. Also, this pattern needs to be distinguished from the following cold injury.

Distinctive points

This pattern is distinctively characterized by fever, chills, sweating and a floating pulse (an exterior deficient cold syndrome).

Cold invasion

Overview

This pattern manifests a condition following wind–cold (particularly cold) attacking the body surface.

Clinical manifestations

Fever, chills or intolerance of wind, an absence of sweating and a floating tight pulse; alternatively, headache, neck rigidity, ache of the bones and joints, coughing, panting and a thin white tongue coating may also be present.

Analysis

The struggle between wind–cold and *wei* may cause fever. Wind–cold binding *wei* may cause chills or intolerance of wind. Cold closes the striae or pores, resulting in an absence of sweating. A floating pulse is indicative of an exterior syndrome. A tight pulse indicates severe cold invasion. The pulse can also be rapid in the case of fever. Since cold has the property of contracting, impaired free flow of *qi* may cause headache, a general ache and low back pain. Wind–cold affecting the lungs (the lungs open into the nose) may cause coughing and panting. A thin white tongue coating is indicative of contraction of wind–cold.

Differentiation

This pattern should be distinguished from an exterior heat syndrome (see "Wind invasion" for reference). Also, it needs to be distinguished from wind invasion. Both patterns have fever, chills and a floating pulse; however, wind invasion causes sweating and a floating moderate pulse, while this pattern causes an absence of sweating and a floating tight pulse.

Distinctive points

This pattern is distinctively characterized by fever, chills, an absence of sweating and a floating tight pulse (an exterior excess cold syndrome).

Delayed or inappropriate treatment of a *taiyang* disease may cause cold to transform into heat, further developing a *yangming* disease.

Pattern Identification of *Yangming* Disease

A *yangming* disease develops at the climax stage of the struggle between antipathogenic *qi* and pathogenic factors. At this stage, the pathogenic nature has transformed from cold into heat and the location from exterior into interior; more particularly, the *yangming* meridians, large intestine and stomach. The disease is mainly characterized by fever, spontaneous sweating, intolerance of heat, constipation, and abdominal distension and pain. By varying clinical manifestations, *yangming* diseases can be categorized into two types: meridian type and *fu* organ type.

Meridian type

Overview

This pattern manifests a condition of exuberant interior heat due to heat attacking *yangming* meridians.

Clinical manifestations

A high-grade fever, sweating, intolerance of heat instead of cold, thirst, a big surging pulse and a red tongue with a thin white or thin yellow coating; alternatively, the clinical manifestations are summarized as the "four bigs" — big fever, big sweating, big thirst and big pulse.

Analysis

Exuberant interior heat causes a high-grade fever. Heat expelling fluids may cause sweating. Cold transforming into heat in the interior may cause intolerance of heat. Heat consuming fluids may cause thirst. The fierce struggle between antipathogenic *qi* and pathogenic factors may cause a big surging pulse, indicating further progression. A red tongue with a thin white or thin yellow coating is indicative of pathogens staying in the *qi* phase due to exuberance of interior heat.

Differentiation

This pattern should be distinguished from wind invasion of *taiyang* disease. Both patterns have fever and sweating; however, wind invasion causes chills due to an unresolved exterior, while this pattern causes intolerance of heat.

Distinctive points

This pattern is distinctively marked by the four bigs (an interior excessive heat syndrome).

Fu organ type

Overview

This pattern manifests a condition of exuberant interior heat in the large intestine and stomach.

Clinical manifestations

Tidal fever in the afternoon, or fever alone without chills, restlessness, delirium, abdominal fullness, distension and pain, constipation or dry stools, a deep excessive powerful pulse and a red tongue with a yellow greasy or thick greasy coating.

Analysis

Since the *yangming* meridian *qi* reaches peak abundance in the afternoon, tidal fever in the afternoon occurs. Exuberance of interior heat may cause fever alone without chills. Exuberant stomach heat may disturb the heart, leading to restlessness and, in severe cases, delirium. Excessive heat may block intestinal *qi* and cause constipation or dry stools. Exuberant interior heat also causes a deep excessive powerful pulse. A red tongue with a yellow greasy or thick greasy coating is indicative of excessive heat.

Differentiation

This pattern should be distinguished from the previous meridian type. Both patterns can have fever and a red tongue with a yellow greasy coating due to interior excessive heat; however, the meridian type is marked by a high-grade fever, sweating, thirst and a big surging pulse but without constipation, while this pattern is mainly marked by tidal fever in the afternoon and constipation due to excessive heat in the gastrointestine.

Distinctive points

This pattern is distinctively characterized by tidal fever in the afternoon and constipation (an interior excessive heat syndrome).

As mentioned before, the stage of *yangming* disease experiences the fiercest struggle between antipathogenic *qi* and pathogenic factors. As the condition progresses, a gradual deficiency of antipathogenic *qi* may occur simultaneously with a decline of pathogenic factors. Afterward, a *shao-yang* disease may occur.

Pattern Identification of *Shaoyang* Disease

Overview

A *shaoyang* disease manifests a condition of relative weakness of both antipathogenic *qi* and pathogenic factors. The pathogenic nature is still heat. The location mainly involves the gallbladder and the gallbladder meridian. The stomach can also be affected. This disease is mainly characterized by alternating chills and fever.

Clinical manifestations

A bitter taste, a dry throat, blurred vision, alternating fever and chills, fullness of the chest and hypochondriac regions, a poor appetite, restlessness, nausea, vomiting and a wiry thready pulse.

Analysis

Heat consuming fluids may cause a bitter taste and a dry throat. The gallbladder meridian starts from the inner canthus, and heat ascending along the pathway of the meridian may cause blurred vision. The seesaw struggle between antipathogenic *qi* and pathogenic factors may cause alternating chills and fever. Since the gallbladder meridian passes through the chest and hypochondriac regions, heat attacking the meridian may cause fullness of the chest and hypochondriac regions. A poor appetite, nausea and vomiting occur as a result of pathogenic heat affecting the stomach.

Differentiation

This pattern should be distinguished from the *taiyang* and *yangming* diseases. A *taiyang* disease causes fever, chills and an exterior syndrome, while a *yangming* disease causes fever alone with an interior excessive heat syndrome. This pattern, however, causes alternating chills and fever. Also, the fullness of the chest and hypochondriac regions in this pattern needs to be distinguished from liver *qi* stagnation. Liver *qi* stagnation often results from internal injury and is associated with emotions, while this pattern results from external contraction and also causes fever.

Distinctive points

This pattern is distinctively characterized by alternating chills and fever (an interior excessive heat syndrome).

A *shaoyang* disease develops at the last stage of the three yang diseases. Heat transforming into cold with further weakening of antipathogenic *qi* may result in further development of *taiyin* diseases.

Pattern Identification of *Taiyin* Disease

Overview

A *taiyin* disease is the mild one among the three yin diseases. It occurs as a result of cold–dampness attacking the interior, especially the spleen and stomach, along with weakness of antipathogenic *qi*. It is mainly characterized by diarrhea, abdominal pain, vomiting and a weak pulse. A *taiyang* disease can develop either directly or gradually from one of the three yang diseases.

Clinical manifestations

Thin clear watery diarrhea mixed with white mucus, intermittent abdominal distension and pain with a preference for warmth and pressure, a poor appetite, nausea, vomiting, a pale tongue with a white greasy coating and a weak pulse.

Analysis

Cold–dampness affecting the transportation and transformation of the spleen and stomach may cause abnormal conduction of the large intestine, leading to thin clear watery diarrhea or this mixed with white mucus. Cold–dampness obstructing the *qi* flow of the spleen and stomach may cause intermittent abdominal distension and pain with a preference for warmth and pressure, and a poor appetite. Adverse ascending of stomach *qi* may cause nausea and vomiting. A pale tongue with a white greasy coating and a weak pulse are signs of deficiency and cold.

Differentiation

This pattern should be distinguished from diarrhea due to heat. Both can have diarrhea and abdominal pain; however, heat diarrhea is marked by strong-smelling feces mixed with yellow mucus or blood, coupled with thirst and a red tongue with a yellow greasy coating.

Distinctive points

This pattern is distinctively characterized by deficient cold diarrhea (an interior deficient cold syndrome).

With further weakness of antipathogenic *qi*, a *taiyin* disease may develop into a *shaoyin* disease.

Pattern Identification of *Shaoyin* Disease

A *shaoyin* disease develops at the later, critical stage of externally contracted febrile conditions. It can develop either from a *taiyin* disease or from one of the three yang diseases. The pathogenic nature can be cold or heat. The location mainly involves the heart and kidneys. According to the pathogenic nature, *shaoyin* diseases can be categorized into two types: cold transformation and heat transformation.

Cold transformation

Overview

This pattern manifests a condition of internal yin cold due to yang–*qi* deficiency.

Clinical manifestations

A low spirit, cold limbs, diarrhea mixed with undigested food, an absence of fever, intolerance of cold, lassitude, pallor, clear profuse urine, a faint thready pulse and a pale tongue with a white coating.

Analysis

Internal exuberance of yin cold due to failure of yang–*qi* may affect the heart–mind, resulting in a low spirit and lassitude. Failure of yang–*qi* to warm the four extremities and skin may cause cold limbs and pallor. Yang deficiency of the spleen and kidneys may cause diarrhea mixed with undigested food. Failure of yang of the spleen and kidneys to constrain water may cause clear profuse urine. Weakness of yang–*qi* in defending against pathogenic factors may cause intolerance of cold alone without fever. Deficiency of yin and yang causes a faint thready weak pulse. A pale tongue with a white coating is indicative of deficiency and cold.

Differentiation

This pattern should be distinguished from *taiyin* disease. Both patterns can have diarrhea and intolerance of cold due to interior deficient cold; however, *taiyin* disease mainly involves the spleen and stomach and may not cause symptoms due to yin preponderance due to yang deficiency, such as a low spirit, cold limbs and a faint thready pulse.

Distinctive points

This pattern is distinctively characterized by a faint thready pulse, a low spirit, cold limbs, diarrhea mixed with undigested food and exuberance of internal yin cold.

Heat transformation

Overview

This pattern manifests a condition of hyperactivity of fire due to yin deficiency following heat damaging yin.

Clinical manifestations

Restlessness, palpitations, an inability to lie flat, insomnia and a thready rapid pulse; alternatively, fever that is more severe at night than during the day, a dry mouth and throat with a desire to drink water and a red or dark-red tongue with a scanty, peeled or no coating.

Analysis

Malnourishment of the heart due to heat damaging yin may cause restlessness, palpitations, an inability to lie flat and insomnia. Heat entering *ying* may cause fever that is more severe at night than during the day. Heat consuming fluids may cause a dry mouth and throat with a desire to drink water. Heat severely damaging yin may cause a red or dark-red tongue and a thready rapid pulse. A scanty, peeled or no coating is indicative of severe damage to yin.

Differentiation

This pattern should be distinguished from a general yin deficiency syndrome. Both can have yin deficiency and fever; however, general yin deficiency often gradually develops from an internal condition and may not cause fever.

Distinctive points

This pattern is distinctively characterized by fever that is more severe at night than during the day, restlessness, insomnia, a thready rapid pulse and a red or dark-red tongue with a scanty coating (an interior deficient heat syndrome).

Pattern Identification of *Jueyin* Disease

A *jueyin* disease develops at the terminal stage of externally contracted febrile conditions. At this stage, the struggle between antipathogenic *qi* and pathogenic factors has become quite complicated. Either prevailing of pathogenic factors over antipathogenic *qi* or prevailing of antipathogenic *qi* over pathogenic factors is possible. The pathogenic nature can also be complicated, manifesting combined cold and heat. The location mainly involves the liver and kidneys. *Jueyin* diseases can be categorized into two types: combined cold and heat; alternating cold limbs and fever.

Combined cold and heat

Overview

This pattern manifests a condition of disordered *qi* activity due to combined cold and heat.

Clinical manifestations

Wasting thirst, rising (liver) *qi* affecting the heart, heartburn, hunger but no appetite and vomiting of food or ascarids after meals.

Analysis

Heat consuming fluids may cause wasting thirst. Retention of heat may obstruct the flow of *qi*, resulting in rising *qi* affecting the heart and heartburn. Cold retention may cause hunger but no appetite. Deficiency and cold in the spleen and stomach may cause ascarids to enter the diaphragm, leading to vomiting of ascarids after eating.

Differentiation

This pattern should be distinguished from combined cold and heat in the spleen and stomach. Both patterns can have *qi* disorder and no appetite; however, combined cold and heat in the spleen and stomach mainly causes vomiting and diarrhea, while this pattern is mainly characterized by wasting thirst, rising *qi* affecting the heart, heartburn and hunger with no appetite.

Distinctive points

This pattern is distinctively marked by combined cold (in the lower body) and heat (in the upper body).

Alternating cold limbs and fever

Overview

This pattern manifests a condition of yin–yang struggle at the later stages of externally contracted febrile conditions.

Clinical manifestations

Alternating cold limbs and fever can occur either before or after the other, coupled with restlessness and a deep pulse.

Analysis

Prevailing of yin over yang–*qi* causes cold limbs. Restoration of yang–*qi* causes fever. Fever following cold limbs indicates antipathogenic *qi* prevailing over pathogens and therefore a subsequent favorable prognosis, while cold limbs following fever indicates pathogens prevailing over antipathogenic *qi* and therefore a subsequent unfavorable prognosis.

Differentiation

This pattern should be distinguished from a simple cold extremity syndrome, which occurs as a result of yang deficiency and yin preponderance and does not cause fever.

Distinctive points

This pattern is distinctively characterized by alternating cold limbs and fever.

Combination of Diseases

Combination of diseases refers to a condition where two or more yang meridians are simultaneously attacked by external pathogens. It is usually termed "two-yang combination of diseases" or "triple-yang combination of diseases." For example, combination of diseases of *taiyang* and *yangming* includes symptoms of both *taiyang* disease and *yangming* disease from the very beginning. Likewise, triple-yang combination of diseases includes symptoms of *taiyang*, *yangming* and *shaoyang* diseases. Combination of diseases often indicates simultaneous conditions of two or three yang diseases.

Overlap of Diseases

Overlap of diseases refers to a condition where symptoms of one meridian follow those of another meridian. It is usually termed "two-yang overlap of diseases." For example, overlap of diseases of *taiyang* and *yangming* includes symptoms of *taiyang* disease first, followed by those of *yangming* disease. Overlap of diseases also indicates consecutive conditions of two or three yang diseases.

Combination of *Yin–Yang* Diseases

Combination of yin–yang diseases refers to a condition where one yin meridian and one yang meridian are simultaneously attacked by external pathogens. These two meridians are often internally–externally connected. For example, combination of *taiyang* and *shaoyin* diseases includes symptoms of both *taiyang* disease and *shaoyin* disease.

Review

QUESTIONS

1. Describe the clinical manifestations of *taiyang* disease.
2. Distinguish wind invasion from cold invasion (of *taiyang* disease) from the clinical manifestations and pathogenesis.
3. Describe the clinical manifestations of *yangming* disease.
4. Distinguish the meridian type from the *fu* organ type (of *yangming* disease) from the clinical manifestations and pathogenesis.
5. Describe the clinical manifestations and pathogenesis of *shaoyang* disease.
6. Describe the clinical manifestations and pathogenesis of *taiyin* disease.
7. Describe the clinical manifestations and pathogenesis of two main types of *shaoyin* disease.
8. How do you understand "combination of diseases," "overlap of diseases" and "combination of yin–yang diseases"?

Pattern identification of the 12 regular meridians

Meridians	Clinical Manifestations
Lung	Fevers, chills, sweating, pain in the shoulder and back with a cold sensation, pain in the collarbone, lung distension, coughing, panting, chest fullness, restlessness, scanty frequent urination, shortness of breath and feverish sensations on the palms and soles
Large intestine	Toothache, a sore throat, nosebleed, a runny nose, swelling of the neck, a dry mouth, pain on the anterior aspect of the shoulder and the anterior border of the extensor aspect of the upper limbs, numbness, pain and impaired flexion and extension of the thumbs and index fingers, abdominal pain, bowel sounds and diarrhea or constipation
Stomach	Fever (especially on the front part of the body), a swollen sore throat, nosebleed, toothache, deviated mouth and eyes, pain in the chest, abdomen and along the lateral aspects of the lower limbs, pain on the dorsum of the feet, numbness and impaired movement of the middle toes, gastric pain, vomiting, fast hunger even with an increased appetite, abdominal distension and fullness, edema, panic and mania
Spleen	Stiffness and pain of the tongue, vomiting after eating food, gastric pain, bloating, frequent belching, a heavy sensation, fatigue, impaired movement, swelling, pain and a cold sensation along the medial aspect of the thigh, numbness and impaired movement of the great toes, physical inactivity, a poor appetite, restlessness, loose stools or diarrhea, edema and jaundice
Heart	A dry throat, thirst with a desire to drink water, pain in the axillary or along the medial aspect of the arm, warmth and pain of the palms, cardiac pain, palpitations, insomnia and abnormal mental activities
Small intestine	Deafness, yellow eyes, swelling of the cheeks, a swollen sore throat, a stiff neck, pain in the shoulder and medial brachial muscle, distending pain of the lower abdomen, frequent urination and diarrhea or constipation

(Continued)

Meridians	Clinical Manifestations
Urinary bladder	Chills, fever, nasal congestion, nosebleed, headache, pain of the eyes, pain along the neck, low back, buttocks and along the posterior aspect of the lower limbs, numbness of the small toes, lower abdominal distension and fullness, dysuria and enuresis
Kidney	Pain on the posterior border of the medial aspect of the thigh, warmth and pain of the soles, a dry tongue, a swollen sore throat, restlessness, cardiac pain, hemoptysis, panting, a dark complexion, panic, enuresis, nocturnal emissions and irregular menstruation
Pericardium	A warm sensation on the palms, spasm of the arms and elbows, swelling of the axilla (armpit), chest fullness, cardiac pain, palpitations, a red face, restlessness and mania
Sanjiao	Deafness, pain behind the ears, a swollen sore throat, pain on the outer canthus, swollen painful cheeks, pain in the shoulder and arm and along the lateral aspect of the elbow, impaired movement of the small and index fingers, bloating, edema, enuresis and dysuria
Gallbladder	Headache, forehead pain, blurred vision, pain on the outer canthus, swollen painful collarbone, swollen painful armpit, pain in the chest, thighs and along the lateral aspect of the lower limbs and impaired movement of the small and fourth toes, a bitter taste, jaundice, pain in the hypochondriac regions, frequent sighing, malaria, anger, panic, timidity and insomnia
Liver	Low back pain with an inability to bend or look up, fullness and distension of the chest and hypochondriac regions, lower (lateral) abdominal pain, hernia, parietal headache, a dry throat, vertigo, a bitter taste and emotional depression or irritability

Pattern identification of the 8 extra meridians

Meridians	Clinical Manifestations
Du	Opisthotonos, stiffness of the neck and back, trismus, headache, convulsions of the four extremities, coma, fever, a white or yellow tongue coating and a wiry or rapid pulse; dizziness, a heavy sensation of the head, vertigo, a poor memory, tinnitus, deafness, lumbar soreness and weakness, rickets, a pale tongue and a thready weak pulse; cold intolerance on the back and spine, impotence, low sperm counts, nocturnal emissions, a falling sensation of the lower abdomen with infertility, lumbar soreness, a pale tongue and a deficient weak pulse
Ren	Amenorrhea, infertility, white leukorrhea, lower abdominal masses with fullness, distension and migratory pain, distending pain of the testes and hernia; increased fetal movement, a falling sensation of the lower abdomen, vaginal bleeding, possible miscarriage, a delayed period, amenorrhea, dribbling menstruation, dizziness, blurred vision, lumbar soreness and weakness of the low back and knee joints, a pale tongue and a thready weak pulse
Chong	A sudden *qi* ascending from the lower abdomen, nausea, vomiting, coughing, hematemesis, abdominal cramp, gushing pain in the epigastric region and severe morning sickness due to pregnancy; scanty menstruation in a pale color, amenorrhea, infertility, delayed menarche, premature menopause, lower abdominal pain, dizziness, blurred vision, palpitations, insomnia, maldevelopment of the male reproductive organs, thin beard or pubic hair, sterility, a pale tongue and a thready weak pulse; unsmooth menstruation, scanty menstruation, a delayed period, breast pain or distension, insufficient lactation and migratory lower abdominal masses
Dai	Lingering white leukorrhea, uterine prolapse, miscarriage, abdominal distension and fullness, pain around the umbilicus, low back and spine, lumbar soreness and weakness, a pale tongue with a white coating and a weak pulse
Yinwei/ Yangwei	Dull cardiac or chest pain, restlessness, emotional depression, mental fatigue, pain in the hypochondriac regions, low back pain, flaccidity of the limbs and persistent irregular fever
Yinqiao/ Yangqiao	Muscle wasting, paralysis or weakness of the legs, unstable walking, weakness of the feet, drowsiness or insomnia, prolapse of the eyelids, abnormal closing and opening of the eyes, a pale tongue with a white coating and a deficient pulse

Pattern identification of the 6 meridians

Meridians	Clinical Manifestations
Taiyang disease	Wind invasion may cause fever, chills, intolerance of wind, sweating and a floating moderate pulse; alternatively, headache, a general pain, low back pain, a stuffy and runny nose and a thin white tongue coating may also be present; cold invasion may cause fever, chills or intolerance of wind, an absence of sweating and a floating tight pulse; alternatively, headache, neck rigidity, ache of the bones and joints, coughing, panting and a thin white tongue coating may also be present
Yangming disease	The meridian type may cause a high-grade fever, sweating, intolerance of heat instead of cold, thirst, a big surging pulse and a red tongue with a thin white or thin yellow coating; alternatively, the clinical manifestations are summarized as the "four bigs" — big fever, big sweating, big thirst and big pulse; the *fu* organ type may cause tidal fever in the afternoon, or fever alone without chills, restlessness, delirium, abdominal fullness, distension and pain, constipation or dry stools, a deep excessive powerful pulse and a red tongue with a yellow greasy or thick greasy coating
Shaoyang disease	A bitter taste, a dry throat, blurred vision, alternating fever and chills, fullness of the chest and hypochondriac regions, a poor appetite, restlessness, nausea, vomiting and a wiry thready pulse
Taiyin disease	Thin clear watery diarrhea mixed with white mucus, intermittent abdominal distension and pain with a preference for warmth and pressure, a poor appetite, nausea, vomiting, a pale tongue with a white greasy coating and a weak pulse
Shaoyin disease	A low spirit, cold limbs, diarrhea mixed with undigested food, an absence of fever, intolerance of cold, lassitude, pallor, clear profuse urine, a faint thready pulse and a pale tongue with a white coating
Jueyin disease	Combined cold and heat may cause wasting thirst, rising (liver) affecting the heart, heartburn, hunger but no appetite and vomiting of food or ascarids after meals; alternating cold limbs and fever can occur either before or after the other, coupled with restlessness and a deep pulse

PATTERN IDENTIFICATION OF *WEI, QI, YING* AND BLOOD

Pattern identification of *wei*, *qi*, *ying* and blood is a method to differentiate externally contracted febrile conditions developed by Ye Tian-shi (1666–1746), a distinguished physician in the Qing dynasty (1636–1912). This method further developed the theories in the *Inner Classic* (*Nèi Jīng*) and *Treatise on Cold Damage* (*Shāng Hán Lùn*).

This method generalizes clinical manifestations of externally contracted febrile conditions into four phases: *wei* phase, *qi* phase, *ying* phase and blood phase. A pericardium pattern is also covered in the method. These phases manifest varying stages of externally contracted febrile conditions as well as the strength between antipathogenic *qi* and pathogenic factors. Along with pattern identification of the six meridians, this method has greatly enriched pattern identification for externally contracted febrile conditions.

Wei phase pattern

Overview

This pattern develops at the early stage of externally contracted febrile conditions following damp-heat attacking the exterior. Since the lungs dominate *qi* and govern the skin and skin hair, lung *qi*, i.e. *wei qi*, is the first line of defense against pathogenic invasion. As a result, a group of signs and symptoms due to an exterior excessive heat syndrome may occur at this stage.

Clinical manifestations

Fever, mild intolerance of wind–cold, mild thirst, an absence of or scanty sweating, headache, a general body ache, coughing, a red swollen sore throat, redness on the tip of the tongue and a floating rapid pulse.

Analysis

The struggle between *wei qi* and pathogenic warm-heat in the body surface may cause a fever. Warm-heat binding the *wei* may cause mild intolerance of wind–cold. Warm-heat damaging fluids may cause a mild thirst. Abnormal closing and opening of the striae and pores may cause an absence of scanty sweating. Ascending of warm-heat may cause headache. Warm-heat affecting the flow of meridian *qi* may cause a general ache. Warm-heat impairing the dispersing and descending of lung *qi* may cause coughing. Since the throat is the gate of the lungs, warm-heat attacking the lungs may cause a red swollen sore throat. A red tongue tip and a floating rapid pulse are signs of warm-heat.

Differentiation

This pattern should be distinguished from an exterior cold syndrome and *taiyang* disease. Both *taiyang* disease and an exterior cold syndrome occur as a result of contracting wind–cold, causing significant chills, headache and a general body ache; however, they may not cause thirst, a red swollen sore throat and a red tongue tip. This pattern is characterized by mild intolerance of wind–cold, thirst and a red swollen sore throat.

Distinctive points

This pattern is distinctively characterized by warm-heat attacking the *wei*.

Clinically, warm-heat is liable to mix with other pathogens to attack the exterior, manifesting as wind–heat attacking the *wei*, summer heat dampness attacking the *wei*, damp-heat attacking the *wei* and dry heat attacking the *wei*. These subpatterns can be identified according to the specific clinical signs and symptoms.

Qi **Phase Pattern**

Overview

This pattern develops at the midstage of externally contracted febrile conditions following warm-heat entering the *qi* phase. At this stage, the fierce struggle between antipathogenic *qi* and pathogenic factors results in dysfunctions of the *zang–fu* organs (an interior excessive heat syndrome). Also, subpatterns may vary, depending on the nature of pathogenic factors and involvement of the *zang–fu* organs.

Clinical manifestations

Fever, intolerance of heat instead of cold, restlessness, sweating, thirst, a red tongue with a yellow coating and a rapid pulse; heat disturbing the chest and diaphragm may cause restlessness and insomnia; heat accumulating in the lungs may cause coughing with yellow thick sputum, panting and chest pain; heat accumulating in the gastrointestine may cause afternoon fever, delirium, abdominal fullness, distension and pain, constipation and a deep excessive powerful pulse; heat blocking *shaoyang* may cause an intermittent fever, a bitter taste, a dry throat, and distension, fullness and pain in the chest and hypochondriac regions.

Analysis

The fierce struggle between antipathogenic *qi* and pathogenic factors may cause a fever. Pathogenic warm-heat entering the interior may cause intolerance of heat instead of cold. Heat expelling fluids may cause sweating. Heat consuming fluids may cause thirst and restlessness. A red tongue with a yellow coating and a rapid pulse are signs of interior exuberant heat. Heat disturbing the chest or diaphragm may cause restlessness and insomnia. Heat impairing the dispersing and descending of lung–*qi* may cause coughing with yellow thick sputum, panting and chest pain. Heat accumulating in the gastrointestine may block the flow of stomach *qi* and result in afternoon fever, delirium, abdominal fullness, distension and pain, constipation and a deep excessive powerful pulse. Heat blocking *shaoyang* may cause alternating prevailing of antipathogenic *qi* and pathogenic factors, causing an intermittent fever, a bitter taste, a dry throat, and distension, fullness and pain in the chest and hypochondriac regions.

Differentiation

This pattern should be distinguished from *yangming* disease, which also causes intolerance of heat instead of cold, restlessness, sweating and thirst in the meridian type. The *fu* organ type of *yangming* disease causes similar symptoms, with heat accumulating in the gastrointestine in this pattern. However, they have different means of transmission: *yangming* disease develops from *taiyang* disease, while this pattern develops from the *wei* phase.

Distinctive points

This pattern is distinctively characterized by an interior excessive heat syndrome in externally contracted febrile conditions.

Ying Phase Pattern

Overview

This pattern manifests a condition of pathogenic warm-heat entering the *ying* phase, causing a severe stage of externally contracted febrile conditions. At this stage, a group of signs and symptoms occur as a result of heat disturbing the heart–mind. Despite the presence of deficiency symptoms, this pattern is still ascribed to an interior excessive heat syndrome.

Clinical manifestations

A fever (especially at night), thirst, restlessness, insomnia, a dark-red tongue and a thready rapid pulse; coma, delirium and subcutaneous maculae may also be present.

Analysis

Warm-heat damaging the *ying* may cause fever at night. Warm-heat damaging fluids may cause thirst. Heat disturbing the heart–mind may cause restlessness, insomnia, and possibly coma with delirium. Heat in the *ying* may affect the blood as well, leading to subcutaneous maculae and a dark-red tongue. A thready rapid pulse is indicative of excessive heat with presence of deficiency.

Differentiation

This pattern should be distinguished from the *qi* phase pattern. Both patterns can have interior excessive heat; however, the *qi* phase pattern is characterized by fever, intolerance of heat instead of cold, and sweating, while this pattern is marked by fever (especially at night), a dark-red tongue and subcutaneous maculae.

Distinctive points

This pattern is distinctively marked by fever at night, a dark-red tongue and visible subcutaneous maculae.

Blood Phase Pattern

Overview

This pattern manifests a condition of pathogenic heat entering blood, involving concurrent interior excessive heat and deficiency. This is the most critical stage of externally contracted febrile conditions.

Clinical manifestations

Fever (especially at night), a burning sensation on the skin, restlessness, insomnia, mania or coma, a dark-purple tongue and a thready rapid pulse; alternatively, skin rashes, hematemesis, bloody urine, bloody stools, convulsions and cold extremities may also be present.

Analysis

Heat entering the *ying* and blood may cause fever at night and a burning sensation on the skin. Heat disturbing the heart–mind may cause restlessness, insomnia, mania and coma. Heat accelerating the flow of blood may cause skin rashes, hematemesis, bloody urine and bloody stools. Extreme heat causes a dark-purple tongue. A thready rapid pulse indicates excess containing deficiency. Heat stirring wind may cause convulsions. Heat staying in the interior may cause failure of yang–*qi* to warm the body, leading to cold limbs.

Differentiation

This pattern should be distinguished from the *ying* phase. Both patterns can have signs and symptoms in the *ying* phase; however, the pattern of the *ying* phase may not cause blood phase symptoms, while this pattern has additional bleeding symptoms, such as skin rashes and hematemesis.

Distinctive points

This pattern is distinctively characterized by heat entering the *ying* and blood, heat consuming and moving blood, and disturbance of the heart–mind.

Pericardium Pattern

Overview

This pattern manifests a critical condition of pathogenic factors entering the pericardium. It is mainly caused by heat, phlegm heat or turbid dampness.

Clinical manifestations

Fever, coma, delirium, alternating mental consciousness and confusion, a stiff tongue, cold limbs and phlegm sounds in the throat.

Analysis

Exuberant heat entering the pericardium may cause coma or delirium. Turbid dampness misting the pericardium may cause alternating mental consciousness and confusion. Since the heart opens into the tongue, disturbance of the heart–mind may cause a stiff tongue. Heat staying inside may cause failure of yang–*qi* to warm the body and result in cold limbs. Internal phlegm dampness may cause phlegm sounds in the throat.

Distinctive points

This pattern is distinctively marked by coma and delirium. In addition, it is necessary to distinguish heat blockage from phlegm misting the mind.

Heat blockage is characterized by exuberant heat and a red tongue, while phlegm misting the mind is characterized by a white greasy or white slippery tongue coating and phlegm sounds in the throat.

Transmission of the Patterns of *Wei, Qi, Ying* and Blood

As four patterns in the process of externally contracted febrile conditions, the patterns of the *wei* phase, *qi* phase, *ying* phase and blood phase are independent but interconnected. An externally contracted febrile condition often begins with the *wei* phase. An unresolved pattern of the *wei* phase can transmit sequentially into the *qi* phase or reversely into the pericardium. A pattern of the *qi* phase can transmit into the *ying* and blood. However, a pattern of the *wei* phase can transmit directly into the *ying* and blood. Also, a pattern of the *ying* phase can transmit back into the *qi* phase.

Clinically, patterns involving two phases can be present; for example, patterns involving the *wei* phase and *qi* phase may cause fever and mild intolerance of wind–cold (*wei* phase), coupled with restlessness, thirst, sweating and dark-yellow urine (*qi* phase); patterns involving the *qi* phase and *ying* phase may cause a high-grade fever and restlessness (*qi* phase), coupled with subcutaneous maculae and a dark-red tongue (*ying* phase); and patterns involving the *qi* phase and blood phase may cause a high-grade fever and restlessness (*qi* phase), coupled with skin rashes and bleeding symptoms. Consequently, it is important to make comprehensive analysis prior to a final diagnosis.

QUESTIONS

1. Describe the clinical manifestations of the pattern of the *wei* phase. How do you distinguish it from an exterior cold syndrome and *taiyang* disease?
2. Describe the clinical manifestations and pathogenesis of the pattern of the *qi* phase.
3. How do you distinguish the pattern of the *ying* phase from the blood phase?
4. Describe the clinical manifestations of the pericardium pattern. How do you distinguish heat blockage from phlegm misting the mind?

PATTERN IDENTIFICATION OF *SANJIAO* (TRIPLE ENERGIZER)

Pattern identification of *sanjiao* is a method to differentiate externally contracted febrile conditions developed by Wu Ju-tong (1758–1836), a distinguished physician in the Qing dynasty (1636–1912). This method is based on the *Inner Classic* (*Nèi Jīng*) and ideas of other physicians, including Ye Tian-shi.

This method generalizes the clinical manifestations in the process of externally-contracted febrile conditions into three stages: the pattern of the upper *jiao* (early stage), the pattern of the middle *jiao* (mid or climax stage) and the pattern of the lower *jiao* (terminal stage). Pattern identification of *sanjiao* is based on the nature of pathogenic factors, individualized constitutions, and the strength between antipathogenic *qi* and pathogenic factors.

Pattern of the Upper *Jiao*

Overview

This pattern develops at the early stage of externally contracted febrile conditions. It often causes symptoms involving the lung defense. It can either sequentially transmit into a pattern of the middle *jiao* or reversely into the pericardium. As a result, this pattern is characterized by signs and symptoms due to warmth attacking the lung meridian and warmth affecting the pericardium. The head, face and chest may also be involved.

Clinical manifestations

Fever, mild intolerance of wind–cold, an absence of sweating or scanty sweating, mild thirst, coughing, a red sore throat, redness on the tip of the tongue with a thin white coating and a floating rapid pulse; alternatively, coma, delirium, a stiff tongue, cold limbs and a red or dark-red tongue may also be present.

Analysis

The struggle between antipathogenic *qi* and pathogenic warm–heat may cause a fever with mild intolerance of wind–cold. Since the lungs dominate the skin and skin hair, failure of lung *qi* to disperse and descend may cause an absence of sweating or scanty sweating. Warm–heat consuming fluids may cause a mild thirst. Warm–heat impairing the dispersing and descending of lung *qi* may cause coughing. Since the throat is the gate of the lungs, warm–heat attacking the lungs may cause a red sore throat. Warm–heat attacking the body surface may cause a red tongue tip with a white coating and a floating rapid pulse. Warm–heat reversely transmitting into the pericardium may cause coma or delirium. Since the heart opens into the tongue, disturbance of the heart–mind may cause a stiff tongue. Heat staying in the interior may cause failure of yang–*qi* to warm the body and may cause cold limbs. Exuberant heat affecting the *ying* phase may cause a red or dark-red tongue.

Differentiation

Since the lung defense symptoms in this pattern are similar to the pattern of the *wei* phase, it should be distinguished from an exterior cold syndrome and *taiyang* disease. Both an exterior cold syndrome and *taiyang* disease result from contraction of wind–cold and are characterized by severe chills, headache and an obvious general body ache; however, they do not cause thirst, a red swollen sore throat and a red tongue tip. This pattern results from contraction of warm–heat and is, therefore, marked by heat symptoms. Since the symptoms involving the heart–mind in this pattern are similar to the pericardium pattern, it is necessary to be clear about the difference between heat blockage and phlegm misting the mind.

Distinctive points

This pattern is distinctively characterized by symptoms involving the lung defense and pericardium.

Remark. The pattern of the upper *jiao* may cause other signs and symptoms. Heat disturbing the chest and diaphragm may cause fever, a feverish sensation on the chest and restlessness. Heat accumulating in the lungs may cause fever, sweating, thirst with a desire to drink water, coughing and panting. Ascending of toxic heat may cause facial puffiness or swollen cheeks, most commonly seen in infectious swollen head, mumps, scarlet fever and acute laryngeal infection.

Pattern of the Middle *Jiao*

Overview

This pattern manifests a condition of pathogenic warm–heat transmitting from the upper *jiao* into the middle *jiao*, manifesting as disorders of the spleen, stomach and large intestine. The spleen and stomach reside in the middle *jiao*. The stomach is yang earth, while the spleen is yin earth. The spleen likes dryness and spleen *qi* ascends, while the stomach likes moistening and stomach *qi* descends. The pattern of the middle *jiao* often manifests as dry heat in the stomach or damp–heat in the spleen.

Clinical manifestations

Fever (especially in the afternoon), tolerance of heat instead of cold, red face and eyes, fast breathing, abdominal fullness, distension and pain, constipation, a dry mouth and throat, hesitant urination, a red tongue with a yellow coating or a charcoaled dark thorny tongue and a deep excessive pulse; alternatively, a low-grade fever, distension of the head, a general heavy sensation, chest tightness, gastric discomfort, dysuria, a sense of incomplete voiding after bowel movements or loose stools, a greasy or yellow-greasy tongue coating and a soft rapid pulse.

Analysis

Exuberant interior heat due to warm–heat entering the stomach may cause a fever with intolerance of heat. Since *yangming* meridian *qi* reaches peak abundance in the afternoon, exuberant heat in the stomach may cause an aggravated fever in the afternoon. Since the stomach meridian passes through the head and face, heat in the stomach meridian may cause a red face and eyes. Exuberant heat affecting lung *qi* may cause fast breathing. Excessive heat accumulating in the gastrointestine may cause abdominal fullness, distension and pain, and constipation. Heat consuming fluids may cause a dry mouth and throat and hesitant urination. A red tongue with a yellow coating or a charcoaled dark thorny tongue is indicative of interior excessive heat. Damp–heat may cause a low-grade fever. Dampness obstructing the flow of *qi* may cause distension of the head, a general heavy sensation, chest tightness and gastric discomfort. Damp–heat affecting the *qi* transformation of the urinary bladder may cause dysuria. Failure of the spleen to transport and transform may cause a sense of incomplete voiding after bowel movements or loose stools. A greasy or yellow greasy tongue coating and a soft rapid pulse are signs of internal accumulation of damp–heat.

Differentiation

The dryness in the stomach in this pattern is similar to the *fu* organ pattern of *yangming* disease. It should be distinguished from the meridian type of *yangming* disease. Both patterns are ascribed to an interior excessive heat syndrome and can cause fever and a red tongue with a yellow coating; however, the meridian type of *yangming* disease is marked by big fever, big sweating, big thirst and big pulse, while this pattern is marked by severe afternoon fever and constipation.

The dampness in the spleen in this pattern needs to be distinguished from spleen *qi* deficiency. Spleen *qi* deficiency is characterized by a thin greasy tongue coating, spleen *qi* deficiency symptoms and gastric distension after eating food (but the distension can be relieved with an empty stomach), while this pattern is marked by persistent gastric distension or discomfort, a thick greasy tongue coating and the presence of damp–heat symptoms.

Distinctive points

This pattern is distinctively characterized by dryness of the stomach and dampness in the spleen.

The pattern of the middle *jiao* may cause other signs and symptoms. Warm–heat attacking the *yangming* meridians may cause a high-grade fever, sweating, tolerance of heat instead of cold, thirst with a desire to drink water, a big surging pulse and a red tongue with a thin white or thin yellow coating. Damp–heat retention may cause bright orange jaundice, a poor appetite, nausea, vomiting and dysuria. Cold–dampness retention may cause dark-gray jaundice, intolerance of cold, bloating, loose stools and dysuria. Damp–heat spreading over the three *jiao* may cause persistent fever, sweating, a red face, chest tightness, gastric discomfort, thirst with no desire to drink much water, nausea, vomiting, diarrhea or dry stools, dark-yellow urine, a red tongue with a white greasy or yellow greasy coating and a soft rapid pulse.

Pattern of the Lower *Jiao*

Overview

This pattern manifests a condition of pathogenic warm–heat entering the lower *jiao*, manifesting disorders of the liver and kidneys. Since the liver and kidneys have the same source and both reside in the lower *jiao*, warm–heat attacking the lower *jiao* may damage yin of the liver and kidneys.

Clinical manifestations

Fever, a red face, feverish sensations on the palms and soles, night fever abating at dawn, a dry mouth and tongue, mental fatigue and a deficient big pulse; alternatively, twitching of the hands and feet, palpitations, a dark-red tongue with a scanty coating and a deficient pulse may also be present.

Analysis

Damp–heat consuming kidney yin may cause deficient fire, leading to fever, a red face and feverish sensations on the palms and soles. Warm–heat entering the lower *jiao* (yin) may cause warm soles and soles warm at night but cold in the morning. Heat damaging yin may cause a dry mouth and tongue. Mental fatigue and a deficient big pulse are signs of deficiency of antipathogenic *qi* with yin damage. Warm–heat consuming yin fluids may cause malnourishment of the tendons and muscles, leading to twitching of the hands and feet. Malnourishment of the heart–mind may cause palpitations. A dark-red tongue with a scanty coating and a deficient pulse are signs of damage to yin fluids.

Differentiation

This pattern should be distinguished from general yin deficiency and hyperactivity of fire due to yin deficiency. All three patterns can have yin deficiency; however, a general yin deficiency syndrome and hyperactivity of fire due to yin deficiency are ascribed to internal injuries and free from warm–heat invasion. A general yin deficiency syndrome is characterized by heat or dryness, hyperactivity of fire due to yin deficiency is marked by additional fire hyperactivity and this pattern is marked by additional warm–heat invasion coupled with yin fluid consumption.

Distinctive points

This pattern is distinctively characterized by warm–heat entering the lower *jiao* and insufficiency of yin liquids of the liver and kidneys.

The pattern of the lower *jiao* may cause other signs and symptoms. Downward flow of damp–heat into the lower *jiao* may cause fever, lower abdominal fullness and discomfort, constipation, dysuria, a red tongue with a greasy coating and a rapid pulse. Blood accumulation in the lower *jiao* may cause lower abdominal hardening and fullness, urinary incontinence and black stools.

Transmission of the Patterns of *Sanjiao*

As three stages in the process of externally contracted febrile conditions, the three *sanjiao* patterns are independent but interconnected. An externally contracted febrile condition often begins with the pattern of the upper *jiao*, starting from the lung meridian. Then it may sequentially transmit into the middle and lower *jiao*. However, with preponderant pathogens and a weak body constitution, pathogenic factors may reversely transmit into the pericardium. In some cases, transmission may never occur thanks to a prompt treatment and subsequent fast recovery. Some febrile conditions may directly start with a pattern of the middle *jiao* or lower *jiao*. In addition, two or triple *jiao* can be simultaneously affected.

QUESTIONS

1. Describe the subpatterns and clinical manifestations of the upper *jiao*.
2. Describe the subpatterns and clinical manifestations of the middle *jiao*.
3. Distinguish the pattern of the lower *jiao* from yin deficiency and hyperactive fire due to yin deficiency.

REVIEW

Pattern Identification of wei, qi, ying and blood

Phases	Clinical Manifestations	Pathogenesis
Wei	Fever, mild intolerance of wind–cold, mild thirst, an absence of sweating or scanty sweating, headache, a general body ache, coughing, a red swollen sore throat, redness on the tip of the tongue and a floating rapid pulse	Warmth attacking the body surface
Qi	Fever, intolerance of heat instead of cold, restlessness, sweating, thirst, a red tongue with a yellow coating and a rapid pulse; heat disturbing the chest and diaphragm may cause restlessness and insomnia; heat accumulating in the lungs, heat accumulating in the gastrointestine or heat blocking *shaoyang* may cause other signs and symptoms	Exuberant heat in the *qi* phase
Ying	Fever (especially at night), thirst, restlessness, insomnia, a dark-red tongue and a thready rapid pulse; coma, delirium and subcutaneous maculae may also be present	Heat entering the *ying*
Blood	Fever (especially at night), a burning sensation on the skin, restlessness, insomnia, mania or coma, a dark-purple tongue and a thready rapid pulse; alternatively, skin rashes, hematemesis, bloody urine, bloody stools, convulsions and cold extremities may also be present	Fast blood flow due to heat entering the blood
Pericardium pattern	Fever, coma, delirium, alternating mental consciousness and confusion, a stiff tongue, cold limbs and phlegm sounds in the throat	Heat entering the pericardium

Pattern identification of sanjiao

Locations	Clinical Manifestations	Pathogenesis
Upper *jiao*	Fever, mild intolerance of wind–cold, an absence of sweating or scanty sweating, mild thirst, coughing, a red sore throat, redness on the tip of the tongue with a thin white coating and a floating rapid pulse; alternatively, coma, delirium, a stiff tongue, cold limbs and a red or dark-red tongue may also be present	Warmth attacking the exterior involving the pericardium
Middle *jiao*	Fever (especially in the afternoon), tolerance of heat instead of cold, a red face and eyes, fast breathing, abdominal fullness, distension and pain, constipation, a dry mouth and throat, hesitant urination, a red tongue with a yellow coating or a charcoaled dark thorny tongue and a deep excessive pulse; alternatively, a low-grade fever, distension of the head, a general heavy sensation, chest tightness, gastric discomfort, dysuria, a sense of incomplete voiding after bowel movements or loose stools, a greasy or yellow greasy tongue coating and a soft rapid pulse	Exuberant interior heat in the middle *jiao*
Lower *jiao*	Fever, a red face, feverish sensations on the palms and soles, warm soles and soles warm at night but cold in the morning, a dry mouth and tongue, mental fatigue and a deficient big pulse; alternatively, twitching of the hands and feet, palpitations, a dark-red tongue with a scanty coating and a deficient pulse may also be present	Heat damaging yin fluids in the lower jiao

CHAPTER 5

Identification of Common Signs and Symptoms

Both signs and symptoms are something abnormal, relevant to a potential medical condition, but a *symptom* is experienced and reported by the patient, while a *sign* is discovered by the physician during examination of the patient.

The concept of a *syndrome* in Chinese medicine is different from that of signs and symptoms. It is a generalization of the causative factors, pathogenesis, signs, symptoms and location of a medical condition. A syndrome can tell about the nature of a disease and is, therefore, essential for the treatment.

There are varieties of medical conditions. Clinical signs and symptoms of these conditions can be numerous and complicated. Syndrome differentiation (i.e. pattern identification) aims to categorize the complicated clinical manifestations into varying patterns, thus providing the basis for effective treatments.

Some symptoms can tell about the nature of a disease, while some can tell about the location. As a result, it is extremely important to identify common signs and symptoms.

FEVER

Fever is a common medical sign characterized by an elevation of temperature above the normal range. It was considered by ancient physicians as a subjective feverish sensation. Fever can also be discovered by a physician during examination of the patient. It can occur as a result of either an externally contracted or an internally damaged condition.

Different syndromes can be identified according to the types of fever coupled with accompanying signs and symptoms.

Fever and Chills

Overview

This refers to a condition of concurrent fever and chills (including intolerance of cold or wind). It is a key diagnostic point for an *exterior syndrome*. Fever and chills are commonly seen in externally contracted febrile conditions. When wind, cold, summer heat, dampness, dryness or fire attacks the body surface, the binding of *wei qi* causes intolerance of cold or wind, and the struggle between *wei qi* and pathogens causes fever. Different subpatterns can be identified by the accompanying signs and symptoms.

Subpatterns

Subpatterns	Accompanying Signs and Symptoms	Pathogenesis
Exterior cold (*taiyang* wind invasion)	Headache, spontaneous sweating and a floating moderate pulse	Wind–cold disturbing the *ying* and *wei*
Exterior cold (*taiyang* cold invasion)	Headache, a general body ache, pain of the bones and joints, no sweating, a floating tight pulse	Wind–cold binding the *ying* and yin
Exterior heat (*wei* phase)	Headache, thirst, coughing, a red swollen sore throat, a red tongue tip and a floating rapid pulse	Warm–heat attacking the lung defense
Dampness blocking the *wei* phase	Fever in the afternoon, headache, a general heavy sensation, chest tightness and discomfort, a white greasy tongue coating and a soft moderate pulse	Dampness attacking the *wei qi*
Dryness attacking the exterior (often seen in autumn)	Headache, scanty sweating, unproductive coughs or coughing with scanty sticky sputum, a dry nose, thirst, a dry throat, a red tongue with a white coating and a rapid pulse	Dryness attacking the lung defense (can be further categorized into warm dryness and cool dryness)
Summer heat attacking the exterior (often seen in summer)	A general heavy sensation, pain, sweating, thirst and a wiry thready hollow deep pulse	Summer heat attacking the *wei qi*

Strong Fever

Overview

A strong fever is also known as a high-grade fever, often accompanied by intolerance of heat instead of cold. It is also described as "fever alone without cold intolerance" or "fever with intolerance of heat instead of cold." It is a key diagnostic point for an *interior excessive heat syndrome*. A strong fever occurs as a result of the fierce struggle between the antipathogenic *qi* and pathogenic factors. It is often seen in the mid or later stages of an externally contracted condition.

Subpatterns

Subpatterns	Accompanying Signs and Symptoms	Pathogenesis
Yangming meridian type (*qi* phase)	Profuse sweating, a red face, thirst with a desire to drink cold water, a red tongue with a yellow coating and a big surging or slippery rapid pulse	Exuberant heat in the *qi* phase of *yangming*
Pericardium pattern	Coma, delirium, unconsciousness, a stiff tongue and cold limbs	Heat entering the pericardium
Heat stirring wind	Distending headache, restlessness, dry mouth and lips, convulsions, coma, a red tongue with a dry yellow coating and a wiry rapid pulse	Heat disturbing the mind and malnourishment of the tendons or muscles
A dual blaze of *qi* and blood	Fever at night, headache, thirst, subcutaneous maculae or visible skin rashes, hematemesis, bloody urine, a dark-red tongue with a yellow coating and a rapid pulse	Exuberant interior heat disturbing the *ying* and blood
Heat accumulating in the lungs	Chest pain and tightness, coughing with profuse yellow sticky sputum, a red tongue with a yellow greasy coating and a slipper rapid pulse	Heat affecting the dispersing and descending of lung *qi*

Tidal Fever

Overview

Tidal fever can be seen in both externally contracted febrile and internally damaged conditions. It is caused by the struggle between antipathogenic *qi* and pathogenic factors. It occurs at a certain time regularly.

Subpatterns

Subpatterns	Accompanying Signs and Symptoms	Pathogenesis
Yangming fu organ pattern	Fever in the afternoon, abdominal distension and pain, constipation or diarrhea, restlessness, delirium, a red tongue with a dry yellow coating and a deep excessive powerful pulse	Excessive heat accumulating in the gastrointestine
Damp–heat retention in the *qi* phase	Afternoon tidal fever, a heavy sensation of the head and body, chest or gastric fullness and discomfort, bloating, loose stools, thirst with no desire to drink water, nausea, a thick greasy tongue coating and a soft rapid pulse	Persistent damp–heat in the *qi* phase
Internal heat due to yin deficiency	Afternoon tidal fever, rosy cheeks, a dry mouth and throat, feverish sensations on the palms and soles, mental fatigue, restlessness, a dry red tongue and a thready rapid pulse	Deficient heat due to yin deficiency
Yin deficiency of the liver and kidneys	Afternoon tidal fever, unproductive coughs or coughing with scanty sputum, insomnia, night sweats, dizziness, tinnitus, feverish sensations on the palms, soles and chest, a dry red tongue with a scanty coating and a thready rapid pulse	Damage to yin liquids of the liver and kidneys

Alternating Chills and Fever

Overview

Alternating chills and fever occurs as result of the struggle between antipathogenic *qi* and pathogenic factors. It is commonly seen in externally contracted febrile conditions.

Subpatterns

Subpatterns	Accompanying Signs and Symptoms	Pathogenesis
Shaoyang disease	Fullness in the chest and hypochondriac regions, loss of appetite, restlessness, vomiting, a bitter taste, a dry throat, blurred vision and a wiry thready pulse	Pathogens entering *Shaoyang*
Malaria	Intermittent high-grade fever and chills, general soreness, fatigue, headache, thirst with a desire to drink water, fever abating after sweating and a wiry pulse	Plasmodium attacking the body

Fever with Restlessness

Overview

Fever with restlessness can occur in both externally contracted febrile and internally damaged conditions.

Subpatterns

Subpatterns	Accompanying Signs and Symptoms	Pathogenesis
Heat disturbing the chest or diaphragm	A burning sensation on the chest or diaphragm, restlessness, a dry mouth with a desire to drink water, a red tongue with a dry yellow coating and a rapid pulse	Heat retention in the chest or diaphragm
Hyperactivity of fire due to yin deficiency	Fever, restlessness, insomnia, a red tongue with a yellow coating and a thready rapid pulse	Kidney yin deficiency with heart fire

Mild Fever

Overview

A mild fever is often seen in internally damaged conditions or a remission stage of externally contracted febrile conditions.

Subpatterns

Subpatterns	Accompanying Signs and Symptoms	Pathogenesis
Yin damage of the lungs and stomach	Unproductive coughs or coughing with scanty sputum, a dry mouth, a dry red tongue and a deficient pulse	Retention of heat in the lungs and stomach
Yin damage of the liver and kidneys	Persistent unresolved mild fever, feverish sensations on the palms, soles and chest, a dry mouth and throat, mental fatigue, a dark-red tongue with a scanty coating and a deficient rapid pulse	Unresolved pathogens damaging yin of the liver and kidneys
Fever due to *qi* deficiency	Recurrent mild fever triggered or aggravated by fatigue, mental fatigue, restlessness, lack of energy, reluctance to talk, spontaneous sweating, a poor appetite, a pale tongue and a deficient pulse	*Qi* deficiency of the spleen and stomach

---

QUESTIONS

1. Describe the clinical manifestations of fever and chills, strong fever, tidal fever and alternating fever and chills. List the patterns that may cause these four types of fever.
2. List the key diagnostic points and patterns that may cause fever with restlessness and mild fever.

SWEATING

This refers to abnormal sweating in a medical condition. Sweating can occur either all over the body or in specific body parts.

Sweating All over the Body

Overview

Sweating all over the body can occur in externally contracted febrile or internally damaged conditions. In externally contracted febrile conditions, wind, cold or other pathogenic factors may disturb the *ying* and *wei*, leading to sweating. Heat may expel fluids and result in sweating as well. In internally damaged conditions, yin–yang disorder may cause sweating.

Subpatterns

Subpatterns	Accompanying Signs and Symptoms	Pathogenesis
Taiyang wind invasion	Scanty sweating, fever, chills, a general body ache, a floating moderate pulse	Wind–cold attacking the exterior
Yangming meridian type or heat in the *qi* phase	Profuse sweating, a strong fever, intolerance of heat, thirst with a desire to drink cold water, a red face, a red tongue with a yellow coating and a big surging pulse	Exuberant interior heat expelling fluids
Yang deficiency	Profuse sweating, intolerance of cold, scanty urine, dysuria, contracture of the extremities and impaired flexion and extension of the joints	Weakened yang–*qi*
Yang depletion	Profuse or oily sweating, panting, pallor, cold limbs and an extremely faint pulse	Collapse of yang–*qi*
Shiver sweating	Chills and restlessness occur first, followed by fever and sweating	Struggle between antipathogenic *qi* and pathogens
Summer heat	Persistent profuse sweating, thirst, a strong fever, chest or gastric discomfort, a red tongue with a yellow coating and a big surging powerful pulse	Heat expelling fluids
Yin deficiency	Night sweats, soreness and weakness of the low back and knee joints, low back pain, nocturnal emissions or spermatorrhea, feverish sensations on the palms, soles and chest, a red tongue with a scanty coating and a thready rapid pulse	Deficient fire due to yin deficiency
Qi deficiency	Sweating upon mild exertion, mental fatigue, shortness of breath, reluctance to talk, a bright pale complexion, a pale tongue and a deficient pulse	Spleen *qi* deficiency

Sweating in Specific Body Parts

Overview

This refers to sweating only in specific areas of the body.

Subpatterns

Sweating on the Head	Accompanying Signs and Symptoms	Pathogenesis
Sweating due to exuberant heat	Fever, a general heavy sensation, fatigue, chest tightness, a red tongue with a yellow coating and a rapid pulse	Interior heat impairing the *qi* activity
Sweating due to damp–heat	Yellow eyes and body skin, dysuria, abdominal fullness, a red tongue with a yellow greasy tongue coating and a rapid pulse	Damp–heat impairing *qi* flow of the liver and gallbladder
Spontaneous sweating due to *qi* deficiency	A bright pale complexion, cold limbs, shortness of breath, reluctance to talk, mental fatigue, a pale tongue and a weak pulse	Spleen *qi* deficiency

Sweating on the Hands and Feet	Accompanying Signs and Symptoms	Pathogenesis
Sweating due to spleen deficiency	Cold limbs, mental fatigue, a poor appetite, loose stools, a pale tongue and a weak pulse	Spleen *qi* deficiency
Sweating due to yin deficiency	Feverish sensations on the palms, soles and chest, a dry mouth and throat, a red tongue with a scanty coating and a deficient pulse	Internal heat (due to yin deficiency) expelling fluids

Hemilateral Sweating	Accompanying Signs and Symptoms	Pathogenesis
Deficiency of *qi* and blood	A bright pale complexion, mental fatigue, palpitations, a pale tongue and a deficient pulse	Failure of *qi* to distribute fluids

(Continued)

(*Continued*)

Hemilateral Sweating	Accompanying Signs and Symptoms	Pathogenesis
Yang–*qi* deficiency	Sweating on the upper body, pallor, cold limbs, intolerance of cold and a pale tongue with a white coating	Failure of yang–*qi* to regulate fluids
Internal heat due to yin deficiency	Sweating on the upper body, soreness and weakness of the low back and knee joints, nocturnal emissions or spermatorrhea, feverish sensations on the palms, soles and chest, a red tongue with a scanty coating and a thready rapid pulse	Internal heat (due to yin deficiency) impairing the *qi* activity and subsequent leaking of fluids
Wind stroke	Hemiplegia and a dark tongue with ecchymosis	Internal stagnant blood obstructing the meridians

COUGHING

Overview

Coughing is one of the most common symptoms of respiratory system conditions. It is often caused by external pathogens attacking the lungs or impaired flow of lung *qi* due to dysfunction of the *zang–fu* organs.

Subpatterns

Subpatterns	Accompanying Signs and Symptoms	Pathogenesis
Contraction of wind–cold	Chills, fever, headache, a runny nose, production of thin white sputum, a thin white tongue coating and a floating pulse	Wind–cold impairing the dispersing and descending of lung *qi*
Contraction of wind–heat	Chills, fever, thirst, a sore throat, sweating, production of yellow thick sputum, a red tongue with a yellow coating and a floating rapid pulse	Wind–heat impairing the dispersing and descending of lung *qi*

(*Continued*)

(Continued)

Subpatterns	Accompanying Signs and Symptoms	Pathogenesis
Liver fire attacking the lungs	Paroxysmal coughing with pain in the chest and hypochondriac regions, scanty or thick sputum, a red face, a dry throat, a red tongue with a thin yellow coating and a wiry rapid pulse	Liver fire impairing the dispersing and descending of lung *qi*
Phlegm dampness attacking the lungs	Production of profuse white sputum, chest and gastric fullness and discomfort, a poor appetite, loose stools, mental fatigue, a white greasy tongue coating and a soft slippery pulse	Phlegm dampness impairing the dispersing and descending of lung *qi*
Lung *qi* deficiency	Production of profuse thin clear sputum, mental fatigue, a bright pale complexion, sweating upon mild exertion, a pale tongue and a deficient pulse	Weakness of lung *qi*
Lung abscesses	Production of sputum containing foul-smelling pus, chest pain, fever, shivering, restlessness, thirst, a red tongue with a thin yellow coating and a slippery rapid pulse	Toxic heat accumulating in the lungs and subsequent pus formation
Lung atrophy	Production of turbid saliva, weight loss, fatigue, shortness of breath, a red tongue with a scanty coating and a deficient rapid pulse	Failure of lung yin to nourish the lungs
Lung yin deficiency	Unproductive coughs or production of scanty blood-stained sputum, hemoptysis, afternoon low-grade fever, night sweats, thirst, a dry throat, a red tongue with a scanty or no coating and a thready rapid pulse	Deficient fire (due to lung yin deficiency) damaging the lung collaterals
Dryness attacking the lungs (often seen in autumn)	Paroxysmal coughing with no or scanty sputum, a dry scratchy throat, a dry mouth, a dry nose, fever, mild intolerance of wind and cold, cough-induced chest pain, a dry thin yellow tongue coating and a floating rapid pulse	Dry heat consuming the fluids

PANTING

Overview

Panting is one of the most common symptoms of respiratory system conditions. Patients can experience fast breathing, more exhalation than inhalation or breathing with an open mouth and raised shoulders. It is often associated with the lungs and kidneys.

Subpatterns

Subpatterns	Accompanying Signs and Symptoms	Pathogenesis
Wind–cold attacking the lungs	Coughing with sputum, chest tightness, fever, chills, sweating or an absence of sweating, a thin white tongue coating and a floating tight pulse	Wind–cold impairing the dispersing and descending of lung *qi*
Wind–heat attacking the lungs	Coughing with yellow thick sputum, nostril flares, fever, chills, thirst with a desire to drink water, sweating, a red tongue with a thin yellow coating and a floating rapid pulse	Wind–heat impairing the dispersing and descending of lung *qi*
Phlegm fluid retention in the lungs	Fast breathing, coughing with profuse foamy sputum, a poor appetite, nausea, chest tightness, a white greasy tongue coating and slippery pulse	Phlegm fluid impairing the dispersing and descending of lung *qi*
Cold fluid retention in the lungs	Breathing with an open mouth and raised shoulders, an inability to lie flat, coughing with production of foamy sputum, a white greasy tongue coating and a slippery pulse; the symptoms can be induced or aggravated by acute external contraction	Impaired lung *qi* due to pre-existent phlegm coupled with acute external contraction
Lung *qi* deficiency	Coughing with scanty sputum, mental fatigue, a low voice, spontaneous sweating, shortness of breath, a dry throat, a pale tongue with a white coating and a deficient pulse	Weakness of lung *qi*

(Continued)

(Continued)

Subpatterns	Accompanying Signs and Symptoms	Pathogenesis
Pleural fluid retention	Fullness and distension in the chest and hypochondriac regions, cough-induced pain, a white tongue coating and a deep wiry pulse	Pleural fluid impairing the dispersing and descending of lung *qi*
Failure of the kidneys to receive *qi*	More exhalation than inhalation which can be aggravated by fatigue, breathing with an open mouth and raised shoulders, weight loss, mental fatigue, cold limbs, a bluish or dark complexion, soreness and weakness of the low back and knee joints, a pale tongue and a deep thready pulse	Kidney *qi* deficiency affecting lung *qi*

QUESTIONS

1. What are the two categories of abnormal sweating? How do you identify their patterns?
2. What conditions can cause coughing? How do you identify their natures?
3. What conditions can cause panting? How do you identify their natures?

BLEEDING

Bleeding (also known as hemorrhaging) refers to loss of blood or blood escape from the vessels. It can be differentiated into cold, heat, deficiency and excess. Bleeding may occur in different areas of the body.

Epistaxis

Overview

This refers to subcutaneous bruises and bleeding from the nostrils, at the gums or from the external auditory canal.

Subpatterns

Subpatterns	Accompanying Signs and Symptoms	Pathogenesis
Nosebleed due to wind–heat or dryness attacking the lungs	Scanty nosebleed, a dry nose and throat, fever, mild intolerance of wind and cold, coughing with scanty sputum, thirst with a desire to drink water, a red tongue with a thin yellow coating and a rapid pulse	Lung heat affecting the nose
Nosebleed due to stomach heat	Profuse nosebleed in a bright red color, thirst with a desire to drink water, a foul breath, constipation, swelling and pain of the gums, a red tongue with a yellow coating and a rapid pulse	Ascending of stomach heat along the meridian to affect the nose
Nosebleed due to ascending of deficient fire	Scanty nosebleed, coughing with scanty thick sputum, night sweats, mild fever in the afternoon, dizziness, tinnitus, a red tongue with a scanty coating and a thready rapid pulse	Deficient fire (due to yin deficiency of the liver and kidneys) consuming fluids
Nosebleed due to liver fire	Scanty nosebleed, restlessness, irritability, red eyes, distending headache, pain in the hypochondriac regions, a red tongue and a wiry rapid pulse	Liver *qi* stagnation transforming into fire to affect the lung collaterals
Nosebleed due to nasal furuncles	Scanty nosebleed, visible furuncles inside and outside of the nasal cavity with redness, swelling, warmness and pain, presence of purulent blood on the tip of the furuncles, a red tongue with a yellow coating and a rapid pulse	Toxic heat damaging the lung collaterals
Nosebleed due to nasal vestibulitis	Scanty nosebleed, scratchy nostrils with ulceration and pain, a red tongue and a rapid pulse (this pattern is often seen in children)	Heat attacking the lungs
Gum bleeding due to stomach heat	Scanty gum bleeding in a bright red color, redness, swelling and pain of the gums, constipation, a foul breath, thirst with a desire to drink water, a red tongue with a yellow coating and a rapid pulse	Ascending of excessive heat in the stomach

(Continued)

(Continued)

Subpatterns	Accompanying Signs and Symptoms	Pathogenesis
Gum bleeding due to kidney deficiency and hyperactivity of fire	Scanty gum bleeding in a pale color, swelling, pain or loosening of the gums, a dry mouth with a desire to drink water, dizziness, tinnitus, a red tongue with a scanty coating and a thready rapid pulse	Ascending of deficient fire (due to kidney yin deficiency) to damage collaterals
Subcutaneous bruises due to *qi* deficiency	Presence of bruises or purpura, dizziness, blurred vision, mental fatigue, pallor, mild or severe palpitations, a pale tongue and a thready weak pulse	Failure of *qi* to hold blood
Bleeding due to furuncles or carbuncles of the external ear	Bleeding from the external auditory canal coupled with a stabbing pain, fever, headache and discharge of pus or blood, a red tongue and a rapid pulse	Toxic heat accumulating in the ear region
Nosebleed due to vicarious menstruation	Nosebleed before, during and after menstrual periods	Blood heat affecting the menstruation

Hematemesis

Overview

Hematemesis is the vomiting of blood mixed with gastric contents. The source is generally the upper gastrointestinal tract. This condition can be differentiated into deficiency, excess, cold and heat.

Subpatterns

Subpatterns	Accompanying Signs and Symptoms	Pathogenesis
Stomach heat	Vomiting of purple or dark blood mixed with food residues, gastric pain, distension and tightness, a dry mouth with a foul breath, dry black stools, a yellow greasy tongue coating and a rapid pulse	Exuberant stomach heat affecting the flow of stomach *qi* and accelerating blood flow

(Continued)

(Continued)

Subpatterns	Accompanying Signs and Symptoms	Pathogenesis
Spleen deficiency	Vomiting of pale or dark blood, gastric pain with a preference for warmth and pressure, pallor, cold limbs, tarry stools, a pale tongue and a thready pulse	Failure of spleen *qi* to control blood with the vessels
Liver fire attacking the stomach	Vomiting of purple or bright red blood mixed with gastric contents, distending headache, pain in the hypochondriac regions, a bitter taste, restlessness, irritability, a red tongue and a wiry rapid pulse	Liver *qi* stagnation transforming into fire to affect the stomach

Hemoptysis

Overview

Hemoptysis is the expectoration (coughing up) of blood or foamy blood-stained sputum from the respiratory tract. It is closely associated with the lungs and can be seen in both externally contracted and internally damaged conditions.

Subpatterns

Subpatterns	Accompanying Signs and Symptoms	Pathogenesis
Dry heat attacking the lungs	Blood-stained sputum, unproductive coughs or coughing with scanty sputum, a dry throat and nose, thirst with a desire to drink water, fever, mild intolerance of wind and cold, a red tongue with a dry scanty coating and a rapid pulse	Dry heat affecting the lung collaterals
Heat accumulating in the lungs	Blood-stained sputum, coughing with profuse yellow sputum, thirst, a sore throat, fever, intolerance of wind and cold, a red tongue with a thin yellow coating and a floating rapid pulse	Heat damaging the lung collaterals

(Continued)

(Continued)

Subpatterns	Accompanying Signs and Symptoms	Pathogenesis
Deficient fire due to lung yin deficiency	Coughing up of bright red blood (containing blood clots), weight loss, afternoon tidal fever, rosy cheeks, production of profuse yellow sputum, a red tongue with a scanty coating and a thready rapid pulse	Deficient fire damaging the lung collaterals
Liver fire attacking the lungs	Coughing up of blood, blood-stained sputum, cough-induced chest and hypochondriac pain, restlessness, irritability, a dry mouth with a bitter taste, dry stools, a red tongue with a yellow coating and a wiry rapid pulse	Liver fire damaging the lung collaterals
Qi and yin deficiency of the heart and lungs	Coughing up of blood and foamy blood stained sputum, panting, an inability to lie flat, chest tightness, palpitations, rosy cheeks, a dry throat, a red tongue and a thready rapid or regularly/irregularly intermittent pulse	Failure of *qi* to control blood plus deficient fire due to yin deficiency

Bloody stools

Overview

Bloody stools (also known as melena) often indicate an injury or disorder in the digestive tract. They include black, tarry or red stools.

Subpatterns

Subpatterns	Accompanying Signs and Symptoms	Pathogenesis
Deficiency and cold in the spleen and stomach	Black or tarry stools, mental fatigue, lassitude, dull gastric pain, a poor appetite, a pale tongue and a thready pulse	Failure of spleen *qi* to control blood
Hemorrhoids	Bloody stools in a bright red color, pain or swelling around the anus and presence of hemorrhoids	Damp–heat affecting the collaterals
Heat damaging the intestinal collaterals	Bloody stools in a bright red color, yellow urine, constipation, a bitter taste, a red tongue with a yellow coating and a rapid pulse	Heat expelling blood from the vessels

Bloody Urine

Overview

Blood in the urine (also known as hematuria) can be either gross or microscopic.

Subpatterns

Subpatterns	Accompanying Signs and Symptoms	Pathogenesis
Heart fire transmitting into the small intestine	Bright red blood in the urine with a burning sensation in the urethra, restlessness, insomnia, thirst, mouth or tongue ulcerations, a red painful tip of the tongue and a rapid pulse	Downward transmission of heart fire to damage the collaterals
Blood stranguria	Blood or clots in the urine with a burning sensation and hesitant urination, restlessness, a red tongue with a yellow coating and a rapid pulse	Downward flow of damp–heat into the urinary bladder to accelerate blood flow
Stone stranguria	Blood or stones in the urine, dysuria, interrupted urination, urgency of urination, referred low back pain, a thin yellow tongue coating and a rapid pulse	Damp–heat forming into stones to damage the collaterals
Fire hyperactivity due to yin deficiency	Blood in the urine, scanty dark-yellow urine, blurred vision, tinnitus, soreness and weakness of the low back and knee joints, a red tongue and a thready rapid pulse	Hyperactive deficient fire damaging the collaterals
Spleen *qi* deficiency	Frequent urination with light-red blood in the urine, mental fatigue, lassitude, a sallow complexion, a poor appetite, a pale tongue and a deficient pulse	Failure of spleen *qi* to control blood within the vessels

Metrorrhagia and Metrostaxis

Overview

This refers to abnormal vaginal bleeding between periods. Acute profuse bleeding is known as metrorrhagia (*bēng* in Chinese), while scanty bleeding that persists for an extended period is known as metrostaxis (*lòu* in Chinese).

Subpatterns

Subpatterns	Accompanying Signs and Symptoms	Pathogenesis
Qi deficiency of the heart and spleen	Sudden profuse or lingering vaginal bleeding in a pale color, pallor, palpitations, shortness of breath, reluctance to talk, cold limbs, a poor appetite, a tongue with tooth marks and a thin moistening coating, and a thready pulse	Failure of *qi* to control blood within the vessels
Kidney yin deficiency	Scanty or lingering vaginal bleeding in a bright red color, dizziness, tinnitus, soreness and weakness of the low back and knee joints, rosy cheeks, night sweats, feverish sensations on the palms, soles and chest, a red tongue with a scanty coating and a thready rapid pulse	Disorder of the *chong* and *ren* due to kidney yin deficiency
Blood stasis	Lingering or profuse vaginal bleeding, presence of blood clots, lower abdominal pain, a dark-red tongue and a wiry pulse	Stagnant blood obstructing the vessels
Liver *qi* stagnation transforming into fire	Sudden profuse or lingering vaginal bleeding in a bright red color, restlessness, irritability, distending pain in the chest and hypochondriac regions, a dry mouth with a desire to drink water, blurred vision, a red tongue with a yellow coating and a wiry pulse	Disorder of the *chong* and *ren* due to liver *qi* stagnation transforming into fire
Downward flow of damp–heat	Profuse or lingering vaginal bleeding in a red color, scanty dark-yellow urine, thirst, mental fatigue, lassitude, constipation or diarrhea, a yellow greasy tongue coating and a rapid pulse	Damp–heat accelerating the flow of blood

---

QUESTIONS

1. How many categories of bleeding are these? How do you identify its patterns?
2. Describe the causative factors and pathogenesis of blood in the urine.

PAIN

Pain is a subjective sensation felt by patients and one of the most common clinical symptoms. It can occur in varying positions of the body, manifesting as headache, chest and hypochondriac pain, gastric pain, low back pain, abdominal pain, and muscle and joint pain. It can be associated with the *zang–fu* organs, meridians, *qi*, blood, yin, yang, cold, heat, deficiency and excess.

Headache

Overview

A headache is pain anywhere in the region of the head or neck. It can be a symptom of a number of different conditions. It can be seen in both externally contracted and internally damaged conditions.

Subpatterns

Subpatterns	Accompanying Signs and Symptoms	Pathogenesis
Contraction of wind–cold	Pain radiating to the neck, intolerance of wind and cold, general bone and joint pain, preference for a wrapping up of the head, a thin white tongue coating and a floating tight pulse	Wind–cold impairing the flow of meridian *qi*
Contraction of wind–heat	Fever, intolerance of wind and cold, sweating, thirst, a red tongue with a thin yellow coating and a floating rapid pulse	Wind–heat impairing the flow of meridian *qi*
Contraction of wind–dampness	Headache with a sense of being wrapped up, a general heavy sensation, chills, fever, chest tightness, a poor appetite, a white greasy tongue coating and a soft pulse; this pattern is especially common on cloudy rainy days	Wind–dampness affecting the head
Yangming headache	Pain of the forehead, fever, sweating, thirst, restlessness, a red tongue and a rapid or big surging pulse	Ascending of heat along the stomach meridian
Shaoyang headache	Pain in the bilateral temples, alternating fever and chills, fullness of the chest and hypochondriac regions, a poor appetite, restlessness, vomiting, a bitter taste, a dry throat, blurred vision and a wiry thready pulse	Ascending of heat along the *shaoyang* meridian

(Continued)

(Continued)

Subpatterns	Accompanying Signs and Symptoms	Pathogenesis
Jueyin headache	Parietal headache, nausea, salivation, intolerance of cold, cold limbs, a pale tongue and a wiry pulse	Ascending of heat along the *jueyin* meridian
Hyperactivity of liver yang	Distending headache, tinnitus, blurred vision, a red face, insomnia, a poor memory, numbness and tremor of the limbs, a red tongue with a yellow coating and a wiry thready pulse	Hyperactive liver yang disturbing the head
Ascending of turbid phlegm	Distending headache, chest and gastric fullness, a general heavy sensation, lassitude, nausea, salivation, a white greasy tongue coating and a wiry slippery pulse	Turbid phlegm disturbing the head
Qi deficiency	Dull headache, lassitude, lack of energy and reluctance to talk that can be aggravated by fatigue, a bright pale complexion, a poor appetite, a pale tongue and a deficient pulse	Failure of the spleen to provide nutrients to nourish the brain
Blood stasis	Persistent stabbing headache in a fixed position, possibly a history of trauma, a dark tongue or a tongue with ecchymosis and a thready hesitant pulse	Stagnant blood obstructing the meridians
Blood deficiency	Dull headache, palpitations, insomnia, numbness of the hands and feet, a lusterless complexion, a pale tongue and a deficient pulse	Failure of blood to nourish the brain
Migraine	Sudden severe headache on one side and a wiry pulse	Ascending of wind–fire along the liver meridian
Kidney deficiency	Empty headache, vertigo, tinnitus, soreness and weakness of the low back and knee joints, nocturnal emissions, leukorrhea, a red tongue with a scanty coating and a deep thready weak pulse	Failure of kidney essence to supplement the brain marrow
Swollen head infection	Distending headache, swollen cheeks, facial boils, fever, coughing, a dry throat, thirst, a red tongue with a yellow coating and a rapid pulse	Toxic heat obstructing the meridians

Chest and Hypochondriac Pain

Overview

Chest pain occurs in the heart or lung regions. Hypochondriac pain is often associated with the liver and gallbladder. Chest and hypochondriac pain can be differentiated into deficiency, excess, cold and heat.

Subpatterns

Subpatterns	Accompanying Signs and Symptoms	Pathogenesis
Blockage of chest yang	Chest pain radiating to the shoulder and back, palpitations, shortness of breath, an inability to lie flat, pallor, cold sweats, cold limbs, a white tongue coating and a deep slow pulse	Chest yang being blocked
Phlegm damp-ness obstruct-ing chest yang	Chest pain radiating to the shoulder and back, panting, coughing with profuse white sputum, a poor appetite, a white greasy tongue coating and a deep wiry pulse	Phlegm dampness affecting chest yang
Blood stasis	A stabbing chest pain in a fixed position, chest tightness and discomfort, a dark tongue and a hesitant or regularly/irregularly intermittent pulse	Blood stasis obstructing chest yang
Qi stagnation	Wandering pain in the hypochondriac regions that is associated with emotions, restlessness, irritability, insomnia, belching, a thin white tongue coating and a wiry pulse	*Qi* stagnation affecting the hypochondriac regions
Phlegm heat accumulating in the lungs	Chest pain with coughs and panting, production of foul-smelling sputum, chills, fever, restlessness, a red tongue with a yellow coating and a floating rapid pulse	Phlegm heat impairing the flow of lung *qi*
Pleural fluid retention	Distending chest and hypochondriac pain that can be aggravated by coughs, along with distension and fullness in the hypochondriac regions, a white greasy or moistening tongue coating and a deep wiry pulse	Pleural fluid impairing the free flow of meridian *qi*

(Continued)

(Continued)

Subpatterns	Accompanying Signs and Symptoms	Pathogenesis
Lung yin deficiency	Chest pain with unproductive coughs or production of scanty blood-stained sputum, afternoon tidal fever, rosy cheeks, night sweats, a red tongue and a thready rapid pulse	Internal disturbance of deficient heat due to lung yin deficiency
Liver yin deficiency	Dull lingering pain in the hypochondriac regions, dizziness, blurred vision, feverish sensations on the palms, soles and chest, mental fatigue, a red tongue with a scanty coating and a thready rapid pulse	Internal disturbance of deficient fire due to liver yin deficiency
Damp–heat in the liver and gallbladder	Hypochondriac pain and discomfort, fever, a bitter taste, chest tightness, a poor appetite, nausea, vomiting, red eyes, yellow urine, possibly jaundice, a red tongue with a yellow greasy coating and a wiry rapid pulse	Damp–heat affecting the liver collaterals
Heart *qi* deficiency	Dull left chest pain, mild or severe palpitations, shortness of breath, reluctance to talk, a bright pale complexion, insomnia, a pale tongue and a deficient or regularly/irregularly intermittent pulse	Failure of heart *qi* to circulate blood

Low Back Pain

Overview

Low back pain can occur on one or both sides. Since the lumbus houses the kidneys, low back pain is closely associated with the kidneys. Either contraction of external pathogens or dysfunctions of the *zang–fu* organs can contribute to low back pain.

Subpatterns

Subpatterns	Accompanying Signs and Symptoms	Pathogenesis
Cold–dampness	Low back pain with a cold sensation that can be aggravated on cold rainy days and alleviated by warmth, impaired movement, intolerance of cold, cold limbs, a pale tongue with a white greasy coating and a deep tight pulse	Cold–dampness obstructing the flow of *qi* and blood

(Continued)

(Continued)

Subpatterns	Accompanying Signs and Symptoms	Pathogenesis
Kidney deficiency	Soreness and weakness of the low back and knee joints that can be aggravated by fatigue. Kidney yang deficiency causes a bright pale complexion, cold limbs, lower abdominal cramp, a pale tongue and a thready pulse. Kidney yin deficiency causes restlessness, insomnia, rosy cheeks, feverish sensations on the palms, soles and chest, a dry mouth and throat, a red tongue with a scanty coating and a thready rapid pulse	Failure of kidney yang to warm or failure of kidney yin to nourish the meridians
Downward flow of damp–heat	Low back and hip pain with a warm sensation, scanty dark-yellow urine, a red tongue with a yellow greasy coating and a thready rapid pulse	Damp–heat affecting the meridians
Blood stasis	Stabbing low back pain in a fixed position from impaired movement to an inability to roll over, a dark tongue and a thready pulse	Stagnant blood affecting *qi* and blood flow
Urinary calculi	Stabbing or dull low back pain on the posterior aspect or one side, hesitant painful urination, presence of stones in the urine, interrupted urine, blood in the urine, alleviated low back pain after passing of stones, a thin white tongue coating and a wiry pulse	Damp–heat forming into stones to obstruct the *qi* flow of meridians

Gastric Pain

Overview

This refers to pain in the epigastric region. Gastric pain can be differentiated into cold, heat, deficiency and excess.

Subpatterns

Subpatterns	Accompanying Signs and Symptoms	Pathogenesis
Cold attacking the stomach	Sudden gastric pain with a preference for warmth (the pain can be alleviated by local hot compression), intolerance of cold, watery vomiting, cold limbs, a desire to drink warm water, a thin white tongue coating and a deep pulse	Cold affecting the stomach due to ingestion of cold food

(Continued)

(*Continued*)

Subpatterns	Accompanying Signs and Symptoms	Pathogenesis
Food retention	Gastric distension and pain, acid reflux, belching, vomiting of undigested food, alleviated gastric pain after vomiting, a sense of incomplete voiding after bowel movements, a red tongue with a thick greasy coating and a slippery pulse	Food retention affecting the descending of stomach *qi*
Liver *qi* attacking the stomach	Gastric distension, fullness and scurry pain involving the hypochondriac regions, belching, acid reflux, a poor appetite, hesitant bowel movements, a thin white tongue coating and a wiry pulse	Liver *qi* stagnation blocking the flow of stomach *qi*
Deficiency and cold in the spleen and stomach	Dull gastric pain (especially with an empty stomach; the pain can be alleviated after eating food), preference for warmth and pressure, watery vomiting, cold limbs, loose stools, a bright pale complexion, a pale tongue with a white coating and a deep thready pulse	Impaired *qi* flow of the middle *jiao* due to weakness of the spleen and stomach
Blood stasis	Stabbing or pricking gastric pain in a fixed position (especially after eating food), black stools, hematemesis, a dark tongue or a tongue with ecchymosis and a deep hesitant pulse	Stagnant blood blocking the collaterals
Stomach yin deficiency	Gastric pain with a feverish sensation, a poor appetite, gastric distension after eating food, thirst, feverish sensations on the palms, soles and chest, dry stools, a red tongue with a scanty coating and a thready rapid pulse	Failure of stomach yin to nourish the stomach
Stomach heat	Burning gastric pain, a dry mouth with a desire to drink cold water, dry stools, dark-yellow urine, a red tongue with a yellow coating and a rapid pulse	Stomach heat obstructing the *qi* activity
Fluid retention in the middle *jiao*	Gastric pain with splashing sounds, a bright pale complexion, intolerance of cold, cold limbs, watery vomiting, a poor appetite, a pale tongue with a thin white coating and a deep pulse	Fluid retention affecting the water distribution

Abdominal Pain

Overview

This refers to pain below the gastric region. Making a definitive diagnosis of the cause of abdominal pain can be difficult, because many diseases inside the abdominal cavity can produce this symptom. It is, therefore, important to identify the specific organs and differentiate the condition into cold, heat, deficiency and excess.

Subpatterns

Subpatterns	Accompanying Signs and Symptoms	Pathogenesis
Qi stagnation	Wandering, distending, emotion-related abdominal pain that can radiate to the lower abdomen, chest tightness, belching, a thin tongue coating and a wiry pulse	*Qi* stagnation blocking the meridians
Blood stasis	Persistent abdominal pain in a fixed position, tenderness, possibly palpable masses, a dark tongue or a tongue with ecchymosis and a deep hesitant pulse	Stagnant blood entering the collaterals
Excessive heat in the gastrointestine	Burning abdominal pain with a preference for cold, tenderness, thirst with a desire to drink water, constipation, a red tongue with a yellow coating and a rapid pulse	Excessive heat blocking the flow of *qi*
Worm accumulation (often seen in children)	Intermittent abdominal pain, gastric upset, a lusterless complexion, a poor appetite, scratchy nostrils, grinding teeth during sleep, millet-sized spots on the lips or white patches on the face, abdominal masses during episodes and a deep tight pulse	*Qi* disorder due to worm accumulation
Ascariasis in the biliary tract	Sudden severe drilling pain in the right upper abdomen, nausea, vomiting, cold limbs, pallor, restlessness, a tight pulse (restored to normal during intermission)	Ascarids entering the biliary tract

(Continued)

(Continued)

Subpatterns	Accompanying Signs and Symptoms	Pathogenesis
Damp–heat in the intestine	Abdominal pain with a falling sensation, fever, chest tightness, a poor appetite, thirst, diarrhea mixed with blood or mucus, tenesmus, a burning sensation around the anus, scanty dark-yellow urine, a red tongue with a yellow coating and a rapid pulse	Damp–heat obstructing the flow of *qi*
Contraction of cold–damp-ness	Sudden abdominal pain, fever, chills, chest tight-ness, a poor appetite, a general heavy sensation, lassitude, no thirst, loose stools, clear urine, a white greasy tongue coating and a floating or tight pulse	Cold–dampness impairing the flow of *qi*
Deficiency and cold in the spleen and stomach	Intermittent dull abdominal pain with a preference for warmth and pressure, mental fatigue, cold limbs, loose stools, intolerance of cold, pain that can be aggravated by hunger or fatigue, a pale tongue with a white coating and a deep thready pulse	Internal cold–dampness obstructing the flow of meridian *qi*
Intestinal abscess (appendici-tis)	Severe abdominal pain with spasm of the abdomi-nal wall, a palpable mass in the abdomen or right lower abdomen, tenderness, impaired flexion and extension of the right lower limb, fever, sweat-ing, scanty dark-yellow urine, a red tongue with a yellow greasy coating and a wiry rapid pulse	Stagnation of *qi* and blood in the intestine
Food retention	Abdominal pain, distension and fullness, tender-ness, constipation, loss of appetite, belching, acid reflux, a foul breath, nausea, vomiting (the symptoms can be alleviated after vomiting or bowel movements), a white greasy tongue coat-ing and a slippery excessive pulse	Dysfunction of the spleen and stomach due to binge eating
Dysmenorrhea	Intolerable lower abdominal pain before, during or after the period, pallor, cold limbs, nausea, a thin tongue coating and a wiry pulse	Disorder of the *chong* and *ren* meridians
Hernia	Periumbilical pain that radiates or transmits to the perineum, cold hands and feet, hypochondriac pain, impotence and a deep wiry pulse	Cold *qi* affect-ing the *ren* meridian
Excessive cold	Abdominal pain and distension, constipation, cold limbs, intolerance of cold, a white tongue coat-ing and a deep wiry pulse	Yin cold block-ing the flow of *qi*

Muscle and Joint Pain

Overview

This refers to pain involving muscle, joints and also the entire body. It is most commonly caused by contraction of external pathogens. However, it can also be seen in other miscellaneous conditions.

Subpatterns

Subpatterns	Accompanying Signs and Symptoms	Pathogenesis
Wind *bi* (impediment)	Migratory muscle and joint pain coupled with impaired flexion and extension of the joints, fever, chills, a thin white tongue coating and a floating or tight pulse	Wind attacking the joints and muscles
Cold *bi* (impediment)	Severe muscle and joint pain in a fixed position (such as the shoulder or knee), fever, chills, impaired flexion and extension of the joints, a white tongue coating and floating tight or wiry tight pulse	Cold attacking the joints and muscles
Damp-*bi* (impediment)	Heavy muscle and joint pain in a fixed position (especially on the low back and lower limbs), fever, chills, heaviness and numbness of the limbs, a white tongue coating and a soft moderate pulse	Dampness attacking the joints and muscles
Wind–damp–heat *bi* (impediment)	Redness, swelling, warmth and pain of the muscles and joints, fever, thirst, impaired flexion and extension of the joints, a red tongue with a yellow coating and a slippery rapid pulse	Wind–damp–heat attacking the joints and muscles
Bi impediment due to blood stasis mixed with heat	Stabbing muscle and joint pain in a fixed position with localized redness and swelling, joint deformity with impaired flexion and extension, feverish sensations on the palms, soles and chest, thirst with a desire to drink water, a red tongue or a tongue with ecchymosis and a yellow coating and a wiry or deep hesitant pulse	Blood stasis and heat affecting the joints and muscles

(Continued)

(*Continued*)

Subpatterns	Accompanying Signs and Symptoms	Pathogenesis
Yang deficiency	Muscle and joint pain, cold limbs, intolerance of cold on the shoulder and back, a bright pale complexion, a deep or deep thready pulse	Failure of yang *qi* to warm the joints and muscles
Deficiency of *qi* and blood	Persistent muscle and joint pain, a lusterless complexion, shortness of breath, fatigue, mild or severe palpitations, sweating upon mild exertion, a pale tongue and a deficient pulse	Failure of *qi* and blood to nourish the meridians

QUESTIONS

1. How many categories of pain are there? How do you identify the patterns of headache, chest and hypochondriac pain, and low back pain?
2. Describe the causative factors and pathogenesis of low back pain.
3. How do you identify the patterns of gastric pain, abdominal pain, and muscle and joint pain?
4. Describe the causative factors and pathogenesis of muscle pain.

VOMITING

Overview

Vomiting (also known medically as emesis and informally as throwing up) is the forceful expulsion of the contents of one's stomach through the mouth. It can be caused by either contraction of external pathogens or an improper diet.

Subpatterns

Subpatterns	Accompanying Signs and Symptoms	Pathogenesis
External pathogens attacking the stomach	Sudden vomiting, chills, fever, headache, chest tightness, vexation, gastric pain, abdominal diarrhea, a white tongue coating and a floating rapid pulse	External pathogens affecting the descending of stomach *qi*

(*Continued*)

(Continued)

Subpatterns	Accompanying Signs and Symptoms	Pathogenesis
Food retention	Vomiting, acid reflux, gastric or abdominal distension, fullness and pain with tenderness, belching, loss of appetite, constipation or loose stools, a thick greasy tongue coating and a slippery excessive pulse	Food retention affecting the descending of stomach *qi*
Liver *qi* attacking the stomach	Vomiting, acid reflux, gastric or abdominal distension and fullness, pain in the hypochondriac regions, frequent belching, a red tongue with a thin greasy coating and a wiry pulse	Liver *qi* stagnation causing ascending of stomach *qi*
Fluid retention in the middle *jiao*	Vomiting of watery saliva, gastric fullness, a poor appetite, dizziness, blurred vision, palpitations, a white or moistening tongue coating and a deep pulse	Fluid retention affecting the *qi* activity in the middle *jiao*
Deficiency of the spleen and stomach	Gastric discomfort and distension after eating food, nausea, vomiting, mental fatigue, a bright pale complexion, thirst, preference for warmth, cold limbs, loose stools, a pale tongue with a white greasy coating and a weak pulse	Abnormal transportation and transformation of the spleen and stomach causing stomach *qi* to rise
Stomach yin deficiency	Recurrent vomiting, retching, a dry mouth with a desire to drink water, hunger but no appetite, a red tongue with a scanty coating and a thready rapid pulse	Failure of stomach yin to nourish the stomach causing abnormal *qi* activity
Deficiency and cold in the liver and stomach	Retching, salivation, parietal headache, cold limbs, a poor appetite, preference for warmth, a white greasy tongue coating and a deep pulse	Ascending of turbid yin due to deficient cold in the liver and stomach
Combined cold and heat	Nausea, vomiting, epigastric fullness, bowel sounds, diarrhea, a red tongue with a yellow coating and a wiry pulse	Combined cold and heat affecting the *qi* activity in the middle *jiao*

DIARRHEA

Overview

Diarrhea is the condition of having increased loose or liquid bowel movements per day. It can be differentiated into cold, heat, deficiency and excess.

Subpatterns

Subpatterns	Accompanying Signs and Symptoms	Pathogenesis
Cold–dampness	Abdominal pain, bowel sounds, thin, clear or watery stools, chills, fever, headache, a general body ache, a white or white greasy tongue coating and a floating rapid pulse	Cold–dampness affecting the stomach and intestine
Downward flow of damp–heat	Urgent watery diarrhea mixed with foul-smelling dark-brown stools following abdominal pain, a burning sensation around the anus, restlessness, thirst, scanty dark-yellow urine, a red tongue with a yellow greasy coating and a rapid pulse	Damp–heat causing abnormal conduction of the large intestine
Food retention	Abdominal pain, bowel sounds, diarrhea mixed with foul-smelling stools, alleviated pain after bowel movements, gastric fullness, belching, acid reflux, a turbid tongue coating and a rapid pulse	Food retention obstructing the *qi* activity of the large intestine
Weakness of the spleen and stomach	Recurrent loose stools and diarrhea mixed with undigested food, increased bowel movements after eating fatty food, a poor appetite, abdominal distension after eating food, mental fatigue, a pale tongue with a white or white greasy coating and a deficient pulse	Failure of the spleen and stomach to transport and transform water and food affecting the functions of the large intestine
Kidney yang deficiency	Diarrhea before dawn, periumbilical pain, diarrhea following bowel sounds, cold limbs, preference for warm drinks, a pale tongue with a white coating and a deep thready pulse	Kidney yang deficiency causing abnormal conduction of the large intestine

(Continued)

(*Continued*)

Subpatterns	Accompanying Signs and Symptoms	Pathogenesis
Disharmony between the liver and the spleen	Abdominal pain and diarrhea following mental stress, chest or hypochondriac fullness, belching, a light-red tongue with a white coating and a wiry pulse	Liver *qi* affecting the transportation and transformation of the spleen
Excessive heat in the gastrointestine	Tidal fever, delirium, abdominal fullness, distension and pain, diarrhea mixed with foul-smelling stools, a red tongue with a yellow greasy coating and a deep excessive powerful pulse	Excessive heat affecting the *qi* activity of the stomach and large intestine
Combined cold and heat	Bowel sounds, gastric discomfort, nausea, vomiting, fever, abdominal pain, a white greasy tongue coating and a wiry pulse	Combined cold and heat impairing the conduction of the large intestine
Internal build-up of toxic heat	Tenesmus, fever, thirst with a desire to drink cold water, a red tongue with a yellow greasy coating and a wiry rapid pulse	Internal toxic heat impairing the *qi* activity of the gastrointestine
Yang deficiency of the spleen and kidneys	Persistent diarrhea mixed with pus and blood in a pale color, fecal incontinence, cold limbs, abdominal pain with a preference for warmth and pressure, a pale tongue with a white coating and a deep pulse	Internal cold–dampness (due to yang deficiency) affecting the large intestine
Preponderance of yin due to yang deficiency	Diarrhea mixed with undigested food, cold limbs, chills, a pale tongue with a white coating and a faint thready pulse	Deficient cold affecting the large intestine
Cholera	Sudden vomiting and diarrhea, fever, chills, abdominal pain, restlessness, thirst with a desire to drink water, a white tongue coating and a floating or deep pulse	External pathogens attacking the stomach and large intestine
Epidemic pathogens	Sudden diarrhea mixed with pus and blood in a purple color, high-grade fever, headache, restlessness, thirst, severe abdominal pain, coma, convulsions, a dark-red tongue with a dry yellow coating and a slippery rapid pulse	Epidemic toxins damaging the intestinal collaterals

CONSTIPATION

Overview

Constipation refers to bowel movements that are infrequent and/or stools that are hard to pass. It is caused by abnormal conduction of the large intestine and can be differentiated into cold, heat, deficiency and excess.

Subpatterns

Subpatterns	Accompanying Signs and Symptoms	Pathogenesis
Excessive heat	Constipation, scanty dark-yellow urine, a red face, fever, abdominal fullness, distension and pain, restlessness, a dry mouth, a red tongue with a dry yellow coating and a slippery excessive pulse	Excessive heat blocking the *qi* flow of the large intestine
Liver *qi* stagnation	Constipation, frequent belching, chest and hypochondriac fullness, a poor appetite, bloating, a thin greasy tongue coating and a wiry pulse	Liver *qi* affecting the stomach and intestine
Qi deficiency	Constipation or difficulty in passing stools, strain during bowel movements, sweating, shortness of breath, a bright pale complexion, a pale tongue with a thin white coating and a deficient pulse	Failure of *qi* to push the conduction of the large intestine
Blood deficiency	Constipation or difficulty in passing stools, a lusterless complexion, palpitations, dizziness, a dry mouth with a desire to drink water, a red tongue with a scanty coating and a thready rapid pulse	Failure of blood to nourish the intestine
Excessive cold	Constipation, abdominal fullness and pain, cold limbs, intolerance of cold, soreness and a cold sensation in the low back and knee joints, profuse clear urine, preference for warmth, a pale tongue with a white coating and a deep excessive pulse	Excessive cold blocking the *qi* activity of the large intestine
Intestine dryness	Extremely dry stools, dry mouth and lips with a desire to drink water, a red tongue with a scanty coating and a thready pulse	Lack of fluids in the large intestine

QUESTIONS

1. How do you identify the patterns of vomiting?
2. How do you identify the patterns of diarrhea?
3. How do you identify the patterns of constipation?

DYSURIA

Overview

Dysuria refers to difficult urination, scanty urine or urine retention. It is important to identify the relevant *zang–fu* organs and differentiate cold, heat, deficiency and excess prior to treatment.

Subpatterns

Subpatterns	Accompanying Signs and Symptoms	Pathogenesis
Damp–heat	Dripping of urine in a dark-yellow color, lower abdominal fullness and distension, thirst with no desire to drink water, irregular bowel movements, a red tongue with a yellow greasy coating and a thready rapid pulse	Damp–heat impairing the *qi* transformation of the urinary bladder
Heat accumulating in the lungs	Urine retention, fast breathing, a dry throat, thirst with a desire to drink water, a red tongue with a yellow coating and a rapid pulse	Heat affecting the lungs and urinary bladder
Taiyang water retention	Scanty urine, lower abdominal fullness, fever, chills, thirst but drinking little, a thin white tongue coating and a floating pulse	Pathogens entering the bladder from *taiyang*
Wind–water	Scanty urine, fever, chills, coughs, facial puffiness in the morning, general pitting edema upon pressure, a white tongue coating and a floating rapid pulse	External pathogens affecting the lungs and urinary bladder

(Continued)

(*Continued*)

Subpatterns	Accompanying Signs and Symptoms	Pathogenesis
Yang deficiency	Scanty urine, facial puffiness, edema in the limbs (especially the lower limbs), mental fatigue, cold limbs, loose stools, a general heavy sensation, lumbar soreness, intolerance of cold, preference for warmth, a pale swollen tongue with a white coating and a deep pulse	Failure of yang–*qi* to maintain the *qi* transformation of the urinary bladder
Stranguria	Stabbing pain during urination or with frequency and urgency, lower abdominal cramp that can radiate to the low back, blood or stones in the urine, a thin tongue coating and a rapid pulse	Damp–heat or stones affecting the urinary bladder
Heat damaging yin	Scanty urine, a strong fever, profuse sweating, a dry mouth, restlessness, constipation, a red tongue with a dry yellow coating and a big surging pulse	Insufficiency of body fluids

EDEMA

Overview

Edema is an abnormal accumulation of fluid beneath the skin or in one or more cavities of the body. It can occur in the head, face, eyelids, four extremities, abdomen or even the entire body. It is important to identify yang edema from yin edema and differentiate the related *zang–fu* organs prior to treatment.

Subpatterns

Subpatterns	Accompanying Signs and Symptoms	Pathogenesis
Wind–cold attacking the lungs	Facial puffiness, edema of the eyelids, possibly edema of the entire body, dysuria, scanty urine; edema often follows an exterior syndrome (fever, chills, headache, joint pain, coughs, a sore throat, a thin white tongue coating and a floating rapid pulse)	Wind–cold affecting the function of the lungs in regulating water passage

(*Continued*)

(Continued)

Subpatterns	Accompanying Signs and Symptoms	Pathogenesis
Dampness obstructing the spleen	General pitting edema (especially in the abdomen and lower limbs), scanty urine, a general heavy sensation, lassitude, chest tightness, nausea, a greasy tongue coating and a soft pulse	Dampness affecting the transportation and transformation of the spleen
Spleen yang deficiency	Severe pitting edema in the lower limbs, gastric or abdominal distension, a poor appetite, loose stools, a sallow complexion, mental fatigue, cold limbs, scanty urine, a pale tongue with a white slippery coating and a deep pulse	Failure of spleen yang to warm and transform water
Kidney yang deficiency	General edema (especially below the low back), lumbar soreness and pain, scanty urine, cold limbs, mental fatigue, a gray or bright pale complexion, a pale swollen tongue with a white coating and a deep thready pulse	Water–dampness retention due to kidney yang deficiency
Yang deficiency of the heart and kidneys	General edema, palpitations, panting, an inability to lie flat, cold limbs, cold intolerance, scanty urine, pallor or a bluish complexion, a white tongue coating and a deep thready or regularly/irregularly intermittent pulse	Failure of heart and kidney yang to warm and transform water
Collapse of yang–*qi*	General edema, palpitations, severe panting, an inability to lie flat, restlessness, profuse sweating, cold limbs, scanty urine, a white moistening tongue coating and a deep thready faint pulse	Water retention due to yang deficiency and yin preponderance
Deficiency of yin and yang	A gray-dark complexion with facial puffiness, a low spirit, chest tightness, abdominal distension, a poor appetite, nausea, vomiting, scanty urine, palpitations, shortness of breath, restlessness, coma, convulsions, a pale swollen tongue with a white greasy coating and a deep thready pulse	Internal toxic dampness due to yin–yang deficiency
Spleen deficiency	Progressive general edema, especially facial puffiness in the morning and edema in the lower limbs in the afternoon, mental fatigue, a poor appetite, a pale swollen tongue with a thin greasy coating and a soft pulse	Water–dampness retention due to spleen deficiency

JAUNDICE

Overview

Jaundice is a yellowish pigmentation of the skin, the conjunctival membranes over the sclera (the whites of the eyes), and urine. It is caused by dysfunction of the liver and gallbladder and subsequent overflow of bile. It is important to distinguish yin jaundice from yang jaundice, and deficiency from excess, prior to treatment.

Subpatterns

Subpatterns	Accompanying Signs and Symptoms	Pathogenesis
Yang jaundice	Jaundice in a bright orange color, fever, thirst, thirst with a desire to drink water, nausea, vomiting, abdominal distension with hypochondriac pain, constipation, a red tongue with a yellow greasy coating and a wiry rapid pulse	Internal damp–heat (more heat) affecting the liver and gallbladder
Yin jaundice	Jaundice in a gray-dark color, fever, headache, a general heavy sensation, lassitude, chest tightness, gastric discomfort, a poor appetite, abdominal distension, loose stools, a thick greasy tongue coating and a soft pulse	Internal damp–heat (more dampness) affecting the liver and gallbladder
Yang jaundice with an exterior syndrome	Jaundice in a bright color, fever, chills, no sweating, abdominal distension with hypochondriac pain, constipation, nausea, vomiting, a red tongue with a yellow greasy coating and a floating rapid pulse	Internal damp–heat with an unresolved exterior syndrome
Severe yang jaundice	Severe jaundice in a golden color, a high fever, restlessness, chest and abdominal distension and fullness, coma, delirium, nosebleed, bloody urine, skin rashes, a red tongue with a yellow greasy coating and a wiry rapid pulse	Internal exuberance of toxic heat affecting the liver and gallbladder

(Continued)

(*Continued*)

Subpatterns	Accompanying Signs and Symptoms	Pathogenesis
Yang jaundice due to liver *qi* stagnation	Jaundice in a bright color, hypochondriac distension and pain, gastric or abdominal distension, nausea, belching, a poor appetite, a red tongue with a white coating and a wiry pulse	Failure of the liver to coordinate bile secretion and discharge
Yin jaundice due to cold–dampness	Jaundice in a gray-dark color, a poor appetite, bloating, loose stools, mental fatigue, cold intolerance, a pale tongue with a white greasy coating and a soft moderate pulse	Cold–dampness affecting the liver and gallbladder
Severe yin jaundice	Jaundice in a gray-dark color, restlessness, chest and abdominal distension and fullness, cold limbs, cold sweating, loose stools, coma, delirium, a pale swollen tongue with a white greasy coating and a deep thready pulse	Internal cold–dampness affecting the liver and gallbladder
Deficiency of the spleen and stomach	Jaundice, dry skin, mental fatigue, restlessness, palpitations, insomnia, abdominal fullness, a poor appetite, loose stools, a pale tongue with a thin coating and a soft thready pulse	Insufficiency of *qi* and blood to supply the liver/gallbladder

---

QUESTIONS

1. How do you identify the patterns of dysuria?
2. How do you identify the patterns of edema?
3. How do you identify the patterns of jaundice?

VERTIGO

Overview

Vertigo is a type of dizziness, where there is a feeling of motion when one is stationary. It is important to identify the causative factors and involved *zang–fu* organs prior to treatment.

Subpatterns

Subpatterns	Accompanying Signs and Symptoms	Pathogenesis
Hyperactivity of liver yang	Tinnitus and distending headache that can be triggered or aggravated by emotions, a red face, restlessness, irritability, insomnia or dream-disturbed sleep, tremor of the hands and feet, a red tongue with a thin yellow coating and a wiry pulse	Liver *qi* stagnation developing into hyperactive liver yang
Ascending of liver fire	Tinnitus, distending headache, a red face, a bitter taste, red eyes, restlessness, hypochondriac pain, a red tongue with a yellow coating and a wiry or wiry rapid pulse	Ascending of liver fire along the meridian
Internal damp–heat	Headache with a heavy sensation, chest tightness, gastric distension, hypochondriac pain, restlessness, irritability, numbness of the limbs, a red tongue with a white greasy or yellow greasy coating and a wiry rapid pulse	Damp–heat obstructing the ascending of clean yang
Yin deficiency of the liver and kidneys	Distending headache, a red face, red eyes, hypochondriac pain, low back pain, soreness and weakness of the low back and knee joints, feverish sensations on the palms, soles and chest, a red tongue with a yellow coating and a wiry thready pulse	Failure of liver and kidney yin to constrain liver yang
Kidney yang deficiency	Tinnitus, soreness and weakness of the low back and knee joints, cold limbs, mental fatigue, enuresis, nocturnal emissions, a pale tongue with a white coating and a deep thready pulse	Failure of the kidneys to nourish the brain
Qi deficiency	Mental fatigue, lassitude, shortness of breath, reluctance to talk, sweating upon mild exertion, a bright pale complexion, a poor appetite, a pale tongue with a thin white coating and a deficient pulse	Failure of spleen *qi* to ascend
Blood deficiency	A lusterless complexion, palpitations, shortness of breath, mental fatigue, insomnia, pale lips and nails, a pale tongue with a scanty coating and a thready pulse	Failure of blood to nourish the brain
Phlegm dampness	Headache with a heavy sensation, chest tightness and discomfort, nausea, vomiting, lassitude, profuse sputum, a poor appetite, a white greasy tongue coating and a soft slippery pulse	Phlegm dampness obstructing the ascending of clean yang

PALPITATIONS

Overview

Palpitations are abnormality of heartbeats that cause a conscious aware-ness of the heart's beating, whether it is too slow, too fast, irregular, or at its normal frequency. The word may also refer to this sensation itself, coupled with restlessness. Palpitations can be seen in either externally contracted or internally damaged conditions.

Subpatterns

Subpatterns	Accompanying Signs and Symptoms	Pathogenesis
External contraction	Mild or severe palpitations with a regularly/ irregularly intermittent pulse, chest tightness, fever, chills, headache, shortness of breath, mental fatigue and a thin white tongue coating	Unresolved pathogens entering the heart
Blood stasis	Palpitations with shortness of breath, chest tight-ness or pain, rosy cheeks, purple lips and nails, coughing, panting or hemoptysis, a pale purple tongue or a tongue with ecchymosis and a thready or regularly/irregularly intermittent pulse	An unresolved *qi* impediment affecting the heart
Qi disorder due to fright	Mild or severe palpitations, panic, restlessness, insomnia or dream-disturbed sleep, a poor appetite, a pale tongue and a deficient pulse	Fear or fright caus-ing *qi* disorder
Qi and blood deficiency of the heart	Mild or severe palpitations, a lusterless complexion, dizziness, shortness of breath, mental fatigue, spontaneous sweating, cold limbs, a pale tongue and a thready weak pulse	Failure of *qi* and blood to nourish the heart
Hyperactive heart fire	Palpitations with restlessness, insomnia, dizzi-ness, blurred vision, tinnitus, a bitter taste, soreness and weakness of the low back and knee joints, feverish sensations on the palms, soles and chest, a red tongue with a scanty coating and a thready rapid pulse	Failure of kidney water to constrain heart fire

(Continued)

(*Continued*)

Subpatterns	Accompanying Signs and Symptoms	Pathogenesis
Yang deficiency	Palpitations with chest tightness and panting, cold limbs, general edema, dysuria, a pale tongue with a white coating and a deep thready or regularly/irregularly intermittent pulse	Water retention (due to yang deficiency) affecting the heart
Stagnant blood	Palpitations with chest tightness and pain that can radiate to the shoulder and back, pallor, gray-dark lips, a dark purple tongue or a tongue with ecchymosis and a hesitant or regularly/irregularly intermittent pulse	Stagnant blood obstructing the heart
Phlegm dampness	Palpitations with chest tightness and dull pain, a bright pale complexion, obesity, nausea, a poor appetite, a swollen tongue with a white greasy or moistening coating and a deep or regularly/irregularly intermittent pulse	Phlegm dampness blocking heart yang

INSOMNIA

Overview

Insomnia refers to a chronic inability to fall asleep or remain asleep for an adequate length of time. In mild cases, patients may experience difficulty in falling asleep, waking up frequently during the night with difficulty in returning to sleep, waking up too early in the morning or interrupted sleep. In severe cases, however, patients cannot sleep throughout the night. Insomnia can be associated with the heart, liver, spleen, kidneys and stomach. It is therefore important to identify the involved organs and differentiate deficiency from excess prior to treatment.

Subpatterns

Subpatterns	Accompanying Signs and Symptoms	Pathogenesis
Deficiency of the heart and spleen	Dream-disturbed sleep, frequent waking up, palpitations, a poor memory, mental fatigue, a poor appetite, a lusterless complexion, a pale tongue with a thin coating and a thready pulse	Failure of *qi* and blood to nourish the heart–mind

(*Continued*)

(*Continued*)

Subpatterns	Accompanying Signs and Symptoms	Pathogenesis
Fire hyperactivity due to yin deficiency	Insomnia with restlessness, dizziness, tinnitus, soreness and weakness of the low back and knee joints, feverish sensations on the palms, soles and chest, a dry mouth, nocturnal emissions, a poor memory, palpitations, a red tongue with a scanty coating and a thready rapid pulse	Failure of kidney yin to constrain heart fire
Ascending of liver fire	Dream-disturbed sleep, nightmares, restlessness, irritability, chest or hypochondriac fullness and distension, headache, a bitter taste, red eyes, a red tongue with a yellow coating and a wiry rapid pulse	Liver *qi* stagnation transforming into fire to disturb the heart
Internal phlegm dampness	Dream-disturbed sleep, frequent waking up, chest and hypochondriac fullness and distension, nausea, vomiting, production of profuse yellow or white sputum, a poor appetite, a white greasy or yellow greasy tongue coating and a slippery pulse	Phlegm dampness disturbing the heart–mind
Qi deficiency of the liver and gallbladder	Dream-disturbed sleep, frequent waking up with fright, timidity, emotional depression, a pale tongue and a wiry thready pulse	A restless mind due to liver/gallbladder *qi* deficiency
Stagnant heat disturbing the heart	Poor sleep or sleeplessness throughout the night, mental confusion, incoherent speech, crying or laughing for no apparent reason, a red or dark tongue or a tongue with ecchymosis and a wiry rapid pulse	Blood stasis mixed with heat disturbing the heart–mind

---

QUESTIONS

1. How do you identify the patterns of vertigo?
2. How do you identify the patterns of palpitations?
3. How do you identify the patterns of insomnia?

CONVULSIONS

Overview

A convulsion is a medical condition where body muscles contract and relax rapidly and repeatedly, resulting in an uncontrolled shaking of the body. It is important to identify cold, heat, deficiency and excess prior to treatment.

Subpatterns

Subpatterns	Accompanying Signs and Symptoms	Pathogenesis
Convulsions with no sweating	Opisthotonos, trismus, headache, neck rigidity, fever, chills, no sweating, a white tongue coating and a floating tight pulse	Wind–cold attacking the flow of *qi* and blood
Convulsions with sweating	Opisthotonos, trismus, headache, neck rigidity, fever, chills, sweating, a white tongue coating and a soft moderate pulse	Wind–cold attacking the *wei*
Excessive heat	Neck and back stiffness, an inability to lie down, trismus, spasm of the hands and feet, fever, abdominal fullness, constipation, scanty dark-yellow urine, a yellow greasy tongue coating and a deep excessive powerful pulse	Exuberant interior heat affecting the tendons or muscles
Tetanus	Convulsions of the four extremities, neck and back stiffness, opisthotonos, trismus, a stiff tongue, salivation, facial spasm and a wiry pulse	Trauma or external pathogens attacking the body
Extreme heat stirring wind	Convulsions of the four extremities, neck rigidity, fever, coma, severe headache, vomiting, a burning sensation of the body, cold limbs, a red tongue with a yellow coating and a surging or excessive pulse	Interior heat consuming fluids and affecting the tendons and muscles
Internal stirring of liver wind	Tremors of the hands and feet, vertigo, neck rigidity, slurred speech, numbness of the hands and feet, unstable walking, possibly unconsciousness, hemiplegia, deviation of the mouth and eyes, a red tongue with a white or greasy coating and a wiry powerful pulse	Hyperactive liver yang stirring wind (the liver controls tendons)

(Continued)

(*Continued*)

Subpatterns	Accompanying Signs and Symptoms	Pathogenesis
Yin deficiency of the liver and kidneys	Twitching of the hands and feet, low back pain, soreness and weakness of the low back and knee joints, hypochondriac pain, afternoon tidal fever, restlessness, nocturnal emissions, a red tongue with a scanty coating and a thready rapid pulse	Insufficient essence blood to nourish the tendons and muscles
Deficiency of *qi* and blood	Mild convulsions of the four extremities, dizziness, a bright pale or sallow complexion, mental fatigue, a poor appetite, sweating on mild exertion, pale lips and nails, a pale tongue and a deficient pulse	Failure of *qi* and blood to nourish the tendons and muscles
Blood stasis	Convulsions of the four extremities, neck rigidity, stabbing headache, weight loss, mental fatigue, soreness and weakness of the low back and knee joints, a dark-purple tongue or a tongue with ecchymosis and a deep hesitant pulse	Internal stagnant blood obstructing the flow of *qi* and blood
Infantile convulsions (acute)	Intermittent convulsions of the four extremities, neck rigidity, trismus, a high-grade fever, restlessness and sudden onset of convulsions	Exuberant interior heat
Infantile convulsions (chronic)	Intermittent convulsions of the four extremities, neck rigidity, trismus, slow onset of convulsions, fever, a sallow complexion, lassitude, drowsiness, loose stools and a deficient pulse	Deficiency of *qi* and blood to nourish the tendons and muscles

UNCONSCIOUSNESS

Overview

Unconsciousness is a state in which a person cannot be awakened. It can be fatal and may occur in either an externally contracted or an internally damaged condition.

Subpatterns

Subpatterns	Accompanying Signs and Symptoms	Pathogenesis
Ascending of liver *qi*	Sudden unconsciousness, trismus, gripping of the fist, chest fullness, panting, cold limbs, a thin white tongue coating and a wiry pulse	Liver *qi* ascending to disturb the mind
Deficiency of *qi* and blood	Sudden unconsciousness, pallor, lusterless lips, tremors of the four extremities, sunken eyes with an open mouth, faint breathing, a pale tongue and a thready weak pulse	Failure of *qi* and blood to nourish the mind
Pericardium pattern	Sudden unconsciousness, a strong fever or fever at night, restlessness, delirium, a stiff tongue, cold limbs and a thready rapid pulse	External pathogens entering the pericardium
Stomach heat disturbing the heart	Unconsciousness, tidal fever in the late afternoon, abdominal fullness, hardness and pain, constipation, restlessness, delirium, thirst with a desire to drink water, a red tongue with a dry yellow coating and a deep powerful pulse	Exuberant stomach heat disturbing the mind
Internal turbid phlegm	Sudden unconsciousness, presence (or absence) of phlegm sounds in the throat, excessive salivation, a white greasy tongue coating and a slippery or deep pulse	Phlegm dampness misting the mind
Heat entering the *ying* and blood	Unconsciousness, delirium, restlessness, skin rashes or subcutaneous bruises, dark-yellow urine, a red or dark-red tongue and a thready rapid pulse	Heat in the *ying* and blood affecting the pericardium
Damp–heat	Unconsciousness or alternating consciousness and confusion, a low-grade body fever, delirium, a red tongue with a yellow greasy coating and a soft rapid pulse	Damp–heat misting the heart–mind
Edema due to yang deficiency of the spleen and kidneys	Unconsciousness or alternating consciousness and confusion, edema, dizziness, a lusterless complexion, nausea, vomiting, an ammonia breath, a pale swollen tongue and a thready pulse	Internal toxic dampness disturbing the mind

(Continued)

(*Continued*)

Subpatterns	Accompanying Signs and Symptoms	Pathogenesis
Sunstroke (often seen in summer)	Sudden unconsciousness, fever, a red face, profuse sweating, a red tongue with a thin yellow coating and a big surging pulse	Summer heat disturbing the mind
Yang depletion	Sudden unconsciousness, cold limbs, profuse sweating, an open mouth, loosened hands, faint breathing, urinary and fecal incontinence, a pale tongue and a faint pulse	Sudden collapse of yang–*qi*
Wind stroke	Sudden unconsciousness, hemiplegia, fever, a red face, trismus, fast breathing, phlegm sounds in the throat, a red tongue with a yellow greasy coating and a wiry pulse	Internal stirring of liver wind
Epilepsy	Sudden unconsciousness, salivation, trismus, jerking of the arms and legs, a white greasy tongue coating and a wiry slippery pulse	Turbid phlegm or liver wind stirring
Stagnant blood	Sudden transient unconsciousness, dizziness, mental fatigue, chest tightness, a dark tongue or a tongue with ecchymosis and a wiry thready or regularly/irregularly intermittent pulse	Stagnant blood obstructing the flow of *qi* and blood

QUESTIONS

1. How do you identify the patterns of convulsions?
2. How do you identify the patterns of unconsciousness?

DYSPHAGIA

Overview

Dysphagia — *ye ge* in Chinese medicine — is the medical term for the symptom of difficulty in swallowing. ("*Ye*" means difficulty in swallowing, while "*Ge*" means diaphragm obstruction.) Difficulty in swallowing can occur alone or as a precursory symptom for diaphragm obstruction. It is important to identify its nature prior to treatment.

Subpatterns

Subpatterns	Accompanying Signs and Symptoms	Pathogenesis
Phlegm *qi* stagnation	Difficulty in swallowing, tightness and dull pain in the chest or diaphragm, dry stools, a dry mouth and throat, gradual weight loss, a red tongue with a white greasy coating and a wiry thready pulse	Liver *qi* stagnation coupled with phlegm dampness affecting the chest or diaphragm
Internal stagnant blood	Chest or diaphragm pain, inability to swallow food or vomiting immediately after eating, possibly an inability to drink water, extremely dry stools, vomiting of a brown liquid, weight loss, dry skin, a dry red tongue or a tongue with ecchymosis and a thready hesitant pulse	Stagnant blood blocking the esophagus
Yang–*qi* deficiency	Chest or diaphragm pain, an inability to eat, a bright pale complexion, cold limbs, shortness of breath, watery vomiting, facial puffiness, edema of the feet, a dry pale tongue and a deep thready weak pulse	Abnormal *qi* activity due to deficiency of yin, yang and *qi*

ABDOMINAL MASSES

Overview

Abdominal masses are known as *ji ju* in Chinese medicine. They can be painful or distending. The *ji* syndrome refers to tangible immobilized masses with pain in fixed positions, whereas the *jù* syndrome refers to intangible mobile masses with migratory pain. It is important to identify their differences and natures prior to treatment.

Subpatterns

Subpatterns	Accompanying Signs and Symptoms	Pathogenesis
Ju syndrome due to liver *qi* stagnation	Mobile abdominal masses with distension and migratory pain, chest and hypochondriac fullness and pain, frequent sighing, a red tongue with a thin white coating and a wiry pulse	Liver *qi* stagnation affecting the free flow of *qi*

(Continued)

(*Continued*)

Subpatterns	Accompanying Signs and Symptoms	Pathogenesis
Ju syndrome due to food retention	Abdominal distension or pain, constipation, a poor appetite, mobile masses with distending pain upon pressure, a greasy tongue coating and a wiry slippery pulse	Food retention blocking the free flow of *qi*
Ji syndrome due to liver *qi* stagnation	Soft immobilized masses in the hypochondrium coupled with distension and pain, a dark tongue or a tongue with ecchymosis and a thin coating, and a wiry pulse	Liver *qi* stagnation affecting the collaterals
Ji syndrome due to *qi* stagnation and blood stasis	Immobilized painful abdominal masses, a dark complexion, weight loss, a poor appetite, fatigue, occasionally chills and fever, amenorrhea, a dark tongue or a tongue with ecchymosis and a white or yellow coating, and a thready hesitant pulse	*Qi* stagnation and blood stasis blocking the collaterals
Ji syndrome due to antipathogenic *qi* deficiency with blood stasis	Solid painful abdominal masses, a sallow or dark complexion, significant weight loss, reduced food ingestion, a pale purple tongue or a mirrored tongue and a thready rapid or wiry thready pulse	Antipathogenic *qi* deficiency coupled with blood stasis

ABDOMINAL TYMPANITES

Overview

Abdominal tympanites often occurs at the later stages of medical conditions, manifesting abdomen bulging in a bluish-yellow color or presence of the abdominal veins. It is often a critical sign, and it is necessary to distinguish deficiency from excess.

Subpatterns

Subpatterns	Accompanying Signs and Symptoms	Pathogenesis
Qi stagnation with dampness	Abdominal distension, hypochondriac fullness or pain, reduced food ingestion, abdominal distension after eating food, belching, scanty urine, a white greasy tongue coating and a wiry pulse	Disharmony between the liver and the spleen

(*Continued*)

(*Continued*)

Subpatterns	Accompanying Signs and Symptoms	Pathogenesis
Phlegm heat in the blood phase	Abdominal fullness and pain, a sallow or dark complexion, yellow eyes and skin, spider nervus on the neck, chest or arms, purple lips, a dry mouth, scanty dark-yellow urine, constipation or loose stools, a purple red tongue with a yellow greasy coating and a wiry rapid pulse	Damp–heat with blood stasis
Yang deficiency of the spleen and kidneys	Abdominal distension and fullness (especially at night), a poor appetite, mental fatigue, cold intolerance, cold limbs, edema in the lower limbs, scanty urine, a sallow or bright pale complexion, a pale purple tongue and a deep thready wiry pulse	Cold water retention due to yang deficiency
Yin deficiency of the liver and kidneys	Abdominal fullness with visible veins, weight loss, a dark complexion, a dry mouth, restlessness, nose or gum bleeding, scanty dark-yellow urine, a dry dark red tongue and a wiry thready rapid pulse	Water retention with blood stasis

ATROPHY–FLACCIDITY

Overview

Atrophy–flaccidity refers to weakness, debilitation or atrophy due to long-term inability to do voluntary movements. It can occur in either externally contracted or internally damaged conditions. Insufficiency of antipathogenic *qi* is a key contributing factor.

Subpatterns

Subpatterns	Accompanying Signs and Symptoms	Pathogenesis
Lung heat damaging fluids	Sudden weakness of the limbs following a fever, coupled with dry skin, restlessness, thirst, choking coughs, scanty dark-yellow urine, dry stools, a red tongue with a yellow coating and a thready rapid pulse	Toxic damp–heat attacking the lungs, causing malnourishment of the limbs

(*Continued*)

(Continued)

Subpatterns	Accompanying Signs and Symptoms	Pathogenesis
Damp–heat	Weakness and flaccidity of the limbs, possibly mild edema and numbness in the lower limbs, fever, scanty dark-yellow urine, a yellow greasy tongue coating and a soft or rapid pulse	Damp–heat affecting the limbs for an extended period
Weakness of the spleen and stomach	Progressive weakness and flaccidity of the lower limbs, a poor appetite, loose stools, facial puffiness, edema in the limbs, a lusterless complexion, a thin white tongue coating and a thready pulse	Insufficient production of *qi* and blood to nourish the tendons or muscles
Yin deficiency of the liver and kidneys	Slow onset of weakness and flaccidity of the limbs, soreness and weakness of the low back and knee joints, vertigo, tinnitus, nocturnal emissions, enuresis, a red tongue with a scanty coating and a thready rapid pulse	Failure of essence blood to nourish the tendons or muscles

QUESTIONS

1. Describe the pattern identification and clinical manifestations of dysphagia.
2. Describe the pattern identification and clinical manifestations of abdominal masses.
3. Describe the pattern identification and clinical manifestations of abdominal tympanites.
4. Describe the pattern identification and clinical manifestations of atrophy–flaccidity.

CHAPTER 6

Syndrome Differentiation and Medical Records

SYNDROME DIFFERENTIATION

Syndrome differentiation and treatment constitute the core of Chinese medicine and an essential paradigm for treatment. They are two closely related steps. The former provides the basis for the latter. As previously discussed, syndrome differentiation is a process for understanding the nature of medical conditions by analyzing the clinical signs and symptoms using the basic theory, four diagnostic methods and syndrome differentiation methods. The focuses of differentiation are as follows:

Differentiation of the Main Signs and Symptoms

The clinical manifestations of a medical condition consist of specific symptoms: some can help to identify the nature, while others can help to identify the location. Differentiation of these symptoms aims to clarify the nature of the disease and thus provide the basis for treatment.

Take fever for example. Fever is a main symptom in externally contracted febrile conditions. It varies in different conditions. Regarding pattern identification of the six meridians, fever and chills are often seen in *taiyang* disease, alternating fever and chills in *shaoyang*, fever without chills in *yangming*, chills without fever in *shaoyin* and tidal fever in the *yangming fu* organ pattern. Further differentiation of associated symptoms can pinpoint the patterns: fever and chills coupled with a floating tight pulse and an absence of sweating indicate a *taiyang* cold invasion; fever and chills coupled with sweating and a floating moderate pulse indicate a *taiyang* wind invasion; fever (without chills) coupled with profuse sweating, extreme thirst and a big surging pulse indicate a *yangming* meridian pattern; and tidal fever coupled with restlessness, delirium, constipation, abdominal fullness, hardness and pain and a deep excessive pulse indicate a *yangming fu* organ pattern.

Differentiation of the Disease Development and Changes

Each medical condition has its own law of occurrence and development. From onset to recovery, each condition passes through varying phases and causes varying clinical manifestations due to the differences in pathogenic nature, individualized constitutions and treatment methods. As a result, it is necessary to observe the patient's signs and symptoms in a dynamic way. For example, *wei*, *qi*, *ying* and blood are four phases of a febrile condition. When one is treating a patient with a febrile condition, it is important to bear in mind the transmission possibility of those four phases. However, it is also worth noting that the transmission may not necessarily follow the sequence. Take pathogenic warmth, for example: it usually attacks the lungs first, but, it may reversely transmit to the pericardium. Same cautionary points should be noted in the transmission of the six meridians.

Differentiation of the Pathogenesis

It is important to identify the pathogenesis prior to treatment. In Chinese medicine, the same condition can be treated with different therapies, while different conditions can be treated with the same therapy. Sometimes, different pathogenesis may cause the same clinical manifestations. For example, both external pathogens attacking the lungs and failure of the kidneys to receive *qi* can cause coughing and panting; however, the former should be treated by removing pathogenic factors and dispersing the lungs, and the latter by tonifying the kidneys. Sometimes, the same pathogenesis may cause different conditions. For example, spleen *qi* sinking may cause rectal prolapse and uterine prolapse. As a result, the two conditions can be treated with the same method — supplementing spleen *qi*.

Differentiation of the Strength Between Antipathogenic Qi and Pathogenic Factors

The struggle between antipathogenic *qi* and pathogenic factors runs through the whole process of a medical condition. Exuberant pathogens and abundant antipathogenic *qi* manifest an excess syndrome. Other manifestations include exuberant pathogens with deficient antipathogenic *qi*, weakened pathogens with deficient antipathogenic *qi* and deficiency of antipathogenic *qi* upon removal of pathogens. The strength between antipathogenic *qi* and pathogenic factors can be identified through signs and symptoms. It is important to evaluate the development tendency of a medical condition and thus take active treatment measures.

Application of Pattern Identification of the Eight Principles and Other Methods

The eight principles are the general paradigm for pattern identification. No matter how complicated, complicated clinical manifestations can always be analyzed and summarized using the eight principles. For example, the categories of a disease can be generalized into a yin syndrome and a yang syndrome; the depth of a disease into an exterior syndrome and an interior syndrome; the nature of a disease into a cold syndrome and a heat syndrome; and the strength between antipathogenic *qi* and pathogenic factors into a deficiency syndrome and an excess syndrome. However, pattern identification of the eight principles emphasizes the common features of medical conditions. Other methods of pattern identification are therefore necessary to combine for a complete pathological analysis. Take jaundice, for example. It can be categorized into yin jaundice and yang jaundice. By pattern identification of the eight principles, yang jaundice is ascribed to an interior excessive heat syndrome, and yin jaundice an interior deficiency cold syndrome. However, this cannot tell about the nature of the jaundice yet. By combining pattern identification of the *zang–fu* organs, yang jaundice is ascribed to damp–heat in the liver and gallbladder, while yin jaundice is ascribed to cold–dampness in the liver and gallbladder.

Differentiation of Externally Contracted Conditions from Miscellaneous Conditions

In a broad sense, medical conditions can be categorized into two types: externally contracted and miscellaneous disease. Generally speaking, the pattern identifications of the six meridians, of *wei*, *qi*, *ying* and blood and of *sanjiao* are indicated for externally contracted conditions. The pattern identifications of the *zang–fu* organs, of *qi*, blood and body fluids and of the meridians are indicated for miscellaneous diseases. However, the pattern identification methods can always be integrated. For example, *yang-ming* disease in pattern identification of the six meridians can be identified a *qi* phase syndrome in pattern identification of *wei*, *qi*, *ying* and blood, and as the middle *jiao* syndrome in pattern identification of *sanjiao*. When one is identifying the strength between antipathogenic *qi* and pathogenic factors, it is also important to identify the exuberance or deficiency of yin and yang of the *zang–fu* organs. To achieve this, the pattern identification of *qi*, blood and body fluids and other methods may also be needed.

MEDICAL RECORDS

A medical record is in general a systematic documentation of a single patient's long-term individual information, including a history of present illness, past medical history, family history and the information regarding pattern identification, diagnosis and treatment. A medical record is the original data for revisits, referrals or case studies. It is also important for disease statistics and medical studies, as well as possible medical malpractice disputes.

The earliest medical records can be traced back to the *Records of the Grand Historian* (*Shi Ji,* 史记) in the Western Han dynasty (202 B.C.–9 A.D.).

Contents of a Medical Record

A medical record should cover the four examination methods, pattern identification, treatment principle and formulas.

Four examination methods

This part should record the medical data collected through inspection, auscultation and olfaction, inquiry and pulse-taking. It is important to record the chief signs and symptoms. It is also necessary to record special negative symptoms or signs to exclude other conditions.

Pattern identification

This part should record the identified etiology, pathogenesis, affected *zang–fu* organs, meridians, yin, yang, deficiency and excess. If necessary, distinguish the identified pattern from other similar patterns to provide the basis for treatment.

Treatment principle

This part should deal with treatment principles based on the previous pattern identification.

Formulas

This part should clarify a formula or integrative therapy including acupuncture or tuina. The formula can be a modified classic one or a completely new one. It is necessary to mark doses for each medicinal as well as decoction method (such as decocting first or later). For acupuncture treatment, it is necessary to write down points. For tuina treatment, it is necessary to write down specific manipulations.

Requirements of a Medical Record

To complete a medical record, one needs to write carefully, correctly and timely, and use standardized terminologies. Clinical manifestations need to be specific and complete. Corrections or revisions should be avoided.

Format of a Medical Record

Inpatient medical record

Hospital admission No.

Name:	Gender:
Age:	Marital status:
Nationality:	Place of birth:
Occupation:	Working institution:
Home address:	Date of admission:
Narrator of case history:	Collection time of medical data:
Season of onset:	Name of next of kin:

Inquiry

Chief complaints. This includes one or more chief complaints regarding the position, nature, characteristics and time.

History of present illness. This includes the time of onset, inducing factors, main clinical manifestations, other associated symptoms, treatment and laboratory findings.

History of past illnesses. This includes the case history.

Personal history. This includes the personal hobbies, life habits, living environment, and menstruation or childbirth for women.

Family history. This includes the health status of family members or the death causes for deceased relatives.

Inspection

For inspection, it is important to record the spirit, complexion, body shape and movement, tongue conditions, luster and discharge.

Auscultation and olfaction

For auscultation and olfaction, it is important to record abnormal sounds and odors.

Pulse-taking and palpation

For pulse-taking and palpation, it is important to record the pulse conditions, skin temperature, tenderness, lumps or pitting edema, etc.

Special physical examination

This refers to surgical or gynecological examinations.

Pattern identification

This part should cover the basis for pattern identification, analysis of the etiology and pathogenesis, the treatment principle and basic formula or other methods (acupuncture or *tuina*) and other medical orders regarding nursing care.

Diagnosis

Identified pattern (or mixed with other patterns)

Signature of physician:

Date:

Inpatient chart

This includes recording the daily treatment, disease changes and modified pattern identification and treatment.

Outpatient medical record

Outpatient No.

Name:	Occupation:
Gender:	Working Institution:
Age:	Date of visit:

Inquiry:
    Chief complaints:
    Case history:
Inspection, auscultation, and olfaction and pulse-taking:
Pattern identification:
Diagnosis:
Treatment principle:
Formula (formula, medicine and dose):
Medical order:
                    Signature of physician:
                    Date:

Part B

CHAPTER 7

Syndrome Differentiation and Treatment for Common Conditions

COMMON RESPIRATORY SYSTEM CONDITIONS

Bronchitis

Overview

Bronchitis is an inflammation of the trachea and bronchi resulting from bacteria, viruses, or physical or chemical irritation. It occurs more in winter and spring, and most commonly affects the elderly. It can be divided into two categories — acute and chronic, according to the duration. Repeated bouts of bronchitis can further result in obstructive emphysema. Some cases may develop bronchiectasis.

In Chinese medicine, bronchitis falls into the categories of "coughing" "phlegm retention" and "shortness of breath." The main contributing factors include invasion by external pathogens and dysfunctions of the lung, spleen and kidneys.

External pathogens, either wind–cold or wind–heat, may affect the dispersing and descending of lung *qi*. Alternatively, those with lung *qi* deficiency are more susceptible to contraction of external pathogens. An aging or debilitating constitution may cause *qi* deficiency of the lungs and spleen, which in turn results in the failure of the spleen to transport and transform, leading to phlegm dampness in the lungs. Over time, deficiency of the lungs and spleen may affect the kidneys, resulting in kidney *qi* deficiency and failure of the kidneys to receive *qi*. All these factors can contribute to bronchitis.

Clinical manifestations

Acute bronchitis is characterized by the development of coughing, which often begins with an irritant unproductive cough coupled with substernal chest pain and a sense of tightness. Production of mucus (sputum), either sticky or clear, may occur after one or two days. Afterward, the cough lingers, along with an increased amount of sticky sputum. In severe cases, patients may develop paroxysmal coughing in the morning or evening. The cough can be worsened by postural changes, inhalation of cold air or physical exertion. Other symptoms may include nonstop coughing, chest pain, abdominal muscle pain, wheezing and shortness of breath. Chills, fever, headache and general discomfort may also be present. The fever may subdue within 3–5 days. However, the cough may linger for several weeks.

Chronic bronchitis is closely associated with acute respiratory tract infections such as acute bronchitis, influenza or pneumonia. In most cases, it is insidious and seen more often in cold weather. It is characterized by the presence of a productive cough, especially in the morning. The sputum often appears white, foamy and sticky. With superimposed infections or cold attack, patients may experience worsened signs and symptoms, along with excessive yellow or bloody sputum. Over time, the signs and symptoms are aggravated. Patients with chronic bronchitis may experience coughing with sputum all year round, particularly in autumn and winter. Repeated bouts may eventually result in emphysema, causing shortness of breath and more exhalation than inhalation upon physical exertion.

Pattern identification and treatment

Wind–cold attacking the lungs

Signs and symptoms

Coughing with white clear sputum, chills, fever, headache, general ache and discomfort, a clear nasal discharge and chest tightness.

Tongue: a thin white coating
Pulse: superficial

Treatment principle

Expel wind, dissipate cold, disperse the lungs and resolve phlegm.

Formula

Modified *Sān Ào Tāng* (三拗汤, "Rough and Ready Three Decoction")

麻黄	*má huáng*	9 g	*Herba Ephedrae*
杏仁	*xìng rén*	12 g	*Semen Armeniacae Amarum*
荆芥	*jīng jiè*	12 g	*Herba Schizonepetae*
防风	*fáng fēng*	12 g	*Radix Saposhnikoviae*
前胡	*qián hú*	9 g	*Radix Peucedani*
款冬花	*kuǎn dōng huā*	9 g	*Flos Farfarae*
紫菀	*zǐ wǎn*	9 g	*Radix et Rhizoma Asteris*
姜半夏	*jiāng bàn xià*	12 g	*Rhizoma Pinelliae Praeparatum*
桔梗	*jié gěng*	6 g	*Radix Platycodonis*
陈皮	*chén pí*	6 g	*Pericarpium Citri Reticulatae*
炙甘草	*zhì gān cǎo*	6 g	*Radix et Rhizoma Glycyrrhizae Praeparata cum Melle*

Modifications

- For severe chills, combine with *xì xīn* (细辛, *Radix et Rhizoma Asari*) 3 g.
- For a thick, greasy tongue coating due to excessive phlegm dampness, combine with *cāng zhú* (苍术, Rhizoma Atractylodis) 9 g and *chuān pò* (川朴, *Cortex Magnoliae Officinalis*) 6 g.

Wind–heat attacking the lungs

Signs and symptoms

Coughing with yellow or sticky, difficult-to-expectorate sputum, fever, sweating, chills, a dry mouth and a sore throat.

Tongue: a thin yellow or concurrently yellow and white coating
Pulse: superficial and rapid

Treatment principle

Expel wind, clear heat, disperse the lungs and resolve phlegm.

Formula

Modified *Sāng Jú Yǐn* (桑菊饮, "Mulberry Leaf and Chrysanthemum Beverage")

桑叶	*sāng yè*	9 g	*Folium Mori*
薄荷	*bò hé*	3 g	*Herba Menthae* (decoct later)
杏仁	*xìng rén*	9 g	*Semen Armeniacae Amarum*
前胡	*qián hú*	9 g	*Radix Peucedani*
连翘	*lián qiào*	12 g	*Fructus Forsythiae*
牛蒡子	*niú bàng zǐ*	9 g	*Fructus Arctii*
桔梗	*jié gěng*	6 g	*Radix Platycodonis*
贝母	*bèi mǔ*	9 g	*Bulbus Fritillaria*
黄芩	*huáng qín*	9 g	*Radix Scutellariae*
鱼腥草	*yú xīng cǎo*	12 g	*Herba Houttuyniae*
炙甘草	*zhì gān cǎo*	6 g	*Radix et Rhizoma Glycyrrhizae Praeparata cum Melle*

Modifications

- For unproductive coughing, combine with *shā shēn* (沙参, *Radix Adenophorae seu Glehniae*) 9 g.
- For profuse phlegm, combine with *zǐ sū zǐ* (紫苏子, *Fructus Perillae*) 9 g and *guā lóu* (瓜蒌, Fructus Trichosanthis) 9 g.

Contraction of cold with fluid retention

Signs and symptoms

Coughing with profuse white foamy phlegm, chest tightness, chills, fever and an absence of sweating.

Tongue: a white slippery coating
Pulse: superficial and tight

Treatment principle

Release the exterior, dissipate cold, warm the lungs and resolve fluid.

Formula

Modified *Xiǎo Qīng Lóng Tāng* (小青龙汤, "Minor Green Dragon Decoction")

麻黄	*má huáng*	6 g	*Herba Ephedrae*
桂枝	*guì zhī*	6 g	*Ramulus Cinnamomi*
细辛	*xì xīn*	3 g	*Radix et Rhizoma Asari*
姜半夏	*jiāng bàn xià*	12 g	*Rhizoma Pinelliae Praeparatum*
干姜	*gān jiāng*	6 g	*Rhizoma Zingiberis*
杏仁	*xìng rén*	9 g	*Semen Armeniacae Amarum*
桔梗	*jié gěng*	6 g	*Radix Platycodonis*
瓜蒌	*guā lóu*	12 g	*Fructus Trichosanthis*
紫菀	*zǐ wǎn*	9 g	*Radix et Rhizoma Asteris*
百部	*bǎi bù*	9 g	*Radix Stemonae*
炙甘草	*zhì gān cǎo*	6 g	*Radix et Rhizoma Glycyrrhizae Praeparata cum Melle*

Modifications

• For severe coughing, combine with *kuǎn dōng huā* (款冬花, *Flos Farfarae*) 9 g.
• For profuse phlegm, combine with *zǐ sū zǐ* (紫苏子, *Fructus Perillae*) 9 g.

Pathogenic heat accumulating in the lungs

Signs and symptoms

Coughing with yellow sticky phlegm, chest tightness, shortness of breath, fever, sweating and thirst with a preference for cold drinks.

Tongue: red, with a yellow or yellow greasy coating
Pulse: rapid or superficial rapid

Treatment principle

Clear heat, disperse the lungs and resolve phlegm.

Formula

Supplemented *Má Xìng Shí Gān Tāng* (麻杏石甘汤, "Ephedra, Apricot Kernel, Gypsum and Licorice Decoction").

麻黄	*má huáng*	6 g	*Herba Ephedrae*
杏仁	*xìng rén*	9 g	*Semen Armeniacae Amarum*
石膏	*shí gāo*	30 g	*Gypsum Fibrosum* (ground, and decoct first)
桑白皮	*sāng bái pí*	12 g	*Cortex Mori*
干姜	*gān jiāng*	6 g	*Rhizoma Zingiberis*
黄芩	*huáng qín*	9 g	*Radix Scutellariae*
贝母	*bèi mǔ*	9 g	*Bulbus Fritillaria*
连翘	*lián qiào*	12 g	*Fructus Forsythiae*
鱼腥草	*yú xīng cǎo*	12 g	*Herba Houttuyniae*
瓜蒌皮	*guā lóu pí*	6 g	*Pericarpium Trichosanthis*
炙甘草	*zhì gān cǎo*	6 g	*Radix et Rhizoma Glycyrrhizae Praeparata cum Melle*

Modifications

- For severe coughing, combine with *zǐ wān* (紫菀, *Radix et Rhizoma Asteris*) 9 g and *kuǎn dōng huā* (款冬花, Flos Farfarae) 9 g.
- For constipation, combine with *dà huáng* (大黄, *Radix et Rhizoma Rhei*) 9 g (decoct later).
- For thirst, combine with *tiān huā fěn* (天花粉, *Radix Trichosanthis*) 12 g.

Phlegm dampness affecting the lungs

Signs and symptoms

Coughing with profuse white sputum, chest tightness, shortness of breath, heavy sensation of the limbs, tastelessness, a poor appetite, abdominal bloating and loose stools.

Tongue: a white greasy coating
Pulse: soft and slippery

Treatment principle

Disperse the lungs, resolve phlegm, dry dampness and strengthen the spleen.

Formula

Modified *Líng Guì Zhú Gān Tāng* (苓桂术甘汤, "*Poria*, Cinnamon Twig, *Atractylodes Macrocephala* and Licorice Decoction) and *Èr Chén Tāng* (二陈汤, "Two Matured Substances Decoction").

茯苓	*fú líng*	12 g	*Poria*
桂枝	*guì zhī*	9 g	*Ramulus Cinnamomi*
白术	*bái zhú*	9 g	*Rhizoma Atractylodis Macrocephalae*
姜半夏	*jiāng bàn xià*	12 g	*Rhizoma Pinelliae Praeparatum*
厚朴	*hòu pò*	9 g	*Cortex Magnoliae Officinalis*
枳实	*zhǐ shí*	9 g	*Fructus Aurantii Immaturus*
陈皮	*chén pí*	6 g	*Pericarpium Citri Reticulatae*
杏仁	*xìng rén*	9 g	*Semen Armeniacae Amarum*
紫菀	*zǐ wǎn*	9 g	*Radix et Rhizoma Asteris*
款冬花	*kuǎn dōng huā*	9 g	*Flos Farfarae*
炙甘草	*zhì gān cǎo*	6 g	*Radix et Rhizoma Glycyrrhizae Praeparata cum Melle*

Modifications

- For dyspnea, combine with *má huáng* (麻黄, *Herba Ephedrae*) 6 g and *zǐ sū zǐ* (紫苏子, *Fructus Perillae*) 9 g.
- For severe chills, combine with *gān jiāng* (干姜, *Rhizoma Zingiberis*) 6 g and *xì xīn* (细辛, *Radix et Rhizoma Asari*) 3 g.
- For scanty, difficult-to-expectorate sputum, combine with *bái jiè zǐ* (白芥子, *Semen Sinapis*) 9 g.

Deficiency of the lungs and spleen

Signs and symptoms

Mental fatigue, lassitude, spontaneous sweating, shortness of breath, a poor appetite, loose stools and bouts of coughing or aggravated symptoms upon contraction of wind–cold.

Tongue: pale, with a white coating
Pulse: thready

Treatment principle

Supplement *qi* and strengthen the spleen.

Formula

Modified *Liù Jūn Zǐ Tāng* (六君子汤, "Six Gentlemen Decoction").

党参	dǎng shēn	12 g	Radix Codonopsis
白术	bái zhú	12 g	Rhizoma Atractylodis Macrocephalae
茯苓	fú líng	12 g	Poria
陈皮	chén pí	6 g	Pericarpium Citri Reticulatae
黄芪	huáng qí	12 g	Radix Astragali
淮山药	huái shān yào	9 g	Rhizoma Dioscoreae
防风	fáng fēng	9 g	Radix Saposhnikoviae
紫菀	zǐ wǎn	9 g	Radix et Rhizoma Asteris
枳壳	zhǐ qiào	9 g	Fructus Aurantii
炙甘草	zhì gān cǎo	6 g	Radix et Rhizoma Glycyrrhizae Praeparata cum Melle

Modifications

- For profuse sputum, combine with *zǐ sū zǐ* (紫苏子, *Fructus Perillae*) 9 g.
- For concurrent dyspnea, combine with *zhì má huáng* (炙麻黄, *Herba Ephedrae Praeparata cum Melle*) 6 g.

Deficiency of the lungs and kidneys

Signs and symptoms

Persistent coughing with dyspnea and more exhalation than inhalation that can be aggravated by physical exertion, profuse white clear sputum, a pale complexion, cold intolerance and cold limbs.

Tongue: pale, with a white and slippery coating
Pulse: deep and thready

Treatment principle

Warm kidney *qi*.

Formula

Modified *Shèn Qì Wán* (肾气丸, "Kidney *Qi* Pill")

制附子	*zhì fù zǐ*	9 g	*Radix Aconiti Lateralis Praeparata* (decoct first)
肉桂	*ròu guì*	6 g	*Cortex Cinnamomi*
熟地黄	*shú dì huáng*	12 g	*Radix Rehmanniae Praeparata*
淮山药	*huái shān yào*	15 g	*Rhizoma Dioscoreae*
山茱萸	*shān zhū yú*	9 g	*Fructus Corni*
茯苓	*fú líng*	12 g	*Poria*
泽泻	*zé xiè*	9 g	*Rhizoma Alismatis*
补骨脂	*bǔ gǔ zhī*	9 g	*Fructus Psoraleae*
紫菀	*zǐ wǎn*	9 g	*Radix et Rhizoma Asteris*
炙甘草	*zhì gān cǎo*	6 g	*Radix et Rhizoma Glycyrrhizae Praeparata cum Melle*

Modifications

- For severe dyspnea, combine with *Hēi Xī Dān* (黑锡丹, *"Galenite Elixir"*) 6 g (swallow).
- For severe deficiency, combine with *qí dài* (脐带, Umbilical Cord) 6 g.

QUESTIONS

1. Describe the two categories of bronchitis and their clinical manifestations.
2. Describe the patterns of bronchitis and treatment principles in Chinese medicine.
3. *Case study.* Try to make pattern identification and give a prescription for the following case:

Mr. Chen, 48, experienced wind intolerance, chills, headache and fever due to a sudden weather change, followed by a scratchy throat, coughing with profuse white sputum, chest tightness and discomfort, and mild shortness of breath. The tongue was light-red with a thin white greasy coating. The pulse was superficial, tight and rapid. In addition, the patient had developed coughing with dyspnea every winter over the past four years.

Bronchial Asthma

Overview

Bronchial asthma (abbreviated to "asthma") is a paroxysmal pulmonary hypersensitive disease. It most commonly occurs in autumn and winter. It can also occur in spring but is often alleviated in summer. Approximately half of the patients experience asthma attacks before the age of 12. In childhood, there are more boys than girls. However, there are indistinguishable differences in adults. Repeated bouts of asthma may result in emphysema or pulmonary heart disease.

In Chinese medicine, asthma falls under the category of "wheezing syndrome." It is understood that hidden phlegm is mainly responsible for this condition. Multiple factors may contribute to hidden phlegm. They include repeated contraction of wind–cold (or wind–heat), over-ingestion of cold drink or hot, spicy, sweet or greasy food, yang–*qi* deficiency of the spleen and kidneys, and deficiency of the lungs and kidneys.

Wind–cold (or wind–heat) may affect the dispersing and descending of lung *qi*, leading to fluid disorder in the upper *jiao* and resultant phlegm. Overintake of cold food or drink may cause internal cold fluid retention to compromise the functions of the lungs. Failure of yang–*qi* of the spleen and kidneys to transform fluid may cause retention of phlegm turbidity to affect the lungs. Over time, lung *qi* deficiency may affect the function of the kidneys to receive *qi* and lead to kidney *qi* deficiency as well. Eventually, phlegm *qi* may ascend and result in difficult breathing.

Clinical manifestations

Prior to asthma attacks, patients may experience precursory symptoms such as coughing, chest tightness or persistent sneezing. During an acute attack, asthma is characterized by shortness of breath, an audible wheezing sound, coughing with profuse sputum, and particularly, difficulty in exhaling. Some patients may have to sit up and raise their shoulders. Some may even experience cold sweating on the forehead. An episode can last minutes or hours. The signs and symptoms can be alleviated after expectoration of sticky sputum, along with disappearance of the wheezing sound and termination of the shortness of breath. After that, the patient feels completely normal. However, fever, chills and sweating can occur as a result of concurrent infections.

Pattern identification and treatment

Cold wheezing

Signs and symptoms

Rapid breathing, an audible wheezing sound in the throat, coughing with scanty foamy clear sputum, chest and diaphragm fullness, a dark bluish complexion and no thirst or thirst with a preference for hot drinks.

Tongue: a white greasy or slippery coating
Pulse: wiry–slippery or superficial–tight

Treatment principle

Warm the lungs, dissipate cold, resolve phlegm and benefit breathing.

Formula

Modified *Shè Gān Má Huáng Tāng* (射干麻黄汤, "Belamcanda and Ephedra Decoction").

麻黄	*má huáng*	9 g	*Herba Ephedrae*
射干	*shè gān*	9 g	*Rhizoma Belamcandae*
生姜	*shēng jiāng*	6 g	*Rhizoma Zingiberis Recens*
细辛	*xì xīn*	3 g	*Radix et Rhizoma Asari*
紫菀	*zǐ wǎn*	9 g	*Radix et Rhizoma Asteris*
款冬花	*kuǎn dōng huā*	9 g	*Flos Farfarae*
五味子	*wǔ wèi zǐ*	3 g	*Fructus Schisandrae Chinensis*
姜半夏	*jiāng bàn xià*	9 g	*Rhizoma Pinelliae Praeparatum*
炒枳壳	*chǎo zhǐ qiào*	9 g	*Fructus Aurantii Praeparatum*
炙甘草	*zhì gān cǎo*	6 g	*Radix et Rhizoma Glycyrrhizae Praeparata cum Melle*

Modifications

- For profuse sputum, combine with *chén pí* (陈皮, *Pericarpium Citri Reticulatae*) 6 g and *bái jiè zǐ* (白芥子, *Semen Sinapis*) 9 g.
- For severe dyspnea, combine with *zǐ sū zǐ* (紫苏子, *Fructus Perillae*) 9 g and *tíng lì zǐ* (葶苈子, *Semen Lepidii*) 9 g.
- For cold limbs, combine with *páo fù zǐ* (炮附子, *Radix Aconiti Lateralis Praeparata*) 6 g (decoct first) and *gān jiāng* (干姜, *Rhizoma Zingiberis*) 6 g.

Heat wheezing

Signs and symptoms

Rapid breathing, an audible wheezing sound in the throat, chest tightness, panting, paroxysmal choking cough, yellow sticky difficult-to-expectorate sputum, a bitter taste, thirst with a desire to drink water, fever and sweating.

Tongue: red, with a yellow greasy coating
Pulse: slippery and rapid

Treatment principle

Disperse the lungs, clear heat, resolve phlegm and benefit breathing.

Formula

Modified *Dìng Chuǎn Tāng* (定喘汤, "Arrest Wheezing Decoction").

麻黄	*má huáng*	9 g	*Herba Ephedrae*
白果	*bái guǒ*	9 g	*Semen Ginkgo*
桑白皮	*sāng bái pí*	9 g	*Cortex Mori*
款冬花	*kuǎn dōng huā*	9 g	*Flos Farfarae*
制半夏	*zhì bàn xià*	9 g	*Rhizoma Pinelliae Praeparata*
紫苏子	*zǐ sū zǐ*	6 g	*Fructus Perillae*
杏仁	*xìng rén*	9 g	*Semen Armeniacae Amarum*
黄芩	*huáng qín*	9 g	*Radix Scutellariae*
葶苈子	*tíng lì zǐ*	9 g	*Semen Lepidii*
炙甘草	*zhì gān cǎo*	6 g	*Radix et Rhizoma Glycyrrhizae Praeparata cum Melle*

Modifications

- For profuse sputum, combine with *guā lóu rén* (瓜蒌仁, *Semen Trichosanthis*) 9 g and *bèi mǔ* (贝母, *Bulbus Fritillaria*) 9 g.
- For exuberant heat, combine with *yú xīng cǎo* (鱼腥草, *Herba Houttuyniae*) 15 g and *shí gāo* (石膏, *Gypsum Fibrosum*) 30 g (ground, and decoct first).
- For constipation, combine with *dà huáng* (大黄, *Radix et Rhizoma Rhei*) 6 g (decoct later).

Lung deficiency

Signs and symptoms

In the intermission stage, patients may experience spontaneous sweating, wind intolerance, coughing with shortness of breath and clear profuse sputum, a bright pale complexion, mental fatigue and susceptibility to the common cold. Sudden weather changes can trigger attacks of asthma.

Tongue: pale, with a thin white coating
Pulse: thready

Treatment principle

Supplement *qi*, tonify the lungs and consolidate the exterior.

Formula

Modified *Yù Píng Fēng Sǎn* (玉屏风散, "Jade Wind-Barrier Powder") and *Guì Zhī Tāng* (桂枝汤, "Cinnamon Twig Decoction").

黄芪	*huáng qí*	15 g	*Radix Astragali*
白术	*bái zhú*	9 g	*Rhizoma Atractylodis Macrocephalae*
防风	*fáng fēng*	9 g	*Radix Saposhnikoviae*
党参	*dǎng shēn*	12 g	*Radix Codonopsis*
桂枝	*guì zhī*	12 g	*Ramulus Cinnamomi*
白芍	*bái sháo*	12 g	*Radix Paeoniae Alba*
姜半夏	*jiāng bàn xià*	9 g	*Rhizoma Pinelliae Praeparatum*
陈皮	*chén pí*	6 g	*Pericarpium Citri Reticulatae*
大枣	*dà zǎo*	7 p	*Fructus Jujubae*
炙甘草	*zhì gān cǎo*	6 g	*Radix et Rhizoma Glycyrrhizae Praeparata cum Melle*

Modifications

- For significant spontaneous sweating, combine with *lóng gǔ* (龙骨, *Os Draconis*) 15 g (decoct first) and *mǔ lì* (牡蛎, *Concha Ostreae*) 15 g (decoct first).
- For a bitter taste and a scanty coating, combine with *běi shā shēn* (北沙参, *Radix Glehniae*) 12 g and *yù zhú* (玉竹, *Rhizoma Polygonati Odorati*) 12 g.
- For profuse sputum, combine with *guā lóu rén* (瓜蒌仁, *Semen Trichosanthis*) 9 g and *bèi mǔ* (贝母, *Bulbus Fritillaria*) 9 g.

Spleen deficiency

Signs and symptoms

In the intermission stage, patients may experience a poor appetite, epigastric discomfort, loose stools, lassitude and a low voice. An improper diet can trigger attacks of asthma.

Tongue: pale, with a thin greasy or white slippery coating
Pulse: thready

Treatment principle

Supplement *qi*, strengthen the spleen and resolve phlegm.

Formula

Modified *Liù Jūn Zǐ Tāng* (六君子汤, "Six Gentlemen Decoction").

党参	dǎng shēn	12 g	Radix Codonopsis
白术	bái zhú	12 g	Rhizoma Atractylodis Macrocephalae
茯苓	fú líng	9 g	Poria
制半夏	zhì bàn xià	9 g	Rhizoma Pinelliae Praeparata
陈皮	chén pí	6 g	Pericarpium Citri Reticulatae
淮山药	huái shān yào	9 g	Rhizoma Dioscoreae
厚朴	hòu pò	6 g	Cortex Magnoliae Officinalis
薏苡仁	yì yǐ rén	9 g	Semen Coicis
炒枳壳	chǎo zhǐ qiào	6 g	Fructus Aurantii Praeparatum
炙甘草	zhì gān cǎo	6 g	Radix et Rhizoma Glycyrrhizae Praeparata cum Melle

Modifications

- For frequent coughing, combine with *zǐ wǎn* (紫菀, *Radix et Rhizoma Asteris*) 9 g and *kuān dōng huā* (款冬花, *Flos Farfarae*) 9 g.
- For profuse sputum, combine with *zǐ sū zǐ* (紫苏子, *Fructus Perillae*) 9 g and *guā lóu rén* (瓜蒌仁, *Semen Trichosanthis*) 9 g.
- For cold intolerance due to constitutional yang deficiency, combine with *gān jiāng* (干姜, *Rhizoma Zingiberis*) 6 g and *bǔ gǔ zhī* (补骨脂, *Fructus Psoraleae*) 9 g.

Kidney deficiency

Signs and symptoms

In the intermission stage, patients with kidney yang deficiency may experience shortness of breath or rapid breathing that can be aggravated by physical exertion, difficult inhalation, soreness and weakness of the low back and knee joints, vertigo, tinnitus, cold intolerance and a pale complexion. Fatigue can trigger attacks of asthma. Patients with kidney yin deficiency may experience rosy cheeks, restlessness, feverish sensations, night sweats and nocturnal emissions.

Tongue: pale with a white coating for kidney yang deficiency; red with a scanty coating for kidney yin deficiency
Pulse: deep and thready for kidney yang deficiency; thready and rapid for kidney yin deficiency

Treatment principle

Tonify the kidneys.

Formula

Modified *Jīn Guì Shèn Qì Wán* (金匮肾气丸, "Golden Cabinet's Kidney *Qi* Pill") for kidney yang deficiency.

熟地黄	shú dì huáng	15 g	Radix Rehmanniae Praeparata
淮山药	huái shān yào	12 g	Rhizoma Dioscoreae
山茱萸	shān zhū yú	9 g	Fructus Corni
泽泻	zé xiè	9 g	Rhizoma Alismatis
茯苓	fú líng	9 g	Poria
牡丹皮	mǔ dān pí	9 g	Cortex Moutan
桂枝	guì zhī	6 g	Ramulus Cinnamomi
制附子	zhì fù zǐ	9 g	Radix Aconiti Lateralis Praeparata (decoct first)
补骨脂	bǔ gǔ zhī	9 g	Fructus Psoraleae
脐带	qí dài	9 g	Umbilical Cord

Modified *Qī Wèi Dū Qì Wán* (七味都气丸, "Seven-Ingredient *Qi*-Restraining Pill") for kidney yin deficiency.

熟地黄	shú dì huáng	15 g	Radix Rehmanniae Praeparata
淮山药	huái shān yào	12 g	Rhizoma Dioscoreae
山茱萸	shān zhū yú	9 g	Fructus Corni
泽泻	zé xiè	9 g	Rhizoma Alismatis
茯苓	fú líng	9 g	Poria
牡丹皮	mǔ dān pí	9 g	Cortex Moutan
麦冬	mài dōng	9 g	Radix Ophiopogonis
沙参	shā shēn	9 g	Radix Adenophorae seu Glehniae
五味子	wǔ wèi zǐ	3 g	Fructus Schisandrae Chinensis
龟板胶	guī bǎn jiāo	9 g	Colla Testudinis Plastri (melted)

Modifications

- For coughing, combine with *zǐ wǎn* (紫菀, *Radix et Rhizoma Asteris*) 9 g and *kuǎn dōng huā* (款冬花, *Flos Farfarae*) 9 g.
- For severe shortness of breath, combine with *zhì má huáng* (炙麻黄, *Herba Ephedrae Praeparata cum Melle*) 6 g and *xìng rén* (杏仁, *Semen Armeniacae Amarum*) 9 g.
- For a poor appetite, combine with *bái zhú* (白术, *Rhizoma Atractylodis Macrocephalae*) 9 g and *jī nèi jīn* (鸡内金, *Endothelium Corneum Gigeriae Galli*) 9 g.

- For insomnia, combine with *suān zǎo rén* (酸枣仁, *Semen Ziziphi Spinosae*) 9 g and *yè jiāo téng* (夜交藤, *Caulis Polygoni Multiflori*) 15 g.

QUESTIONS

1. Describe the clinical manifestations of bronchial asthma.
2. Describe the patterns of bronchitis in Chinese medicine.
3. *Case study.* Try to make a pattern identification and give a prescription for the following case:

Mr. Jin, 41, had been suffering from 17 years of repeated coughing with shortness of breath, and coughing all year round over the past 3–4 years. The signs and symptoms worsened during the week prior to treatment, along with profuse white foamy sputum, a wheezing sound in the throat, nasal flares, inability to lie flat and cyanosis of the lips. The patient also presented with a high fever of 40.1°C, a dry mouth and a sore throat, chest tightness, nausea, scanty dark-yellow urine and no bowel movements within three days. The tongue was red with a yellow greasy coating. The pulse was slippery and rapid.

Lobar Pneumonia

Overview

Lobar pneumonia is an acute inflammation of the lungs, usually caused by bacterial or viral infections. It can occur in all seasons but more often in winter and spring. Young and middle-aged adults are more vulnerable to this condition. *Staphylococci aureus* pneumonia is more common in children. A strong immune system is important for preventing lobar pneumonia. Without prompt treatment, lobar pneumonia may cause severe secondary complications.

In Chinese medicine, lobar pneumonia falls under the category of "coughing with shortness of breath," "lung distension" or "wind–warmth." The contributing factors include deficiency of antipathogenic *qi*, compromised *wei qi* and contraction of external pathogens.

According to Ye Gui, a distinguished physician from the Qing dynasty (1644–1911), "pathogenic warmth attacks the lungs first." After attacking the lungs, wind–heat or wind–cold may affect the dispersing and descending of lung *qi*, leading to a series of symptoms. Heat or phlegm dampness may also accumulate in the lungs and result in symptoms as well. Over time, patients in the later stage may present with signs and symptoms of damage to *qi* and yin or critical conditions due to yang–*qi* collapse.

Clinical manifestations

With 1–2 days of latency, lobar pneumonia often follows an upper respiratory tract infection. The most common symptoms are chills, fever, chest pain, coughing and bloody sputum. The onset of this condition is often quite sudden and may start off with chills and fever. The body temperature can reach 39–49°C within a couple of hours. Headache, fatigue and general muscle pain may also be present. After 2–3 days, the patient start to experience chest pain and frequent coughing with sputum containing pus, bloods or a rusty tint. In severe cases, shortness of breath and cyanosis may occur as a result of anoxia. Some patients may present with digestive tract reactions such as nausea, vomiting, abdominal bloating and diarrhea. After 6–10 days, the fever may be subdued and other symptoms start to be alleviated.

Pattern identification and treatment

Wind–cold attacking the lungs

Signs and symptoms

Coughing with thin white clear sputum, chest pain, chills, fever, absence of sweating, soreness of the bones and joints, a stuffy and runny nose, and headache with a sense of distension.

Tongue: a thin white coating
Pulse: superficial and tight

Treatment principle

Expel wind, dissipate cold, disperse the lungs and resolve phlegm.

Formula

Modified *Xìng Sū Sǎn* (杏苏散, "Apricot Kernel and Perilla Powder")

杏仁	xìng rén	9 g	Semen Armeniacae Amarum
紫苏叶	zǐ sū yè	9 g	Folium Perillae
荆芥	jīng jiè	9 g	Herba Schizonepetae
防风	fáng fēng	9 g	Radix Saposhnikoviae
桔梗	jié gěng	6 g	Radix Platycodonis
前胡	qián hú	9 g	Radix Peucedani
姜半夏	jiāng bàn xià	12 g	Rhizoma Pinelliae Praeparatum
陈皮	chén pí	6 g	Pericarpium Citri Reticulatae
枳壳	zhǐ qiào	9 g	Fructus Aurantii
生姜	shēng jiāng	6 g	Rhizoma Zingiberis Recens

Modifications

- For absence of sweating with severe chills, combine with *má huáng* (麻黄, *Herba Ephedrae*) 6 g.
- For severe coughing, combine with *zǐ wǎn* (紫菀, *Radix et Rhizoma Asteris*) 9 g and *kuǎn dōng huā* (款冬花, *Flos Farfarae*) 9 g.
- For profuse sputum, combine with *zǐ sū zǐ* (紫苏子, *Fructus Perillae*) 9 g.

Wind–heat attacking the lungs

Signs and symptoms

Coughing with yellow sticky sputum, chest pain or tightness, chills, fever, thirst, a sore throat and general ache.

Tongue: red on the tips, with a thin yellow coating
Pulse: superficial and rapid

Treatment principle

Formula

Modified *Yín Qiào Sǎn* (银翘散, "Lonicera and Forsythia Powder").

金银花	*jīn yín huā*	12 g	Flos Lonicerae Japonicae
连翘	*lián qiào*	12 g	Fructus Forsythiae
荆芥	*jīng jiè*	9 g	Schizonepetae
薄荷	*bò he*	3 g	Herba Menthae (decoct later)
前胡	*qián hú*	9 g	Radix Peucedani
桑白皮	*sāng bái pí*	12 g	Cortex Mori
黄芩	*huáng qín*	9 g	Radix Scutellariae
瓜蒌皮	*guā lóu pí*	9 g	Pericarpium Trichosanthis
芦根	*lú gēn*	15 g	Rhizoma Phragmitis
竹叶	*zhú yè*	4 g	Folium Phyllostachydis Henonis

Modifications

- For severe coughing, combine with *zǐ wǎn* (紫菀, *Radix et Rhizoma Asteris*) 9 g and *bǎi bù* (百部, *Radix Stemonae*) 9 g.
- For profuse sputum, combine with *tíng lì zǐ* (葶苈子, *Semen Lepidii*) 9 g and *bèi mǔ* (贝母, *Bulbus Fritillaria*) 9 g.
- For exuberant heat, combine with *zhī zǐ* (栀子, *Fructus Gardeniae*) 9 g and *shí gāo* (石膏, *Gypsum Fibrosum*) 30 g (decoct first).

Phlegm heat accumulating in the lungs

Signs and symptoms

Coughing with yellow, sticky, rusty or bloody sputum and fever with no aversion to cold. Chills, nasal flares, panting, a sore throat, thirst and scanty dark-yellow urine may also be present.

Tongue: dry and red, with a yellow or yellow greasy coating
Pulse: slippery–rapid or surging

Treatment principle

Clear heat, remove toxins, disperse the lungs and resolve phlegm.

Formula

Má Xìng Shí Gān Tāng (麻杏石甘汤, "Ephedra, Apricot Kernel, Gypsum and Licorice Decoction") and *Qiān Jīn Wěi Jìng Tāng* (千金苇茎汤, "Valuable Phragmites Stem Decoction").

麻黄	*má huáng*	9 g	*Herba Ephedrae*
杏仁	*xìng rén*	9 g	*Semen Armeniacae Amarum*
石膏	*shí gāo*	30 g	*Gypsum Fibrosum* (decoct first)
芦根	*lú gēn*	15 g	*Rhizoma Phragmitis*
冬瓜子	*dōng guā zǐ*	12 g	*Semen Benincasae*
鱼腥草	*yú xīng cǎo*	12 g	*Herba Houttuyniae*
桃仁	*táo rén*	9 g	*Semen Persicae*
天竺黄	*tiān zhú huáng*	9 g	*Concretio Silicea Bambusae*
黄芩	*huáng qín*	9 g	*Radix Scutellariae*
炙甘草	*zhì gān cǎo*	6 g	*Radix et Rhizoma Glycyrrhizae Praeparata cum Melle*

Modifications

- For severe chest pain, combine with *chì sháo* (赤芍, *Radix Paeoniae Rubra*) 9 g and *yù jīn* (郁金, *Radix Curcumae*) 9 g.
- For bloody sputum, combine with *qiàn cǎo* (茜草, *Radix et Rhizoma Rubiae*) 9 g and *bái máo gēn* (白茅根, *Rhizoma Imperatae*) 15 g.
- For constipation, combine with *dà huáng* (大黄, *Radix et Rhizoma Rhei*) 9 g (decoct later).

Pathogens entering the pericardium

Signs and symptoms

A high-grade fever, a wheezing sound in the throat, rapid breathing, chest pain, distension and tightness, delirium, cyanosis of the lips and cold limbs.

Tongue: red or dark-red, with a yellow greasy or white greasy coating
Pulse: thready and rapid

Treatment principle

Disperse the lungs, resolve phlegm, clear the heart and open orifices.

Formula

Qīng Gōng Tāng (清宫汤, "Palace-Clearing Decoction") and *Qiān Jīn Wěi Jìng Tāng* (千金苇茎汤, "Valuable Phragmites Stem Decoction").

连翘	*lián qiào*	12 g	*Fructus Forsythiae*
玄参	*xuán shēn*	12 g	*Radix Scrophulariae*
水牛角	*shuǐ niú jiǎo*	30 g	*Cornu Bubali* (decoct first)
麦冬	*mài dōng*	12 g	*Radix Ophiopogonis*
竹叶	*zhú yè*	6 g	*Folium Phyllostachydis Henonis*
薏苡仁	*yì yǐ rén*	12 g	*Semen Coicis*
冬瓜子	*dōng guā zǐ*	9 g	*Semen Benincasae*
桃仁	*táo rén*	9 g	*Semen Persicae*
芦根	*lú gēn*	15 g	*Rhizoma Phragmitis*
安宫牛黄丸	*Ān Gōng Niú Huáng Wán*	1 pill	*"Peaceful Palace Bovine Bezoar Pill"*

Modifications

- For a persistent high-grade fever, combine with *shí gāo* (石膏, *Gypsum Fibrosum*) 30 g (decoct first) and *zhī mǔ* (知母, *Rhizoma Anemarrhenae*) 12 g.
- For profuse sputum, combine with *tiān zhú huáng* (天竺黄, *Concretio Silicea Bambusae*) and *zhú lì yóu* (竹沥油, "Juice of *Succus Bambusae*") 1 g.
- For constipation, combine with *dà huáng* (大黄, *Radix et Rhizoma Rhei*) 9 g (decoct later).

Yang–qi collapse

Signs and symptoms

A pale complexion, profuse sweating, extremely cold limbs, rapid breathing, shortness of breath, cold intolerance and lassitude.

Pulse: faint and thready

Treatment principle

Resuscitate yang and prevent collapse.

Formula

Modified *Shēn Fù Tāng* (参附汤, "Ginseng and Aconite Decoction") and *Shēng Mài Sǎn* (生脉散, "Pulse-Engendering Powder").

人参	*rén shēn*	15 g	*Radix et Rhizoma Ginseng* (decoct separately)
制附子	*zhì fù zǐ*	9 g	*Radix Aconiti Lateralis Praeparata* (decoct first)
干姜	*gān jiāng*	9 g	*Rhizoma Zingiberis*
麦冬	*mài dōng*	12 g	*Radix Ophiopogonis*
五味子	*wǔ wèi zǐ*	9 g	*Fructus Schisandrae Chinensis*
炙甘草	*zhì gān cǎo*	6 g	*Radix et Rhizoma Glycyrrhizae Praeparata cum Melle*
煅龙骨	*duàn lóng gǔ*	30 g	*Os Draconis Praeparatum*
煅牡蛎	*duàn mǔ lì*	30 g	*Concha Ostreae Praeparatum*

Modifications

When yang is resuscitated, combine with the method of dispersing the lungs, resolving phlegm and supplementing *qi* and yin.

Deficiency of qi and yin

Signs and symptoms

In the remission stage, patients may experience coughing, a low-grade fever, spontaneous sweating, feverish sensations on the palms and soles, a poor appetite and mental fatigue.

Tongue: red, with a thin coating
Pulse: thready and rapid

Treatment principle

Supplement *qi*, nourish yin, moisten the lungs and resolve phlegm.

Formula

Modified *Zhú Yè Shí Gāo Tāng* (竹叶石膏汤, "Lophatherum and Gypsum Decoction").

竹叶	*zhú yè*	12 g	*Folium Phyllostachydis Henonis*
石膏	*shí gāo*	15 g	*Gypsum Fibrosum* (decoct first)
麦冬	*mài dōng*	12 g	*Radix Ophiopogonis*
沙参	*shā shēn*	12 g	*Radix Adenophorae seu Glehniae*
天花粉	*tiān huā fěn*	12 g	*Radix Trichosanthis*
贝母	*bèi mǔ*	9 g	*Bulbus Fritillaria*
杏仁	*xìng rén*	9 g	*Semen Armeniacae Amarum*
茯苓	*fú líng*	9 g	*Poria*
太子参	*tài zǐ shēn*	9 g	*Radix Pseudostellariae*
炙甘草	*zhì gān cǎo*	6 g	*Radix et Rhizoma Glycyrrhizae Praeparata cum Melle*

Modifications

- For a persistent low-grade fever, combine with *lián qiào* (连翘, *Fructus Forsythiae*) 9 g and *huáng qín* (黄芩, *Radix Scutellariae*) 9 g.
- For a severe poor appetite, combine with *bái zhú* (白术, *Rhizoma Atractylodis Macrocephalae*) 9 g, *gǔ yá* (谷芽, *Fructus Setariae Germinatus*) 9 g and *mài yá* (麦芽, *Fructus Hordei Germinatus*) 9 g.
- For severe mental fatigue, combine with *dǎng shēn* (党参, *Radix Codonopsis*) 12 g.
- For persistent coughing, combine with *bǎi bù* (百部, *Radix Stemonae*) 9 g and *wǔ wèi zǐ* (五味子, *Fructus Schisandrae Chinensis*) 3 g.

QUESTIONS

1. Describe the clinical manifestations of lobar pneumonia.
2. Describe the pattern identification and treatment of lobar pneumonia in Chinese medicine.
3. *Case study*. Try to make a pattern identification and give a prescription for the following case:

Ms. Xiong, 20, developed fever, chills and absence of sweating four days prior to treatment, followed by a high-grade fever, slight cold intolerance, coughing, difficult breathing, cough-induced chest pain on the left side and some rusty tint sputum one day prior to hospitalization. Other signs and symptoms included headache, fatigue, a poor appetite, a dry mouth, dark-yellow urine, a body temperature of 38.6°C, and audible bronchial breath sounds and scattered dry and moist rales by auscultation. The patient was confirmed by X-ray as having left lower lobar pneumonia.

Bronchiectasis

Overview

Bronchiectasis is an abnormal dilation and deformation of the bronchus caused by destruction of the bronchial wall from chronic inflammations of the bronchus and the surrounding lung tissue. It is more common in children and young adults. Influenza or whooping cough can trigger bronchial or pulmonary infections, causing damage to the bronchial wall and its elastic tissue and leading to bronchiectasis. This condition may further result in pulmonary dysfunction, increase the resistance of the pulmonary circulation and eventually lead to pulmonary heart disease.

In Chinese medicine, bronchiectasis falls under the category of "coughing" or "lung abscesses". The contributing factors include contraction of external pathogens, an improper diet, emotional disturbance, overexertion and deficiency of antipathogenic *qi*.

Pathogenic heat or heat transformed from pathogenic cold may affect the lungs, causing blood stasis and resultant abscesses. Constitutional phlegmheat or damp–heat resulting from overintake of alcohol or hot spicy food may affect the transportation and transformation of the spleen, leading to internal phlegm dampness. Liver *qi* stagnation may transform into fire to affect the lungs, damaging the lung collaterals. Overexertion may consume *qi* and yin of the lungs. Hyperactivity of fire due to yin deficiency may also damage the lung collaterals, leading to this condition.

Clinical manifestations

Bronchiectasis often follows a whooping cough or bronchial pneumonia and involves repeated bouts of respiratory tract infections. It is characterized by persistent coughing which produces profuse smelly purulent sputum (100–400 ml per day) and recurrent hemoptysis. General signs of toxicity may also be present. They include fever, night sweats, a poor appetite, weight loss or anemia. Postural changes like getting up or going to bed may increase the production of sputum. Shortness of breath and cyanosis may occur as a result of concurrent obstructive emphysema.

Pattern identification and treatment

For patterns of wind–cold attacking the lungs, wind–heat attacking the lungs and phlegm heat accumulating in the lungs, refer to lobar pneumonia.

Lung yin deficiency

Signs and symptoms

Unproductive cough, tidal fever, night sweats, and a dry throat and mouth. Some patients may experience bloody or profuse purulent sputum.

Tongue: red, with a scanty coating
Pulse: thready and rapid

Treatment principle

Nourish yin and benefit the lungs.

Formula

Modified *Bǎi Hé Gù Jīn Tāng* (百合固金汤, "Lily Bulb Metal-Securing Decoction").

生地	*shēng dì*	15 g	*Radix Rehmanniae*
沙参	*shā shēn*	12 g	*Radix Adenophorae seu Glehniae*
麦冬	*mài dōng*	9 g	*Radix Ophiopogonis*
百部	*bǎi bù*	9 g	*Radix Stemonae*
百合	*bǎi hé*	12 g	*Bulbus Lilii*
贝母	*bèi mǔ*	9 g	*Bulbus Fritillaria*
黄芩	*huáng qín*	9 g	*Radix Scutellariae*
杏仁	*xìng rén*	9 g	*Semen Armeniacae Amarum*
天花粉	*tiān huā fěn*	12 g	*Radix Trichosanthis*
炙甘草	*zhì gān cǎo*	6 g	*Radix et Rhizoma Glycyrrhizae Praeparata cum Melle*

Modifications

- For hemoptysis, combine with *cè bǎi yè* (侧柏叶, *Cacumen Platycladi*) 12 g and a powder of *bái jí* (白及, *Rhizoma Bletillae*) 9 g (swallow).
- For kidney yin deficiency, combine with *shú dì huáng* (熟地黄, *Radix Rehmanniae Praeparata*) 12 g.
- For hyperactivity of fire due to yin deficiency, combine with *huáng bǎi* (黄柏, *Cortex Phellodendri Chinensis*) 9 g.
- For profuse sweating, combine with *nuò dào gēn* (糯稻根, *Radix Oryzae Glutinosae*) 9 g.

Hyperactivity of fire due to yin deficiency

Signs and symptoms

Unproductive cough, tidal fever in the afternoon, night sweats, dizziness, blurred vision, tinnitus, lumbar soreness, dream-disturbed sleep, nocturnal emissions and scanty dark-yellow urine. Some patients may experience bloody purulent sputum or hemoptysis.

Tongue: red, with a scanty coating
Pulse: thready and rapid

Treatment principle

Nourish yin and reduce fire.

Formula

Modified *Dà Bǔ Yīn Wán* (大补阴丸, "Major Yin-Supplementing Pill") and *Zhī Bǎi Dì Huáng Wán* (知柏地黄丸, "Anemarrhena, Phellodendron and Rehmannia Pill").

熟地黄	*shú dì huáng*	15 g	*Radix Rehmanniae Praeparata*
麦冬	*mài dōng*	12 g	*Radix Ophiopogonis*
知母	*zhī mǔ*	9 g	*Rhizoma Anemarrhenae*
黄柏	*huáng bǎi*	9 g	*Cortex Phellodendri Chinensis*
龟板	*guī bǎn*	12 g	*Plastrum Testudinis* (decoct first)
鳖甲	*biē jiǎ*	12 g	*Carapax Trionycis* (decoct first)

牡丹皮	*mǔ dān pí*	9 g	Cortex Moutan
百部	*bǎi bù*	12 g	Radix Stemonae
黄芩	*huáng qín*	9 g	Radix Scutellariae
侧柏叶	*cè bǎi yè*	12 g	Cacumen Platycladi

Modifications

- For increased blood in the sputum, combine with a powder of *bái jí* (白及, *Rhizoma Bletillae*) 9 g (swallow).
- For profuse sweating, combine with *nuò dào gēn* (糯稻根, *Radix Oryzae Glutinosae*) 9 g.
- For severe internal heat due to yin deficiency, combine with *shēng dì* (生地, *Radix Rehmanniae*) 12 g and *zé xiè* (泽泻, *Rhizoma Alismatis*) 9 g.

Liver fire affecting the lungs

Signs and symptoms

Paroxysmal coughing with sputum containing blood or mucus, cough-induced chest and hypochondriac pain, restlessness, irritability, headache with a sense of distension, dry stools and scanty dark-yellow urine.

Tongue: red, with a thin yellow coating
Pulse: wiry and rapid

Treatment principle

Clear the lungs, soothe the liver, harmonize the collaterals and arrest bleeding.

Formula

Supplemented *Xiè Bái Sǎn* (泻白散, "White-Draining Powder") and *Dài Gé Sǎn* (黛蛤散, "Natural Indigo and Clam Shell Powder").

桑白皮	*sāng bái pí*	15 g	Cortex Mori
地骨皮	*dì gǔ pí*	12 g	Cortex Lycii
黛蛤散	*Dài Gé Sǎn*	12 g	"Natural Indigo and Clam Shell Powder" (wrapped)

生地	shēng dì	12 g	Radix Rehmanniae
黄芩	huáng qín	12 g	Radix Scutellariae
牡丹皮	mǔ dān pí	9 g	Cortex Moutan
白茅根	bái máo gēn	15 g	Rhizoma Imperatae
白芍	bái sháo	15 g	Radix Paeoniae Alba
仙鹤草	xiān hè cǎo	15 g	Herba Agrimoniae
炙甘草	zhì gān cǎo	6 g	Radix et Rhizoma Glycyrrhizae Praeparata cum Melle

Modifications

- For increased blood in the sputum, swallow a powder of *bái jí* (白及, *Rhizoma Bletillae*) 9 g or *sān qī* (三七, *Radix et Rhizoma Notoginseng*) 9 g.
- For constipation, combine with *dà huáng* (大黄, *Radix et Rhizoma Rhei*) 9 g (decoct later).
- For severe coughing, combine with *zǐ wǎn* (紫菀, *Radix et Rhizoma Asteris*) 9 g and *bǎi bù* (百部, *Radix Stemonae*) 9 g.

Qi deficiency of the lungs and spleen

Signs and symptoms

Coughing with production of sputum containing blood or mucus, mental fatigue, lassitude, shortness of breath, chest tightness, a poor appetite, a low voice, a bright pale complexion and cold intolerance.

Tongue: a white greasy coating
Pulse: thready

Treatment principle

Strengthen the spleen and benefit the lungs.

Formula

Supplemented *Sì Jūn Zǐ Tāng* (四君子汤, "Four Gentlemen Decoction").

太子参	tài zǐ shēn	15 g	Radix Pseudostellariae
焦白术	jiāo bái zhú	12 g	Rhizoma Atractylodis Macrocephalae Praepareta
茯苓	fú líng	12 g	Poria

陈皮	chén pí	6 g	Pericarpium Citri Reticulatae
姜半夏	jiāng bàn xià	9 g	Rhizoma Pinelliae Praeparatum
百部	bǎi bù	12 g	Radix Stemonae
杏仁	xìng rén	9 g	Semen Armeniacae Amarum
薏苡仁	yì yǐ rén	12 g	Semen Coicis
黄精	huáng jīng	12 g	Rhizoma Polygonati
炙甘草	zhì gān cǎo	6 g	Radix et Rhizoma Glycyrrhizae Praeparata cum Melle

Modifications

- For spontaneous sweating due to *qi* deficiency, combine with *huáng qí* (黄芪, *Radix Astragali*) 12 g.
- For hemoptysis, combine with *xiān hè cǎo* (仙鹤草, *Herba Agrimoniae*) 15 g.
- For a poor appetite, combine with *jī nèi jīn* (鸡内金, *Endothelium Corneum Gigeriae Galli*) 9 g, *gǔ yá* (谷芽, *Fructus Setariae Germinatus*) 9 g and *mài yá* (麦芽, *Fructus Hordei Germinatus*) 9 g.

Deficiency of qi and yin

Signs and symptoms

Coughing with scanty or bloody-stripped sputum, mental fatigue, spontaneous sweating, night sweats, rosy cheeks, a pale complexion, a poor appetite, a dry mouth and throat, and tidal fever in the afternoon.

Tongue: red, with a scanty or peeled coating

Pulse: thready, rapid and weak

Treatment principle

Supplement *qi* and nourish yin.

Formula

Supplemented *Shēng Mài Sǎn* (生脉散, "Pulse-Engendering Powder").

党参	*dǎng shēn*	15 g	Radix Codonopsis
麦冬	*mài dōng*	12 g	Radix Ophiopogonis
白术	*bái zhú*	12 g	Rhizoma Atractylodis Macrocephalae
黄精	*huáng jīng*	12 g	Rhizoma Polygonati
百合	*bǎi hé*	12 g	Bulbus Lilii
百部	*bǎi bù*	12 g	Radix Stemonae
沙参	*shā shēn*	12 g	Radix Adenophorae seu Glehniae
玉竹	*yù zhú*	12 g	Rhizoma Polygonati Odorati
杏仁	*xìng rén*	9 g	Semen Armeniacae Amarum
炙甘草	*zhì gān cǎo*	6 g	Radix et Rhizoma Glycyrrhizae Praeparata cum Melle

Modifications

- For hemoptysis, combine with *qiàn cǎo gēn* (茜草根, *Radix et Rhizoma Rubiae*) 15 g.
- For constipation, combine with *bǎi zǐ rén* (柏子仁, *Semen Platycladi*) 9 g.

QUESTIONS

1. Describe the clinical manifestations of bronchiectasis.
2. Describe the pattern identification and treatment of bronchiectasis.
3. *Case study*. Try to make pattern identification and give a prescription for the following case:

Mr. Zheng, 55, experienced paroxysmal coughing with production of sputum containing smelly mucus and bright-colored blood, along with a poor appetite, shortness of breath upon mild exertion, and cough-induced chest pain. The tongue coating was thick and greasy. The pulse was soft and rapid.

COMMON DIGESTIVE SYSTEM CONDITIONS

Gastric and Duodenal Ulcers

Overview

Gastric and duodenal ulcers, also known as peptic ulcers, are closely related to gastric acid and pepsin. They can affect people at any age, particularly young and middle-aged adults. The male/female ratio of the peptic ulcer is approximately 2–4:1. Without prompt and effective treatments, this condition may further result in secondary complications such as gastrointestinal bleeding, perforation or pyloric obstruction.

In Chinese medicine, peptic ulcers fall under the category of "gastric pain", "gastric discomfort" or "acid regurgitation." The contributing factors include deficiency of the spleen and stomach, emotional disturbance and an improper diet.

Failure of the spleen and stomach to transport and transform may cause retention of internal cold. Insufficiency of stomach fluid may result in internal stagnant heat. Emotional disturbance may cause liver *qi* stagnation, which can in turn affect the stomach and result in blood stasis. An improper diet may cause disharmony of stomach *qi*, malnourishment of stomach collaterals or internal cold retention. All these factors can contribute to peptic ulcers.

Clinical manifestations

Peptic ulcers are mainly characterized by long-term periodic abdominal pain, with severity relating to mealtimes. Gastric ulcers cause pain on the left side below the xiphoid bone. The pain starts 30 min to 2 h after taking a meal and is relieved after gastric emptying in 1–2 h (food intake → pain → alleviation). Duodenal ulcers cause pain on the right side below the xiphoid bone. The pain starts 2–4 h after taking a meal and is relieved until the next meal (food intake → alleviation → pain). Some patients can wake from the pain during night sleep. The pain due to peptic ulcers is often tolerably dull, distending, pricking or burning. Hunger pain may also be present. Other digestive system and general symptoms include belching, waterbrash, nausea, vomiting, gastric discomfort (fullness, distension or tightness), restlessness, insomnia and profuse sweating.

Pattern identification and treatment

Liver-qi stagnation

Signs and symptoms

Gastric distension and pain, a sense of tightness in the chest and hypo-chondriac regions that can be aggravated by emotions and relieved by belching or flatus; other symptoms include restlessness, frequent sighing, a poor appetite and excessive salivation.

Tongue: a thin white coating
Pulse: wiry

Treatment principle

Soothe the liver, regulate *qi*, harmonize the stomach and relieve pain.

Formula

Modified *Chái Hú Shū Gān Sǎn* (柴胡疏肝散, "Bupleurum Liver-Soothing Powder").

柴胡	*chái hú*	9 g	*Radix Bupleuri*
香附	*xiāng fù*	9 g	*Rhizoma Cyperi*
白芍	*bái sháo*	12 g	*Radix Paeoniae Alba*
枳壳	*zhǐ qiào*	9 g	*Fructus Aurantii*
陈皮	*chén pí*	6 g	*Pericarpium Citri Reticulatae*
川芎	*chuān xiōng*	9 g	*Rhizoma Chuanxiong*
木香	*mù xiāng*	6 g	*Radix Aucklandiae*
煅瓦楞子	*duàn wǎ léng zǐ*	30 g	*Concha Arcae Praeparatum* (decoct first)
甘草	*gān cǎo*	6 g	*Radix et Rhizoma Glycyrrhizae*

Modifications

- For intense pain, combine with *yán hú suǒ* (延胡索, *Rhizoma Corydalis*) 9 g and *chuān liàn zǐ* (川楝子, *Fructus Toosendan*) 9 g.
- For severe gastric comfort and acid reflux, combine with *huáng lián* (黄连, *Rhizoma Coptidis*) 4.5 g and *wú zhū yú* (吴茱萸, *Fructus Evodiae*) 3 g.

- For a dry mouth with a bitter taste, combine with *zhī mǔ* (知母, *Rhizoma Anemarrhenae*) 9 g and *shēng dì* (生地, *Radix Rehmanniae*) 9 g.

Stagnant heat in the liver and stomach

Signs and symptoms

Sudden intense epigastric pain with a burning sensation that cannot be relieved by food intake; other symptoms include a dry mouth with a bitter taste, preference for cold drinks, acid reflux, gastric discomfort, restlessness, irritability and constipation.

Tongue: red, with a yellow coating
Pulse: wiry or rapid

Treatment principle

Clear stomach heat, harmonize the stomach and relieve pain.

Formula

Modified *Huà Gān Jiān* (化肝煎, "Liver-Benefiting Decoction") and *Zuǒ Jīn Wán* (左金丸, "Left Metal Pill").

黄连	*huáng lián*	4.5 g	*Rhizoma Coptidis*
山栀	*shān zhī*	9 g	*Fructus Gardeniae*
牡丹皮	*mǔ dān pí*	9 g	*Cortex Moutan*
白芍	*bái sháo*	9 g	*Radix Paeoniae Alba*
陈皮	*chén pí*	9 g	*Pericarpium Citri Reticulatae*
青皮	*qīng pí*	9 g	*Pericarpium Citri Reticulatae Viride*
知母	*zhī mǔ*	9 g	*Rhizoma Anemarrhenae*
吴茱萸	*wú zhū yú*	3 g	*Fructus Evodiae*
大黄	*dà huáng*	6 g	*Radix et Rhizoma Rhei* (decoct later)
甘草	*gān cǎo*	6 g	*Radix et Rhizoma Glycyrrhizae*

Modifications

- For severe pain, combine with *yán hú suǒ* (延胡索, *Rhizoma Corydalis*) 9 g and *chuān liàn zǐ* (川楝子, *Fructus Toosendan*) 9 g.

- For frequent belching, combine with *xuán fù huā* (旋覆花, *Flos Inulae*) 9 g (wrapped) and *dài zhē shí* (代赭石, *Haematitum*)15 g.
- For constipation, combine with *huǒ má rén* (火麻仁, *Fructus Cannabis*) 9 g.

Stomach yin deficiency

Signs and symptoms

Dull gastric pain (especially with an empty stomach), hunger but no desire to eat food, a dry mouth with no desire to drink water, a poor appetite, retching, and feverish sensations on the palms and soles.

Tongue: dry and red, with cracks and a scanty or peeled coating
Pulse: thready

Treatment principle

Nourish yin, benefit the stomach and relieve pain.

Formula

Modified *Yī Guàn Jiān* (一贯煎, "Effective Integration Decoction").

北沙参	*běi shā shēn*	12 g	*Radix Glehniae*
麦冬	*mài dōng*	9 g	*Radix Ophiopogonis*
生地	*shēng dì*	12 g	*Radix Rehmanniae*
当归	*dāng guī*	9 g	*Radix Angelicae Sinensis*
川楝子	*chuān liàn zǐ*	9 g	*Fructus Toosendan*
石斛	*shí hú*	9 g	*Caulis Dendrobii*
麻仁	*má rén*	9 g	*Fructus Cannabis*
白芍	*bái sháo*	9 g	*Radix Paeoniae Alba*

Modifications

- For severe pain, combine with *yán hú suǒ* (延胡索, *Rhizoma Corydalis*) 9 g and *lù lù tōng* (路路通, *Fructus Liquidambaris*) 9 g.
- For severe retching, combine with *jiāng bàn xià* (姜半夏, *Rhizoma Pinelliae Praeparatum*) 9 g and *jiāng zhú rú* (姜竹茹, *Caulis Bambusae in Taenia Praeparatum*) 9 g.

- For a severe poor appetite, combine with *zhì jī nèi jīn* (炙鸡内金, *Endothelium Corneum Gigeriae Galli Praeparata cum Melle*) 9 g and *shén qū* (神曲, *Massa Medicata Fermentata*) 9 g.

Deficiency and cold in the spleen and stomach

Signs and symptoms

Dull gastric pain with a preference for warmth and pressure; the pain can be triggered by fatigue or contraction of cold, and the pain can be worsened by hunger but relieved after eating food. Other symptoms include mental fatigue, reluctance to talk, cold intolerance, cold limbs, watery vomiting and loose stools.

Tongue: pale and swollen with tooth marks and a thin white coating
Pulse: deep and thready

Treatment principle

Strengthen the spleen, supplement *qi*, warm the middle *jiao* and relieve pain.

Formula

Modified *Huáng Qí Jiàn Zhōng Tāng* (黄芪建中汤, "Astragalus Center-Fortifying Decoction") and *Lǐ Zhōng Wán* (理中丸, "Center-Regulating Pill").

黄芪	*huáng qí*	15 g	*Radix Astragali*
党参	*dǎng shēn*	9 g	*Radix Codonopsis*
白术	*bái zhú*	9 g	*Rhizoma Atractylodis Macrocephalae*
白芍	*bái sháo*	15 g	*Radix Paeoniae Alba*
桂枝	*guì zhī*	6 g	*Ramulus Cinnamomi*
干姜	*gān jiāng*	3 g	*Rhizoma Zingiberis*
陈皮	*chén pí*	6 g	*Pericarpium Citri Reticulatae*
木香	*mù xiāng*	6 g	*Radix Aucklandiae*
炙甘草	*zhì gān cǎo*	6 g	*Radix et Rhizoma Glycyrrhizae Praeparata cum Melle*
大枣	*dà zǎo*	10 P	*Fructus Jujubae*
饴糖	*yí táng*	30 g	*Saccharum Granorum (melted)*

Modifications

- For chest tightness and a greasy tongue coating, combine with *cāng zhú* (苍术, *Rhizoma Atractylodis*) 9 g and *hòu pò* (厚朴, *Cortex Magnoliae Officinalis*) 9 g.
- For cold intolerance and cold limbs, combine with *pào fù zǐ* (炮附子, *Radix Aconiti Lateralis Praeparata*) 6 g (decoct first).
- For severe watery vomiting, combine with *bàn xià* (半夏, *Rhizoma Pinelliae*) 9 g and *wú zhū yú* (吴茱萸, *Fructus Evodiae*) 3 g.

Blood stasis in the stomach collaterals

Signs and symptoms

Stabbing stomach pain in a fixed position, tenderness, cold limbs, sweating; the pain can radiate to the back. This pattern is often associated with a history of hematemesis or black stools.

Tongue: dark, purple or with ecchymosis
Pulse: wiry or thready–hesitant

Treatment principle

Invigorate blood, resolve stasis, regulate *qi* and relieve pain.

Formula

Modified *Huó Luò Xiào Líng Dān* (活络效灵丹, "Effective Channel-Activating Elixir") and *Shī Xiào Sǎn* (失笑散, "Sudden Smile Powder").

丹参	*dān shēn*	15 g	*Radix et Rhizoma Salviae Miltiorrhizae*
当归	*dāng guī*	9 g	*Radix Angelicae Sinensis*
乳香	*rǔ xiāng*	6 g	*Olibanum*
没药	*mò yào*	6 g	*Myrrha*
五灵脂	*wǔ líng zhī*	9 g	*Faeces Trogopterori*
蒲黄	*pú huáng*	9 g	*Pollen Typhae* (wrapped)
陈皮	*chén pí*	9 g	*Pericarpium Citri Reticulatae*
青皮	*qīng pí*	9 g	*Pericarpium Citri Reticulatae Viride*
延胡索	*yán hú suǒ*	9 g	*Rhizoma Corydalis*
川楝子	*chuān liàn zǐ*	9 g	*Fructus Toosendan*

Modifications

- For black stools, combine with *sān qī* (三七, *Radix et Rhizoma Notoginseng*) 9 g and *huā ruǐ shí* (花蕊石, *Ophicalcitum*) 30 g.
- For severe pain, combine with *chuān xiōng* (川芎, *Rhizoma Chuanxiong*) 9 g and *zhǐ shí* (枳实, *Fructus Aurantii Immaturus*) 9 g.
- For gastric discomfort and nausea, combine with *zhī mǔ* (知母, *Rhizoma Anemarrhenae*) 9 g and *jiāng zhú rú* (姜竹茹, *Caulis Bambusae in Taenia Praeparatum*) 9 g.

QUESTIONS

1. How do you distinguish between the pain from gastric ulcers and the pain from duodenal ulcers?
2. Describe the pattern identification and treatment of gastric and duodenal ulcers.
3. *Case study.* Try to make a pattern identification and give a prescription for the following case:

Ms. Zhang, 40, suffered from duodenal ulcers for five years and experienced dull gastric pain, due to recent weather changes, especially with an empty stomach. Her pain could be alleviated by warmth, pressure and eating food. Other symptoms included mental fatigue, cold limbs and loose stools. The tongue was pale and swollen, with tooth marks and a thin white coating. The pulse was soft and thready.

Chronic Gastritis

Overview

Chronic gastritis is a chronic inflammation of the stomach mucosa. It can have multiple causes. By morphological changes, chronic gastritis can be categorized into superficial gastritis, atrophic gastritis and hypertrophic gastritis. By position, chronic gastritis can be categorized into corpus gastritis and antral gastritis.

In Chinese medicine, chronic gastritis falls under the category of "epigastric pain" or "gastric masses". The main contributing factors include constitutional deficiency of the spleen and stomach, an improper diet and liver *qi* affecting the stomach.

Failure of the spleen and stomach to transport and transform may obstruct the *qi* activities. Excessive ingestion of hot spicy food or overconsumption of alcohol may damage the spleen and the stomach, and result in disharmony between the spleen and the stomach. Emotional disturbance may cause liver *qi* stagnation to further affect the descending of stomach *qi*.

Clinical manifestations

This condition progresses slowly. It is clinically characterized by gastric fullness, distension and pain, nausea, vomiting, a poor appetite and belching. Superficial gastritis causes upper abdominal distension and discomfort that can be relieved by belching. Acid reflux, nausea and transient stomachache may also be present. Atrophic gastritis causes dull upper abdominal pain, bloating and discomfort, and a poor appetite. Anemia, unexplained weight loss and diarrhea may also be present. Hypertrophic gastritis causes intractable, irregular upper abdominal pain that can be relieved by eating food or taking basic drugs.

Pattern identification and treatment

Disharmony between the liver and the stomach

Signs and symptoms

Gastric distension and pain radiating to the bilateral hypochondriac regions, chest tightness, belching, frequent sighing and occasional waterbrash. The symptoms can be worsened by emotional disturbance.

Tongue: light red, with a thin white coating
Pulse: wiry

Treatment principle

Soothe the liver, regulate *qi*, harmonize the stomach and relieve pain.

Formula

Sì Nì Săn (四逆散, "Frigid Extremities Powder") and *Jīn Líng Zǐ Săn* (金铃子散, "Toosendan Powder").

柴胡	*chái hú*	9 g	Radix Bupleuri
白芍	*bái sháo*	9 g	Radix Paeoniae Alba
枳壳	*zhǐ qiào*	9 g	Fructus Aurantii
陈皮	*chén pí*	9 g	Pericarpium Citri Reticulatae
半夏	*bàn xià*	9 g	Rhizoma Pinelliae
川楝子	*chuān liàn zǐ*	9 g	Fructus Toosendan
延胡索	*yán hú suǒ*	9 g	Rhizoma Corydalis
甘草	*zhì gān cǎo*	6 g	Radix et Rhizoma Glycyrrhizae
降香	*jiàng xiāng*	6 g	Lignum Dalbergiae Odoriferae

Modifications

- For severe pain, combine with *bā yuè zhā* (八月札, *Fructus Akebiae*) 15 g and *lù lù tōng* (路路通, *Fructus Liquidambaris*) 9 g.
- For severe nausea and waterbrash, combine with *huáng lián* (黄连, *Rhizoma Coptidis*) 4.5 g and *hǎi piāo xiāo* (海螵蛸, *Endoconcha Sepiae*) 15 g.
- For a dry mouth with a bitter taste, combine with *zhī mǔ* (知母, *Rhizoma Anemarrhenae*) 9 g and *shēng dì* (生地, *Radix Rehmanniae*) 9 g.

Damp–heat in the spleen and stomach

Signs and symptoms

Gastric distension and pain with a burning sensation, belching, chest tightness and a sticky bitter taste in the mouth with a foul breath.

Tongue: red, with a yellow greasy coating
Pulse: wiry and slippery

Treatment principle

Clear heat, resolve dampness, harmonize the stomach and relieve pain.

Formula

Supplemented *Qīng Zhōng Tāng* (清中汤, "Middle Jiao–Clearing Decoction").

黄连	huáng lián	6 g	Rhizoma Coptidis
山栀	shān zhī	9 g	Fructus Gardeniae
半夏	bàn xià	9 g	Rhizoma Pinelliae
茯苓	fú líng	9 g	Poria
枳壳	zhǐ qiào	9 g	Fructus Aurantii
白豆蔻	bái dòu kòu	6 g	Fructus Amomi Kravanh
苍术	cāng zhú	9 g	Rhizoma Atractylodis
陈皮	chén pí	9 g	Pericarpium Citri Reticulatae
蒲公英	pú gōng yīng	15 g	Herba Taraxaci
厚朴	hòu pò	9 g	Cortex Magnoliae Officinalis
甘草	zhì gān cǎo	6 g	Radix et Rhizoma Glycyrrhizae

Modifications

- For severe chest discomfort and a greasy tongue coating, combine with *huò xiāng* (藿香, *Herba Agastachis*) 9 g and *pèi lán* (佩兰, *Herba Eupatorii*) 6 g.
- For a bitter taste and constipation due to exuberant heat, combine with *dà huáng* (大黄, *Radix et Rhizoma Rhei*) 9 g (decoct later) or *má rén* (麻仁, *Fructus Cannabis*) 12 g.
- For severe pain, combine with *fó shǒu* (佛手, *Fructus Citri Sarcodactylis*) 9 g and *xiāng yuán pí* (香橼皮, *Cortex Citri*) 9 g.

Deficiency of the spleen and stomach

Signs and symptoms

Dull gastric pain with a preference for warmth and pressure, a poor appetite, abdominal fullness and bloating after eating food, watery vomiting, a lusterless complexion, mental fatigue and cold limbs.

Tongue: pale, with a thin white coating
Pulse: soft and thready

Treatment principle

Strengthen the spleen, supplement *qi*, warm the middle *jiao* and relieve pain.

Formula

Supplemented *Xiāng Shā Liù Jūn Zǐ Tāng* (香砂六君子汤, "Costusroot and Amomum Six Gentlemen Decoction").

党参	*dǎng shēn*	12 g	*Radix Codonopsis*
白术	*bái zhú*	9 g	*Rhizoma Atractylodis Macrocephalae*
茯苓	*fú líng*	9 g	*Poria*
半夏	*bàn xià*	9 g	*Rhizoma Pinelliae*
陈皮	*chén pí*	9 g	*Pericarpium Citri Reticulatae*
木香	*mù xiāng*	6 g	*Radix Aucklandiae*
砂仁	*shā rén*	6 g	*Fructus Amomi* (decoct later)
佛手	*fó shǒu*	9 g	*Fructus Citri Sarcodactylis*
干姜	*gān jiāng*	4.5 g	*Rhizoma Zingiberis*
炙甘草	*zhì gān cǎo*	6 g	*Radix et Rhizoma Glycyrrhizae Praeparata cum Melle*

Modifications

- For cold limbs and excessive salivation, combine with *páo fù zǐ* (炮附子, *Radix Aconiti Lateralis Praeparata*) 6 g (decoct first) and *wú zhū yú* (吴茱萸, *Fructus Evodiae*) 3 g.
- For severe pain, combine with *yán hú suǒ* (延胡索, *Rhizoma Corydalis*) 9 g and *chuān liàn zǐ* (川楝子, *Fructus Toosendan*) 9 g.
- For severe gastric and abdominal distension, combine with *jiāo shén qū* (焦神曲, *Massa Medicata Fermentata Praeparata*) 9 g, *jiāo shān zhā* (焦山楂, *Fructus Crataegi Praeparata*) 9 g and *zhì jī nèi jīn* (炙鸡内金, *Endothelium Corneum Gigeriae Galli Praeparata cum Melle*) 9 g.

Stomach yin deficiency

Signs and symptoms

Dull gastric pain with a burning sensation, thirst with a desire to drink water, a dry mouth and throat, gastric discomfort and constipation.

Tongue: red, with cracks and a scanty coating
Pulse: wiry and thready

Treatment principle

Nourish yin, benefit the stomach and relieve pain.

Formula

Modified *Yì Wèi Tāng* (益胃汤, "Stomach Benefiting Decoction") and *Zhú Yè Shí Gāo Tāng* (竹叶石膏汤, "Lophatherum and Gypsum Decoction").

北沙参	*běi shā shēn*	12 g	*Radix Glehniae*
麦冬	*mài dōng*	9 g	*Radix Ophiopogonis*
生地	*shēng dì*	12 g	*Radix Rehmanniae*
玉竹	*yù zhú*	9 g	*Radix Ophiopogonis*
竹叶	*zhú yè*	9 g	*Folium Phyllostachydis Henonis*
石膏	*shí gāo*	30 g	*Gypsum Fibrosum*
半夏	*bàn xià*	9 g	*Rhizoma Pinelliae*
陈皮	*chén pí*	9 g	*Pericarpium Citri Reticulatae*
川楝子	*chuān liàn zǐ*	9 g	*Fructus Toosendan*
麻仁	*má rén*	9 g	*Fructus Cannabis*
甘草	*gān cǎo*	6 g	*Radix et Rhizoma Glycyrrhizae*

Modifications

- For a gastric upset with a burning sensation, combine with *huáng lián* (黄连, *Rhizoma Coptidis*) 4.5 g and *zhī mǔ* (知母, *Rhizoma Anemarrhenae*) 9 g.
- For a severe dry mouth and throat, combine with *shí hú* (石斛, *Caulis Dendrobii*) 15 g and *tiān huā fěn* (天花粉, *Radix Trichosanthis*) 15 g.
- For severe gastric pain, combine with *bā yuè zhā* (八月札, *Fructus Akebiae*) 15 g and *yán hú suǒ* (延胡索, *Rhizoma Corydalis*) 9 g.

Blood stasis in the stomach collaterals

Signs and symptoms

Persistent stabbing gastric pain in a fixed position, tenderness, gastric upset, acid reflux and occasional black stools.

Tongue: dark-purple or with ecchymosis
Pulse: thready and hesitant

Treatment principle

Resolve stasis, unblock the collaterals, regulate *qi* and relieve pain.

Formula

Modified *Táo Hóng Sì Wù Tāng* (桃红四物汤, "Peach Kernel and Carthamus Four Substances Decoction").

桃仁	*táo rén*	9 g	*Semen Persicae*
红花	*hóng huā*	9 g	*Flos Carthami*
当归	*dāng guī*	9 g	*Radix Angelicae Sinensis*
赤芍	*chì sháo*	9 g	*Radix Paeoniae Rubra*
川芎	*chuān xiōng*	9 g	*Rhizoma Chuanxiong*
枳壳	*zhǐ qiào*	9 g	*Fructus Aurantii*
蒲黄	*pú huáng*	9 g	*Pollen Typhae* (wrapped)
陈皮	*chén pí*	9 g	*Pericarpium Citri Reticulatae*
延胡索	*yán hú suǒ*	9 g	*Rhizoma Corydalis*

Modifications

- For severe pain, combine with *chuān liàn zǐ* (川楝子, *Fructus Toosendan*) 9 g and *wǔ líng zhī* (五灵脂, *Faeces Trogopterori*) 9 g (wrapped).
- For severe acid reflux, combine with *duàn wǎ léng* (煅瓦楞, *Concha Arcae Praeparatum*) and *dài zhě shí* (代赭石, *Haematitum*) 15 g.
- For black stools, combine with *dì yú* (地榆, *Radix Sanguisorbae*) 15 g and *sān qī* (三七, *Radix et Rhizoma Notoginseng*) 9 g.

QUESTIONS

1. How do you understand the causative factors of chronic gastritis?
2. Describe the signs and symptoms of chronic gastritis due to disharmony between the liver and the stomach.
3. *Case study.* Try to make pattern identification and give a prescription for the following case:

Ms. Zheng, 35, suffered from stomach conditions for five years and was once diagnosed with atrophic gastritis, which responded well to Western treatment.

> However, she then started to experience dull gastric pain, coupled with a poor appetite and gastric distension after eating food that could be relieved by warmth and pressure. Other symptoms included mental fatigue and loose stools. The tongue was pale, with a thin white coating. The pulse was soft and thready.

Cholecystitis and Cholelithiasis

Overview

Cholecystitis can be acute or chronic. Cholelithiasis involves gallstones within the gallbladder, common bile duct or hepatic duct. They are two common biliary tract conditions, cholecystitis can be a consequence of cholelithiasis, and vice versa.

In Chinese medicine, these two conditions fall under the category of "pain in the hypochondriac regions", "epigastric pain" or "jaundice". The main contributing factors include an improper diet and emotional disturbance.

Long-term alcohol consumption and overingestion of sweet oily food may cause internal damp–heat in the spleen and stomach, which in turn affects the liver and gallbladder, forming stones. Emotional disturbance may damage the liver, which can further compromise the gallbladder due to the internal–external relationship between the two. This may affect the secretion of bile and lead to stones.

Clinical manifestations

Cholecystitis and cholelithiasis are characterized by pain on the upper right side of the abdomen, fever, jaundice, belching and intolerance of fatty food. Patients with acute episodes can experience paroxysmal colic on the upper right side of the abdomen or referred pain below the right shoulder. Other symptoms include chills, fever, jaundice, nausea, vomiting, gastric or abdominal distension and fullness, and dark-yellow urine. Constipation or diarrhea may also be present. In the remission stage, patients may present with pain or discomfort in the epigastric or right hypochondriac region, belching, a poor appetite, intolerance of fatty food and bloating.

Pattern identification and treatment

Qi stagnation of the liver and gallbladder

Signs and symptoms

Distending or migrating pain in the right hypochondriac region, epigastric fullness, chest tightness or discomfort, frequent belching, nausea, vomiting, a poor appetite and a dry mouth with a bitter taste.

Tongue: a thin-white or thin yellow coating
Pulse: wiry

Treatment principle

Soothe the liver and gallbladder, regulate *qi* and relieve pain.

Formula

Modified *Chái Hú Shū Gān Sǎn* (柴胡疏肝散, "Bupleurum Liver-Soothing Powder").

柴胡	*chái hú*	9 g	*Radix Bupleuri*
枳壳	*zhǐ qiào*	9 g	*Fructus Aurantii*
白芍	*bái sháo*	9 g	*Radix Paeoniae Alba*
赤芍	*chì sháo*	9 g	*Radix Paeoniae Rubra*
川芎	*chuān xiōng*	9 g	*Rhizoma Chuanxiong*
郁金	*yù jīn*	9 g	*Radix Curcumae*
陈皮	*chén pí*	6 g	*Pericarpium Citri Reticulatae*
黄芩	*huáng qín*	9 g	*Radix Scutellariae*
金钱草	*jīn qián cǎo*	30 g	*Herba Lysimachiae*
甘草	*gān cǎo*	6 g	*Radix et Rhizoma Glycyrrhizae*

Modifications

- For fever, combine with *hǔ zhàng* (虎杖, *Rhizoma Polygoni Cuspidati*) 9 g, *pú gōng yīng* (蒲公英, *Herba Taraxaci*) 15 g and *shān zhī* (山栀, *Fructus Gardeniae*) 9 g.
- For nausea and vomiting, combine with *jiāng bàn xià* (姜半夏, *Rhizoma Pinelliae Praeparatum*) 9 g and *zǐ sū gěng* (紫苏梗, *Caulis Perillae*) 9 g.

- For severe pain in the hypochondriac regions, combine with *chuān liàn zǐ* (川楝子, *Fructus Toosendan*) 9 g and *yán hú suǒ* (延胡索, *Rhizoma Corydalis*) 9 g.
- For constipation, combine with *dà huáng* (大黄, *Radix et Rhizoma Rhei*) 9g (decoct later).

Fire–heat in the liver and gallbladder

Signs and symptoms

A burning pain in the right hypochondriac region that can radiate to the shoulder and back, tenderness, bloating, fever, cold intolerance, a dry throat, a bitter taste, and red face and eyes; other symptoms may include yellow sclera, restlessness, nausea, intolerance of fatty food, dark-yellow urine and dry stools.

Tongue: red, with a dry yellow coating
Pulse: wiry and slippery

Treatment principle

Soothe the liver and gallbladder, clear fire and reduce heat.

Formula

Modified *Dà Chái Hú Tāng* (大柴胡汤, "Major Bupleurum Decoction") and *Huáng Lián Jiě Dú Tāng* (黄连解毒汤, "Coptis Toxin-Resolving Decoction").

柴胡	chái hú	9 g	Radix Bupleuri
白芍	bái sháo	9 g	Radix Paeoniae Alba
枳实	zhǐ shí	9 g	Fructus Aurantii Immaturus
半夏	bàn xià	9 g	Rhizoma Pinelliae
黄连	huáng lián	6 g	Rhizoma Coptidis
黄芩	huáng qín	9 g	Radix Scutellariae
黄柏	huáng bǎi	9 g	Cortex Phellodendri Chinensis
山栀	shān zhī	9 g	Fructus Gardeniae
大黄	dà huáng	9 g	Radix et Rhizoma Rhei
甘草	gān cǎo	9 g	Radix et Rhizoma Glycyrrhizae

Modifications

- For severe fire–heat, combine with *mǔ dān pí* (牡丹皮, *Cortex Moutan*) 9 g and *lóng dǎn cǎo* (龙胆草, *Radix et Rhizoma Gentianae*) 12 g.
- For bloating and constipation, combine with *máng xiāo* (芒硝, *Natrii Sulfas*) 9 g and *dà fù pí* (大腹皮, *Pericarpium Arecae*) 9 g.
- For severe jaundice, combine with *yīn chén* (茵陈, *Herba Artemisiae Scopariae*) 15 g and *jīn qián cǎo* (金钱草, *Herba Lysimachiae*) 30 g.
- For severe pain, combine with *yù jīn* (郁金, *Radix Curcumae*) 9 g and *yán hú suǒ* (延胡索, *Rhizoma Corydalis*) 9 g.

Damp–heat in the liver and gallbladder

Signs and symptoms

Persistent pain on the upper right side of the abdomen or paroxysmal colic radiating to the right shoulder and back, palpable masses in the hypochondrium, chills, fever, nausea, vomiting, thirst with no desire to drink water, dark-yellow urine and unsmooth bowel movements.

Tongue: red, with a yellow greasy coating
Pulse: wiry and tight

Treatment principle

Soothe the liver and gallbladder, clear heat and resolve dampness.

Formula

Modified *Sì Nì Sǎn* (四逆散, "Frigid Extremities Powder") and *Lóng Dǎn Xiè Gān Tāng* (龙胆泻肝汤, "Gentian Liver-Draining Decoction").

柴胡	*chái hú*	9 g	*Radix Bupleuri*
枳实	*zhǐ shí*	9 g	*Fructus Aurantii Immaturus*
郁金	*yù jīn*	9 g	*Radix Curcumae*
龙胆草	*lóng dǎn cǎo*	9 g	*Radix et Rhizoma Gentianae*
金钱草	*jīn qián cǎo*	30 g	*Herba Lysimachiae*
黄芩	*huáng qín*	9 g	*Radix Scutellariae*
木通	*mù tōng*	6 g	*Caulis Akebiae*
山栀	*shān zhī*	9 g	*Fructus Gardeniae*
甘草	*zhì gān cǎo*	6 g	*Radix et Rhizoma Glycyrrhizae*

Modifications

- For chest tightness and a thick greasy tongue coating, combine with *cāng zhú* (苍术, *Rhizoma Atractylodis*) 9 g and *hòu pò* (厚朴, *Cortex Magnoliae Officinalis*) 9 g.
- For severe pain, combine with *yán hú suŏ* (延胡索, *Rhizoma Corydalis*) 9 g, *chuān liàn zĭ* (川楝子, *Fructus Toosendan*) 9 g and *mù xiāng* (木香, *Radix Aucklandiae*) 9 g.
- For severe jaundice, combine with *hŭ zhàng* (虎杖, *Rhizoma Polygoni Cuspidati*) 9 g, *chē qián zĭ* (车前子, *Semen Plantaginis*) 15 g (wrapped) and *yīn chén* (茵陈, *Herba Artemisiae Scopariae*) 15 g.
- For severe nausea and vomiting, combine with *bàn xià* (半夏, *Rhizoma Pinelliae*) 9 g, *zhú rú* (竹茹, *Caulis Bambusae in Taenia*) 9 g and *chén pí* (陈皮, *Pericarpium Citri Reticulatae*) 9 g.
- For severe constipation, combine with *dà huáng* (大黄, *Radix et Rhizoma Rhei*) 9 g (decoct later) and *máng xiāo* (芒硝, *Natrii Sulfas*) 9 g.

Blood stasis in the collaterals

Signs and symptoms

Persistent stabbing pain in the upper right hypochondriac region in a fixed position, tenderness, the pain worsening at night, a palpable mass in the hypochondrium, gastric or abdominal distension and fullness, and constipation.

Tongue: dark-purple or with ecchymosis and a thin coating
Pulse: wiry and hesitant

Treatment principle

Invigorate blood, resolve stasis, soothe the liver and remove masses.

Formula

Modified *Táo Rén Chéng Qì Tāng* (桃仁承气汤, "Semen Persicae Purgative Decoction").

桃仁	*táo rén*	9 g	*Semen Persicae*
大黄	*dà huáng*	9 g	*Radix et Rhizoma Rhei* (decoct later)
延胡索	*yán hú suǒ*	9 g	*Rhizoma Corydalis*
川芎	*chuān xiōng*	9 g	*Rhizoma Chuanxiong*
郁金	*yù jīn*	9 g	*Radix Curcumae*
陈皮	*chén pí*	9 g	*Pericarpium Citri Reticulatae*
当归	*dāng guī*	9 g	*Radix Angelicae Sinensis*
金钱草	*jīn qián cǎo*	30 g	*Herba Lysimachiae*
甘草	*zhì gān cǎo*	9 g	*Radix et Rhizoma Glycyrrhizae*

Modifications

- For severe blood stasis, combine with *sān léng* (三棱, *Rhizoma Sparganii*) 9 g, *é zhú* (莪术, *Rhizoma Curcumae*) 9 g and *chuān shān jiǎ* (穿山甲, *Squama Manitis*) 9 g (decoct first).
- For fever, combine with *hóng téng* (红藤, *Caulis Sargentodoxae*) 15 g and *bài jiàng cǎo* (败酱草, Herba Patriniae) 15 g.
- For severe pain in the hypochondriac regions, combine with *xiāng fù* (香附, *Rhizoma Cyperi*) 9 g, *zhǐ qiào* (枳壳, *Fructus Aurantii*) 9 g and *lù lù tōng* (路路通, *Fructus Liquidambaris*) 9 g.
- For a dry mouth with a bitter taste, combine with *shēng dì* (生地, *Radix Rehmanniae*) 9 g and *xuán shēn* (玄参, *Radix Scrophulariae*) 9 g.

Exuberance of toxic pus

Signs and symptoms

Intense colic in the upper right abdomen, tenderness, high fever, chills, restlessness, persistent jaundice, abdominal bloating and fullness, dark-yellow urine and constipation; in severe cases, coma with delirium may also be present.

Tongue: dark-red, with a dry yellow coating
Pulse: wiry and rapid

Treatment principle

Clear heat, remove toxins, resolve stasis and drain pus.

Formula

Modified *Yīn Chén Hāo Tāng* (茵陈蒿汤, "Artemisiae Scopariae Decoction") and *Tòu Nóng Sǎn* (透脓散, "Pus-Expelling Powder").

茵陈	yīn chén	30 g	Herba Artemisiae Scopariae
山栀	shān zhī	9 g	Fructus Gardeniae
大黄	dà huáng	9 g	Radix et Rhizoma Rhei (decoct later)
黄芪	huáng qí	12 g	Radix Astragali
川芎	chuān xiōng	9 g	Rhizoma Chuanxiong
当归	dāng guī	9 g	Radix Angelicae Sinensis
皂角刺	zào jiǎo cì	9 g	Spina Gleditsiae
蒲公英	pú gōng yīng	30 g	Herba Taraxaci
赤芍	chì sháo	9 g	Radix Paeoniae Rubra
金银花	jīn yín huā	9 g	Flos Lonicerae Japonicae

Modifications

- For coma and delirium, combine with *Ān Gōng Niú Huáng Wán* (安宫牛黄丸, "Peaceful Palace Bovine Bezoar Pill"), one pill for one treatment, twice a day.
- For high fever with convulsions, combine with *Zǐ Xuě Dān* (紫雪丹, "Purple Snow Elixir"), 6 g for one treatment.
- For severe pain, combine with *yán hú suǒ* (延胡索, *Rhizoma Corydalis*) 9 g, *chuān liàn zǐ* (川楝子, *Fructus Toosendan*) 9 g, *pú huáng* (蒲黄, *Pollen Typhae*) 9 g (wrapped) and *wǔ líng zhī* (五灵脂, *Faeces Trogopterori*) 9 g (wrapped).
- For severe jaundice, combine with *jīn qián cǎo* (金钱草, *Herba Lysimachiae*) 30 g, *hǔ zhàng* (虎杖, *Rhizoma Polygoni Cuspidati*) 9 g and *chē qián zǐ* (车前子, *Semen Plantaginis*) 15 g (wrapped).

Combined yin deficiency and dampness

Signs and symptoms

Dull pain in the right hypochondriac region with a burning sensation, a persistent low-grade fever, a dry mouth and throat, lassitude, dizziness, blurred vision, dark-yellow urine and dry stools.

Tongue: red, with a thin yellow greasy coating
Pulse: wiry, thready and rapid

Treatment principle

Nourish yin, reduce fire and resolve dampness.

Formula

Zhī Bǎi Dì Huáng Tāng (知柏地黄汤, "Phellodendron and Rehmannia Decoction") and *Gān Lù Yǐn* (甘露饮, "Sweet Dew Beverage").

生地	*shēng dì*	15 g	Radix Rehmanniae
山茱萸	*shān zhū yú*	9 g	Fructus Corni
牡丹皮	*mǔ dān pí*	9 g	Cortex Moutan
茯苓	*fú líng*	12 g	Poria
知母	*zhī mǔ*	9 g	Rhizoma Anemarrhenae
黄柏	*huáng bǎi*	9 g	Cortex Phellodendri Chinensis
泽泻	*zé xiè*	9 g	Rhizoma Alismatis
石斛	*shí hú*	9 g	Caulis Dendrobii
黄芩	*huáng qín*	9 g	Radix Scutellariae
茵陈	*yīn chén*	30 g	Herba Artemisiae Scopariae
柴胡	*chái hú*	9 g	Radix Bupleuri

Modifications

- For severe constipation, combine with *má rén* (麻仁, *Fructus Cannabis*) 9 g and *yù lǐ rén* (郁李仁, *Semen Pruni*) 9 g.
- For significant pain in the hypochondriac regions, combine with *bā yuè zhā* (八月札, *Fructus Akebiae*) 15 g and *lù lù tōng* (路路通, *Fructus Liquidambaris*) 9 g.
- For lassitude and a greasy tongue coating, combine with *cāng zhú* (苍术, *Rhizoma Atractylodis*) 9 g and *chē qián zǐ* (车前子, *Semen Plantaginis*) 15 g (wrapped)
- For severe feverish sensations on the soles and palms, combine with *qīng hāo* (青蒿, *Herba Artemisiae Annuae*) 9 g and *biē jiǎ* (鳖甲, *Carapax Trionycis*) 15 g (decoct first).

QUESTIONS

1. How do you distinguish the causative factors of cholecystitis and cholelithiasis?
2. Describe the main symptoms of cholecystitis and cholelithiasis.
3. *Case study*. Try to make a pattern identification and give a prescription for the following case:

Ms. Zhang, 30, experienced persistent pain in the right upper abdomen for three days, which also radiated to the right shoulder blade, coupled with nausea, vomiting, intolerance of fatty food, fever, a dry mouth with no desire to drink water, dark-yellow urine and unsmooth bowel movements. The tongue was red, with thin yellow greasy coating. The pulse was wiry.

Chronic Nonspecific Ulcerative Colitis

Overview

Chronic nonspecific ulcerative colitis, also known as ulcerative colitis, is a form of chronic colitis with unknown causes. It is specifically limited to the mucosa of the colon, mainly including characteristic ulcers in the rectum and distal colon. However, the proximal or entire colon can be affected. According to progression, this condition can be categorized into four patterns: chronic recurrent type, chronic persistent type, acute onset type and primary type. According to the severity, it can be categorized into mild, moderate or severe patterns. Ulcerative colitis can develop at any age — especially young and middle-aged adults. It is seen slightly more in men than in women.

In Chinese medicine, ulcerative colitis falls under the category of "diarrhea", "dysentery" or "bloody stools". The main contributing factors include an improper diet, contraction of damp–heat, emotional disturbance and chronic conditions.

An improper diet or contraction of damp–heat may block the *qi* flow of the large intestine, leading to stagnation of *qi* and blood, which may further transform into purulent mucus. Emotional disturbance may affect the liver's function in maintaining the free flow of *qi*, which in turn affects the spleen and results in disharmony between the liver and the spleen. Over time, patients may develop deficiency of the spleen and kidneys, followed by failure of clean *qi* to ascend, sinking of spleen *qi* and internal blood stasis.

Clinical manifestations

Typical manifestations of ulcerative colitis are abdominal diarrhea mixed with blood, pus and mucus, as well as paroxysmal abdominal pain or cramping. Normally, patients may experience remission of symptoms a couple of days after the onset. However, the condition can be retriggered by an improper diet, emotions and secondary infections. In some patients, despite regular bowel movements, blood, pus and mucus are still contained in the feces. Over time, some patients may also present with significant weight loss, anemia, a low-grade fever and hepatomegaly. In severe cases, patients may have more than 10–30 bowel movements daily, accompanied by a high-grade fever, vomiting, abdominal pain, bloating and dehydration. Coma or shock may also occur in rare cases.

Pattern identification and treatment

Downward flow of damp–heat

Signs and symptoms

Abdominal pain, diarrhea mixed with blood, pus or mucus, tenesmus, a burning sensation around the anus, fever, a bitter taste, chest tightness, a poor appetite and dark-yellow urine.

Tongue: a yellow greasy coating
Pulse: slippery and rapid

Treatment principle

Clear heat, remove toxins, dry dampness and regulate *qi*.

Formula

Modified *Bái Tóu Wēng Tāng* (白头翁汤, "Pulsatilla Decoction") and *Mù Xiāng Bīng Láng Wán* (木香槟榔丸, "Costus Root and Areca Pill").

白头翁	*bái tóu wēng*	15 g	*Radix Pulsatillae*
黄连	*huáng lián*	6 g	*Rhizoma Coptidis*
黄柏	*huáng bǎi*	9 g	*Cortex Phellodendri Chinensis*
秦皮	*qín pí*	9 g	*Cortex Fraxini*
木香	*mù xiāng*	9 g	*Radix Aucklandiae*
槟榔	*bīng láng*	9 g	*Semen Arecae*
枳壳	*zhǐ qiào*	9 g	*Fructus Aurantii*
莪术	*é zhú*	9 g	*Rhizoma Curcumae*

Modifications

- For significant fever, combine with *jīn yín huā* (金银花, *Flos Lonicerae Japonicae*) 9 g and *lián qiào* (连翘, *Fructus Forsythiae*) 9 g.
- For pus and blood in the feces, combine with *bài jiàng cǎo* (败酱草, *Herba Patriniae*) 15 g, *hóng téng* (红藤, *Caulis Sargentodoxae*) 15 g, *dì yú* (地榆, *Radix Sanguisorbae*) 12 g and *yì yǐ rén* (薏苡仁, *Semen Coicis*) 15 g.
- For chest tightness, a poor appetite and a thick, greasy tongue coating, combine with *cāng zhú* (苍术, *Rhizoma Atractylodis*) 9 g, *hòu pò* (厚朴, *Cortex Magnoliae Officinalis*) 9 g and *chē qián zǐ* (车前子, *Semen Plantaginis*) 15 g (wrapped).

Liver qi stagnation affecting the spleen

Signs and symptoms

Abdominal pain and diarrhea that can be induced by emotions (the pain can be relieved by bowel movements), distending pain in the chest and hypochondriac regions, frequent belching, gastric discomfort, a poor appetite, restlessness and irritability.

Tongue: light-red, with a thin coating
Pulse: wiry

Treatment principle

Soothe the liver, regulate *qi*, strengthen the spleen and harmonize the stomach.

Formula

Supplemented *Tòng Xiè Yào Fāng* (痛泻要方, "Important Formula for Painful Diarrhea").

柴胡	*chái hú*	9 g	Radix Bupleuri
白术	*bái zhú*	9 g	Rhizoma Atractylodis Macrocephalae
白芍	*bái sháo*	9 g	Radix Paeoniae Alba
防风	*fáng fēng*	9 g	Radix Saposhnikoviae
陈皮	*chén pí*	9 g	Pericarpium Citri Reticulatae
茯苓	*fú líng*	9 g	Poria
黄连	*huáng lián*	6 g	Rhizoma Coptidis
山楂	*shān zhā*	9 g	Fructus Crataegi
大黄	*dà huáng*	9 g	Radix et Rhizoma Rhei
枳壳	*zhǐ qiào*	9 g	Fructus Aurantii

Modifications

- For severe restlessness and irritability, combine with *shān zhī* (山栀, *Fructus Gardeniae*) 9 g and *lóng dǎn cǎo* (龙胆草, *Radix et Rhizoma Gentianae*) 12 g.
- For severe abdominal pain, combine with *yán hú suǒ* (延胡索, *Rhizoma Corydalis*) 9 g and *wū yào* (乌药, *Radix Linderae*) 9 g.
- For remarkable bloody stools, combine with *dì yú* (地榆, *Radix Sanguisorbae*) 9 g, *bái jí* (白及, *Rhizoma Bletillae*) 9 g and *huái huā* (槐花, *Flos Sophorae*) 12 g.
- For frequent belching, combine with *xuán fù huā* (旋覆花, *Flos Inulae*) 9 g (wrapped) and *dài zhě shí* (代赭石, *Haematitum*) 15 g (decocted first).

Blood stasis in the intestinal collaterals

Signs and symptoms

Stabbing pain in the lower abdomen with a fixed position, tenderness, diarrhea mixed with blood, pus, blood clots or mucus, a dark-gray complexion, chest tightness and a poor appetite.

Tongue: dark-purple or with ecchymosis and a thin coating
Pulse: thready and hesitant

Treatment principle

Invigorate blood, resolve stasis, regulate *qi* and relieve pain.

Formula

Modified *Shào Fǔ Zhú Yū Tāng* (少腹逐瘀汤, "Lower Abdominal Stasis–Expelling Decoction").

当归	*dāng guī*	9 g	Radix Angelicae Sinensis
川芎	*chuān xiōng*	9 g	Rhizoma Chuanxiong
赤芍	*chì sháo*	9 g	Radix Paeoniae Rubra
蒲黄	*pú huáng*	9 g	Pollen Typhae (wrapped)
五灵脂	*wǔ líng zhī*	9 g	Faeces Trogopterori (wrapped)
小茴香	*xiǎo huí xiāng*	6 g	Fructus Foeniculi
没药	*mò yào*	6 g	Myrrha
地榆	*dì yú*	15 g	Radix Sanguisorbae
枳壳	*zhǐ qiào*	9 g	Fructus Aurantii

Modifications

- For excessive mucus in the feces, combine with *huáng bǎi* (黄柏, *Cortex Phellodendri Chinensis*) 9 g and *qín pí* (秦皮, *Cortex Fraxini*) 9 g.
- For chest tightness and a greasy tongue coating, combine with *cāng zhú* (苍术, *Rhizoma Atractylodis*) 9 g and *hòu pò* (厚朴, *Cortex Magnoliae Officinalis*) 9 g.
- For severe abdominal pain, combine with *táo rén* (桃仁, *Semen Persicae*) 9 g, *hóng huā* (红花, *Flos Carthami*) 9 g and *dà fù pí* (大腹皮, *Pericarpium Arecae*) 9 g.

Deficiency of the spleen and stomach

Signs and symptoms

Bowel sounds, diarrhea mixed with undigested food and mucus, lingering dull abdominal pain, mental fatigue, chest tightness, a poor appetite and a lusterless complexion.

Tongue: pale and swollen, with a thin white coating
Pulse: thready and weak

Treatment principle

Strengthen the spleen, supplement *qi* and relieve pain.

Formula

Modified *Shēn Líng Bái Zhú Sǎn* (参苓白术散, "Ginseng, Poria and Atractylodes Macrocephalae Powder").

党参	*dǎng shēn*	12 g	*Radix Codonopsis*
白术	*bái zhú*	9 g	*Rhizoma Atractylodis Macrocephalae*
茯苓	*fú líng*	9 g	*Poria*
山药	*shān yào*	15 g	*Rhizoma Dioscoreae*
莲子心	*lián zǐ xīn*	9 g	*Plumula Nelumbinis*
砂仁	*shā rén*	6 g	*Fructus Amomi* (decoct later)
焦山楂	*jiāo shān zhā*	9 g	*Fructus Crataegi Praeparata*
陈皮	*chén pí*	6 g	*Pericarpium Citri Reticulatae*
甘草	*gān cǎo*	9 g	*Radix et Rhizoma Glycyrrhizae*

Modifications

- For lassitude and fatigue, combine with *huáng qí* (黄芪, *Radix Astragali*) 15 g and *bái biǎn dòu* (白扁豆, *Semen Lablab Album*) 9 g.
- For chest tightness and a greasy tongue coating, combine with *cāng zhú* (苍术, *Rhizoma Atractylodis*) 9 g and *yì yǐ rén* (薏苡仁, *Semen Coicis*) 9 g.
- For excessive mucus in the feces, combine with *huáng lián* (黄连, *Rhizoma Coptidis*) 6 g, *huáng bǎi* (黄柏, *Cortex Phellodendri Chinensis*) 9 g and *bái tóu wēng* (白头翁, *Radix Pulsatillae*) 15 g.
- For fecal incontinence, combine with *ym yú liáng* (禹余粮, *Limonitum*) 12 g and *hē zǐ* (诃子, *Fructus Chebulae*) 9 g.

Yang deficiency of the spleen and kidneys

Signs and symptoms

Bowel sounds, abdominal pain, diarrhea before dawn mixed with mucus, cold limbs, soreness and weakness of the low back and knee joints, and a pale complexion.

Tongue: pale, with a thin white coating
Pulse: deep and thready

Treatment principle

Warm and tonify the spleen and kidneys, astringe the large intestine and arrest diarrhea.

Formula

Modified *Sì Shén Wán* (四神丸, "Four Spirits Pill") and *Fù Zǐ Lǐ Zhōng Wán* (附子理中丸, "Aconite Center-Regulating Pill")

附子	*fù zǐ*	9 g	*Radix Aconiti Lateralis* (decoct first)
补骨脂	*bǔ gǔ zhī*	9 g	*Fructus Psoraleae*
肉豆蔻	*ròu dòu kòu*	6 g	*Semen Myristicae*
五味子	*wǔ wèi zǐ*	6 g	*Fructus Schisandrae Chinensis*
吴茱萸	*wú zhū yú*	3 g	*Fructus Evodiae*
赤石脂	*chì shí zhī*	15 g	*Halloysitum Rubrum*
白术	*bái zhú*	9 g	*Rhizoma Atractylodis Macrocephalae*
炙甘草	*zhì gān cǎo*	6 g	*Radix et Rhizoma Glycyrrhizae Praeparata cum Melle*

Modifications

- For severe cold intolerance and cold limbs, combine with *ròu guì* (肉桂, *Cortex Cinnamomi*) 6 g and *gān jiāng* (干姜, *Rhizoma Zingiberis*) 6 g.
- For fecal incontinence with a prolapsed rectum, combine with *huáng qí* (黄芪, *Radix Astragali*) 15 g and *shēng má* (升麻, *Rhizoma Cimicifugae*) 9 g.

- For severe soreness and weakness of the low back and knee joints, combine with *ròu cōng róng* (肉苁蓉, *Herba Cistanches*) 9 g and *bā jǐ tiān* (巴戟天, *Radix Morindae Officinalis*) 9 g.

QUESTIONS

1. Describe the main clinical manifestations of chronic nonspecific ulcerative colitis.
2. Describe the pattern identification and treatment of ulcerative colitis in Chinese medicine.
3. *Case study*. Try to make a pattern identification and give a prescription for the following case:

Ms. Wang, 45, suffered from chronic diarrhea for five years and was diagnosed with chronic nonspecific ulcerative colitis. Three days prior to treatment, she experienced diarrhea due to emotional disturbance mixed with mucus. Other symptoms included abdominal pain, fullness and distension (the pain could be relieved after diarrhea), epigastric discomfort, frequent sighing and a poor appetite. The tongue was pale, with a thin white coating. The pulse was wiry and thready.

Cirrhosis of the Liver

Overview

Cirrhosis of the liver is a consequence of chronic progressive diffuse liver disease. It has many possible causes. It is characterized by replacement of liver tissue by fibrosis, scar tissue and regenerative nodules, leading to loss of liver function. According to causative factors, cirrhosis of the liver can be categorized into six patterns: posthepatitis cirrhosis, biliary cirrhosis, stasis cirrhosis, chemical cirrhosis, metabolic cirrhosis and trophic cirrhosis. Posthepatitis cirrhosis is more common in China. Common complications of this condition are heavy bleeding from the upper digestive tract, hepatic coma and liver cancer.

In Chinese medicine, cirrhosis of the liver falls under the category of "abdominal masses" and "abdominal tympanites". The main contributing factors include long-term jaundice, contraction of toxins, an improper diet and excessive consumption of alcohol. All these factors may cause internal accumulation of damp–heat in the liver and spleen, followed by stagnation of *qi* and blood. Over time, the kidneys can also be affected.

Clinical manifestations

Patients with cirrhosis of the liver in the early stages may not have any symptoms. Mild symptoms include a poor appetite, chest tightness, abdominal distension, belching, nausea, vomiting and dull pain in the right abdomen. However, in the later stages, nasal bleeding, gum bleeding, anemia, spider angiomata, palmar erythema, gynecomastia, irregular menstruation, ascites and splenomegaly may be present.

Pattern identification and treatment

Liver qi stagnation with spleen deficiency

Signs and symptoms

Fullness and distension in the hypochondriac regions, chest tightness, belching, a poor appetite, aggravated bloating after eating food, mental fatigue, lassitude and a sallow complexion.

Tongue: a thin white coating
Pulse: wiry

Treatment principle

Soothe the liver, regulate *qi* and strengthen the spleen (*qi*).

Formula

Modified *Chái Hú Shū Gān Sǎn* (柴胡疏肝散, "Bupleurum Liver-Soothing Powder") and *Sì Jūn Zǐ Tāng* (四君子汤, "Four Gentlemen Decoction").

柴胡	*chái hú*	9 g	*Radix Bupleuri*
枳壳	*zhǐ qiào*	9 g	*Fructus Aurantii*
白芍	*bái sháo*	9 g	*Radix Paeoniae Alba*
茯苓	*fú líng*	9 g	*Poria*
白术	*bái zhú*	9 g	*Rhizoma Atractylodis Macrocephalae*
川芎	*chuān xiōng*	9 g	*Rhizoma Chuanxiong*
香附	*xiāng fù*	9 g	*Rhizoma Cyperi*
鸡内金	*jī nèi jīn*	9 g	*Endothelium Corneum Gigeriae Galli*
甘草	*gān cǎo*	6 g	*Radix et Rhizoma Glycyrrhizae*

Modifications

- For chest tightness and a greasy tongue coating, combine with *cāng zhú* (苍术, *Rhizoma Atractylodis*) 9 g and *hòu pò* (厚朴, *Cortex Magnoliae Officinalis*) 9 g.
- For nausea and vomiting, combine with *jiāng bàn xià* (姜半夏, *Rhizoma Pinelliae Praeparatum*) 9 g and *jiāng zhú rú* (姜竹茹, *Caulis Bambusae in Taenia Praeparatum*) 9 g.
- For mental fatigue and lassitude, combine with *dǎng shēn* (党参, *Radix Codonopsis*) and *shān yào* (山药, *Rhizoma Dioscoreae*) 9 g.
- For intense pain in the hypochondriac regions, combine with *chén pí* (陈皮, *Pericarpium Citri Reticulatae*), *huáng lián* (黄连, *Rhizoma Coptidis*) 4.5 g and *chuān liàn zǐ* (川楝子, *Fructus Toosendan*) 9 g.

Qi stagnation and blood stasis

Signs and symptoms

Distending pain in the right hypochondriac region with palpable masses, bloating, frequent belching, a poor appetite, exposed veins in the neck and arms, nasal bleeding, gum bleeding and a dark-gray complexion.

Tongue: dark-red or with ecchymosis
Pulse: wiry and hesitant

Treatment principle

Circulate *qi*, invigorate blood, resolve stasis and unblock collaterals.

Formula

Modified *Huà Yū Tāng* (化瘀汤, "Stasis-Resolving Decoction").

当归	*dāng guī*	9 g	*Radix Angelicae Sinensis*
丹参	*dān shēn*	15 g	*Radix et Rhizoma Salviae Miltiorrhizae*
郁金	*yù jīn*	9 g	*Radix Curcumae*
桃仁	*táo rén*	9 g	*Semen Persicae*
红花	*hóng huā*	9 g	*Flos Carthami*
穿山甲	*chuān shān jiǎ*	15 g	*Squama Manitis* (decoct first)
青皮	*qīng pí*	9 g	*Pericarpium Citri Reticulatae Viride*
牡蛎	*mǔ lì*	30 g	*Concha Ostreae* (decoct first)
白术	*bái zhú*	9 g	*Rhizoma Atractylodis Macrocephalae*
赤芍	*chì sháo*	9 g	*Radix Paeoniae Rubra*
鳖甲煎丸	*Biē Jiǎ Jiān Wán*	9 g	*Turtle Shell Decocted Pill* (wrapped)

Modifications

- For severe pain in the hypochondriac regions, combine with *yán hú suǒ* (延胡索, *Rhizoma Corydalis*) 9 g and *chuān liàn zǐ* (川楝子, *Fructus Toosendan*) 9 g.
- For a dark-purple tongue or a tongue with ecchymosis, combine with *wǔ líng zhī* (五灵脂, *Faeces Trogopterori*) 9 g (wrapped) and *pú huáng* (蒲黄, *Pollen Typhae*) 9 g.
- For severe nasal and gum bleeding, combine with a powder of *sān qī* (三七, *Radix et Rhizoma Notoginseng*) 9 g and *huā ruǐ shí* (花蕊石, *Ophicalcitum*) 15 g, twice a day, 6 g for one treatment.

Damp–heat accumulation

Signs and symptoms

Drumlike abdominal distension with solid fullness by palpation, facial puffiness, edema in the limbs, chest tightness, a poor appetite, restlessness, a bitter taste, scanty dark-yellow urine and constipation or loose stools.

Tongue: red, with a yellow greasy coating
Pulse: wiry and rapid

Treatment principle

Clear heat, resolve dampness, promote urination and resolve edema.

Formula

Modified *Zhōng Mǎn Fēn Xiāo Wán* (中满分消丸, "Abdominal Fullness–Relieving Pill").

黄连	*huáng lián*	6 g	Rhizoma Coptidis
黄芩	*huáng qín*	9 g	Radix Scutellariae
枳实	*zhǐ shí*	9 g	Fructus Aurantii Immaturus
半夏	*bàn xià*	9 g	Rhizoma Pinelliae
陈皮	*chén pí*	9 g	Pericarpium Citri Reticulatae
猪苓	*zhū líng*	15 g	Polyporus
茯苓	*fú líng*	9 g	Poria
泽泻	*zé xiè*	15 g	Rhizoma Alismatis
山栀	*shān zhī*	9 g	Fructus Gardeniae
车前子	*chē qián zǐ*	30 g	Semen Plantaginis (wrapped)

Modifications

- For severe constipation, combine with *dà huáng* (大黄, *Radix et Rhizoma Rhei*) 15 g (decoct later).
- For yellow eyes and face, combine with *yīn chén* (茵陈, *Herba Artemisiae Scopariae*) 15 g and *jīn qián cǎo* (金钱草, *Herba Lysimachiae*) 30 g.
- For ascites with severe edema, combine with *bái chǒu* (白丑, *Semen Pharbitidis*) 6 g.
- For chest tightness and a greasy tongue coating, combine with *cāng zhú* (苍术, *Rhizoma Atractylodis*) 9 g and *hòu pò* (厚朴, *Cortex Magnoliae Officinalis*) 9 g.

Yang deficiency of the spleen and kidneys

Signs and symptoms

Drumlike abdominal distension, a sallow complexion, cold intolerance, cold limbs, mental fatigue, lassitude, a poor appetite, soreness and weakness of the lower back and knee joints, facial puffiness, edema in the limbs, scanty urine and loose stools.

Tongue: pale and swollen, with a thin white coating
Pulse: deep, thready and weak

Treatment principle

Warm and tonify the spleen and kidneys, circulate *qi* and promote urination.

Formula

Modified *Zhēn Wǔ Tāng* (真武汤, "True Warrior Decoction").

炮附子	*páo fù zǐ*	9 g	*Radix Aconiti Lateralis Praeparata* (decoct first)
茯苓	*fú líng*	9 g	*Poria*
白术	*bái zhú*	9 g	*Rhizoma Atractylodis Macrocephalae*
炮姜	*páo jiāng*	6 g	*Rhizoma Zingiberis Praeparatum*
白芍	*bái sháo*	9 g	*Radix Paeoniae Alba*
肉桂	*ròu guì*	3 g	*Cortex Cinnamomi* (decoct later)
车前子	*chē qián zǐ*	30 g	*Semen Plantaginis* (wrapped)
泽泻	*zé xiè*	15 g	*Rhizoma Alismatis*
大腹皮	*dà fù pí*	9 g	*Pericarpium Arecae*

Modifications

- For ascites with severe edema, combine with *zhū líng* (猪苓, *Polyporus*) 15 g and *hú lú* (葫芦, *Fructus Lagenariae*) 15 g.
- For severe cold intolerance and cold limbs, combine with *xiān máo* (仙茅, *Rhizoma Curculiginis*) 9 g and *xiān líng pí* (仙灵脾, *Herba Epimedii*) 12 g.
- For severe mental fatigue and lassitude, combine with *huáng qí* (黄芪, *Radix Astragali*) 15 g and *dǎng shēn* (党参, *Radix Codonopsis*) 9 g.
- For severe bloating, combine with *zhǐ shí* (枳实, *Fructus Aurantii Immaturus*) 9 g and *hòu pò* (厚朴, *Cortex Magnoliae Officinalis*) 9 g.

Yin deficiency of the liver and kidneys

Signs and symptoms

Drumlike abdominal distension, epigastric fullness and pain, soreness and weakness of the low back and knee joints, a dark complexion, feverish sensations on the soles and palms, a dry mouth and throat, nasal bleeding, scanty urine and unsmooth bowel movements.

Tongue: dark-red, with a scanty or peeled coating
Pulse: wiry, thready and rapid

Treatment principle

Nourish and tonify yin of the liver and kidneys, and promote urination.

Formula

Yī Guàn Jiān (一贯煎, "Effective Integration Decoction") and *Zhū Líng Tāng* (猪苓汤, "Polyporus Decoction").

北沙参	*běi shā shēn*	9 g	Radix Glehniae
麦冬	*mài dōng*	9 g	Radix Ophiopogonis
生地	*shēng dì*	12 g	Radix Rehmanniae
枸杞子	*gǒu qǐ zǐ*	9 g	Fructus Lycii
牡蛎	*mǔ lì*	30 g	Concha Ostreae
泽泻	*zé xiè*	15 g	Rhizoma Alismatis
猪苓	*zhū líng*	15 g	Polyporus
茯苓	*fú líng*	9 g	Poria
滑石	*huá shí*	15 g	Talcum (decoct first)
赤芍	*chì sháo*	9 g	Radix Paeoniae Rubra

Modifications

- For mental confusion, combine with *shí chāng pú* (石菖蒲, *Rhizoma Acori Tatarinowii*) 15 g and *yù jīn* (郁金, *Radix Curcumae*) 9 g.
- For unconsciousness, combine with one pill of *Ān Gōng Niú Huáng Wán* (安宫牛黄丸, "Peaceful Palace Bovine Bezoar Pill").

- For severe nasal and gum bleeding, combine with *sān qī* (三七, *Radix et Rhizoma Notoginseng*) 9 g and *bái jí* (白及, *Rhizoma Bletillae*) 9 g.
- For scanty urine, combine with *hú lú* (葫芦, *Fructus Lagenariae*) 15 g and *chē qián zǐ* (车前子, *Semen Plantaginis*) 30 g (wrapped).

QUESTIONS

1. Describe the main causative factors for cirrhosis of the liver in Chinese medicine.
2. Describe the main clinical manifestations of later-stage cirrhosis of the liver.
3. *Case study.* Try to make pattern identification and give a prescription for the following case:

Mr. Wang, 50, who had been suffering from hepatitis B for over 10 years, recently experienced distending pain in the right hypochondriac region with palpable masses. Other symptoms included frequent belching, a poor appetite, mental fatigue, exposed veins in the neck and arms, and a dark-gray complexion. The tongue was dark-purple, with a thin coating. The pulse was wiry and hesitant.

COMMON CIRCULATION SYSTEM CONDITIONS

Hypertension

Overview

Hypertension, or high blood pressure, is a chronic systemic vascular medical condition in which the arterial blood pressure, especially the diastolic pressure, is persistently elevated. It is classified as either primary (essential) or secondary. The cause of hypertension is still unidentified. However, other than genetic factors, there are many factors, such as sedentary lifestyle, smoking, stress, visceral obesity, salt (sodium) sensitivity, alcohol intake and vitamin D deficiency, that increase the risk of developing hypertension. It may also be associated with the age, occupation and environment. According to the onset, progression and duration, hypertension can be categorized into two patterns: chronic hypertension (also known as benign hypertension, affecting most cases) and accelerated hypertension (also known as malignant hypertension, affecting only 1%–5% of cases). Common complications of hypertension are stroke, hypertensive heart disease, heart failure and chronic kidney failure.

In Chinese medicine, hypertension falls under the category of "vertigo" and "headache". The main contributing factors are emotional disturbance, an improper diet and deficiency of the zang–fu organs.

Long-term mental stress or anger may cause liver *qi* stagnation which may over time transform into fire. Overexertion or aging may result in kidney yin deficiency and subsequent hyperactivity of liver yang. Excessive ingestion of sweet fatty food or consumption of alcohol may impair the spleen and stomach, leading to turbid dampness and heat. All these factors may eventually result in hypertension.

Clinical manifestations

The main symptoms of hypertension are dizziness, headache, distension of the head and elevated blood pressure. However, hypertension at the early stages can be asymptomatic. Often, patients realize that they have hypertension during a physical checkup, manifesting as elevation of both the systolic and the diastolic pressure. The condition can be aggravated by emotions and fatigue but is relieved by an adequate rest. In the middle or later stages, the elevation may become stabilized within a certain range, especially the elevation of diastolic pressure. Owing to recurrent spasm of the general small arteries and hardening of the arterial walls due to deposition of lipids, ischemic changes of the heart, brain and kidneys may be present, leading to headache with a sense of distension, dizziness, tinnitus, palpitations, insomnia, restlessness and irritability. In severe cases, severe headache, nausea, vomiting, polyuria or anuria, coma and convulsions may be present.

Pattern identification and treatment

Hyperactivity of liver yang

Signs and symptoms

Headache with a sense of distension, vertigo, tinnitus, restlessness, irritability, red face and eyes, a dry mouth with a bitter taste and constipation.

Tongue: red, with a yellow coating
Pulse: wiry

Treatment principle

Soothe the liver and suppress yang.

Formula

Modified *Tiān Má Gōu Téng Yǐn* (天麻钩藤饮, "Gastrodia and Uncaria Beverage").

天麻	*tiān má*	9 g	*Rhizoma Gastrodiae*
钩藤	*gōu téng*	12 g	*Ramulus Uncariae Cum Uncis* (decoct later)
石决明	*shí jué míng*	30 g	*Concha Haliotidis*
山栀	*shān zhī*	9 g	*Fructus Gardeniae*
黄芩	*huáng qín*	9 g	*Radix Scutellariae*
杜仲	*dù zhòng*	9 g	*Cortex Eucommiae*
牛膝	*niú xī*	9 g	*Radix Achyranthis Bidentatae*
桑寄生	*sāng jì shēng*	15 g	*Herba Taxilli*
茯神	*fú shén*	9 g	*Sclerotium Poriae Pararadicis*
夜交藤	*yè jiāo téng*	30 g	*Caulis Polygoni Multiflori*

Modifications

- For a severe bitter taste, and red face and eyes, combine with *lóng dǎn cǎo* (龙胆草, *Radix et Rhizoma Gentianae*) 12 g and *xià kū cǎo* (夏枯草, *Spica Prunellae*) 9 g.
- For constipation, combine with *dà huáng* (大黄, *Radix et Rhizoma Rhei*) 9 g.
- For coma with convulsions, combine with a powder of *líng yáng jiǎo* (羚羊角, *Cornu Saigae Tataricae*) 3 g.
- For restlessness with insomnia, combine with *zhēn zhū mǔ* (珍珠母, *Concha Margaritiferae Usta*) 30 g and *wǔ wèi zǐ* (五味子, *Fructus Schisandrae Chinensis*) 9 g.

Hyperactivity of yang due to yin deficiency

Signs and symptoms

Headache with a sense of distension, vertigo, tinnitus, palpitations, restlessness, insomnia, poor memory, feverish sensations on the palms and soles, and soreness and weakness of the low back and knee joints.

Tongue: red, with a thin coating
Pulse: wiry, thready and rapid

Treatment principle

Nourish yin and suppress yang.

Formula

Modified *Qǐ Jú Dì Huáng Wán* (杞菊地黄丸, "Lycium Berry, Chrysanthemum and Rehmannia Pill") and *Zhèn Gān Xī Fēng Tāng* (镇肝息风汤, "Liver-Sedating and Wind-Extinguishing Decoction").

枸杞子	*gǒu qǐ zǐ*	9 g	*Fructus Lycii*
熟地黄	*shú dì huáng*	9 g	*Radix Rehmanniae Praeparata*
山茱萸	*shān zhū yú*	9 g	*Fructus Corni*
山药	*shān yào*	15 g	*Rhizoma Dioscoreae*
茯神	*fú shén*	9 g	*Sclerotium Poriae Pararadicis*
牡丹皮	*mǔ dān pí*	9 g	*Cortex Moutan*
钩藤	*gōu téng*	12 g	*Ramulus Uncariae Cum Uncis* (decoct later)
菊花	*jú huā*	9 g	*Flos Chrysanthemi*
炙龟板	*zhì guī bǎn*	12 g	*Plastrum Testudinis Preparata*
牡蛎	*mǔ lì*	30 g	*Concha Ostreae*
桑寄生	*sāng jì shēng*	15 g	*Herba Taxilli*

Modifications

- For a severe headache with vertigo, combine with *tiān má* (天麻, *Rhizoma Gastrodiae*) 9 g and *shí jué míng* (石决明, *Concha Haliotidis*) 30 g (decoct first).
- For dry stools, combine with *má rén* (麻仁, *Fructus Cannabis*) 9 g and *yù lǐ rén* (郁李仁, *Semen Pruni*) 9 g.

- For a dry mouth with a desire to drink water, combine with *shēng dì* (生地, *Radix Rehmanniae*) 15 g and *mài dōng* (麦冬, *Radix Ophiopogonis*) 9 g.
- For a dark-purple tongue, combine with *dān shēn* (丹参, *Radix et Rhizoma Salviae Miltiorrhizae*) 9 g and *yì mǔ cǎo* (益母草, *Herba Leonuri*) 15 g.

Yin deficiency of the liver and kidneys

Signs and symptoms

Dizziness, blurred vision, poor sleep or dream-disturbed sleep, palpitations, tinnitus, feverish sensations of the palms, soles and chest, a dry mouth with a desire to drink water and occasional night sweats.

Tongue: red, with no or a scanty coating
Pulse: wiry, thready and rapid

Treatment principle

Nourish and tonify the liver and kidneys.

Formula

Modified *Liù Wèi Dì Huáng Wán* (六味地黄丸, "Six Ingredients Rehmannia Pill").

熟地黄	*shú dì huáng*	9 g	*Radix Rehmanniae Praeparata*
山茱萸	*shān zhū yú*	9 g	*Fructus Corni*
山药	*shān yào*	15 g	*Rhizoma Dioscoreae*
牡丹皮	*mǔ dān pí*	9 g	*Cortex Moutan*
茯神	*fú shén*	9 g	*Sclerotium Poriae Pararadicis*
泽泻	*zé xiè*	9 g	*Rhizoma Alismatis*
枸杞子	*gǒu qǐ zǐ*	9 g	*Fructus Lycii*
炙龟板	*zhì guī bǎn*	12 g	*Plastrum Testudinis Preparata*
牛膝	*niú xī*	9 g	*Radix Achyranthis Bidentatae*

Modifications

- For severe vertigo, combine with *zhēn zhū mǔ* (珍珠母, *Concha Margaritiferae Usta*) 30 g and *gōu téng* (钩藤, *Ramulus Uncariae Cum Uncis*) 12 g (decoct later).
- For restlessness and insomnia, combine with *lián zǐ xīn* (莲子心, *Plumula Nelumbinis*) 9 g and *yè jiāo téng* (夜交藤, *Caulis Polygoni Multiflori*) 15 g.
- For a severe dry mouth, combine with *mài dōng* (麦冬, *Radix Ophiopogonis*) 9 g and *shí hú* (石斛, *Caulis Dendrobii*) 9 g.
- For dry stools, combine with *má rén* (麻仁, *Fructus Cannabis*) 9 g and *yù lǐ rén* (郁李仁, *Semen Pruni*) 9 g.

Exuberance of phlegm dampness

Signs and symptoms

A heavy cloth-wrapping sensation of the head, dizziness with a sense of distension, chest fullness, restlessness, insomnia, a poor appetite, nausea, vomiting and excessive salivation.

Tongue: swollen, with a greasy coating
Pulse: wiry and slippery

Treatment principle

Dry dampness and resolve phlegm.

Formula

Modified *Bàn Xià Bái Zhú Tiān Má Tāng* (半夏白术天麻汤, "Pinellia, Atractylodes Macrocephala and Gastrodia Decoction").

天麻	tiān má	9 g	Rhizoma Gastrodiae
白术	bái zhú	9 g	Rhizoma Atractylodis Macrocephalae
半夏	bàn xià	9 g	Rhizoma Pinelliae
橘红	jú hóng	9 g	Exocarpium Citri Rubrum
茯苓	fú líng	9 g	Poria
石菖蒲	shí chāng pú	9 g	Rhizoma Acori Tatarinowii
钩藤	gōu téng	12 g	Ramulus Uncariae Cum Uncis (decoct later)
甘草	gān cǎo	9 g	Radix et Rhizoma Glycyrrhizae

Modifications

- For severe nausea and vomiting, combine with *xuán fù huā* (旋覆花, *Flos Inulae*) 9 g (wrapped) and *dài zhē shí* (代赭石, *Haematitum*)15 g (decoct first).
- For coughing with profuse sputum, combine with *dǎn nán xīng* (胆南星, *Arisaema cum Bile*) 9 g and *guā lóu* (瓜蒌, *Fructus Trichosanthis*) 15 g.
- For chest fullness and a greasy tongue coating, combine with *cāng zhú* (苍术, Rhizoma Atractylodis) 9 g and *hòu pò* (厚朴, *Cortex Magnoliae Officinalis*) 9 g.
- For a severe bitter taste and restlessness, combine with *huáng lián* (黄连, *Rhizoma Coptidis*) 4.5 g and *zhú yè* (竹叶, *Folium Phyllostachydis Henonis*) 9 g.

Deficiency of yin and yang

Signs and symptoms

Headache, vertigo, tinnitus (cicada ringing), mild or severe palpitations, shortness of breath upon physical exertion, soreness and weakness of the low back and knee joints, and muscle twitching.

Tongue: pale or red, with a thin coating
Pulse: wiry and thready

Treatment principle

Nourish yin and supplement yang.

Formula

Modified *Èr Xiān Tāng* (二仙汤, "*Chong* and *Ren*–Regulating Decoction").

仙茅	*xiān máo*	9 g	*Rhizoma Curculiginis*
仙灵脾	*xiān líng pí*	15 g	*Herba Epimedii*
当归	*dāng guī*	9 g	*Radix Angelicae Sinensis*
黄柏	*huáng bǎi*	9 g	*Cortex Phellodendri Chinensis*
巴戟天	*bā jǐ tiān*	9 g	*Radix Morindae Officinalis*
绿豆衣	*lǜ dòu yī*	9 g	*Testa Glycinis*
白蒺藜	*bái jí lí*	12 g	*Fructus Tribuli*

Modifications

- For feverish sensations of the hands and feet, and a severe dry mouth and throat, combine with *guī bǎn* (龟板, *Plastrum Testudinis*) 15 g (decoct first) and *gǒu qǐ zǐ* (枸杞子, *Fructus Lycii*) 9 g.
- For cold intolerance and cold limbs, and clear profuse urine, combine with *lù jiǎo* (鹿角, *Cornu Cervi*) 9 g (decoct first) and *dù zhòng* (杜仲, *Cortex Eucommiae*) 9 g.
- For mild or severe palpitations, combine with *duàn lóng gǔ* (煅龙骨, *Os Draconis Praeparatum*) 15 g (decoct first) and *duàn mǔ lì* (煅牡蛎, *Concha Ostreae Praeparatum*) 15 g (decoct first).

QUESTIONS

1. Describe the common complications of hypertension.
2. How do you understand the causative factors of hypertension in Chinese medicine?
3. *Case study*. Try to make a pattern identification and give a prescription for the following case:

Mr. Zhuang, 40, suffered from recent dizziness, headache with a sense of distension, restlessness, irritability, red face and eyes, a dry mouth with a bitter taste and dry stools. The tongue was red, with a thin yellow coating. The pulse was wiry.

Atherosclerotic Coronary Heart Disease

Overview

Atherosclerotic coronary heart disease, also known as coronary artery disease, develops when the coronary arteries become narrowed or hardened, resulting in myocardial ischemia or anoxia. According to the position, extension and severity, this condition can be categorized into five patterns: latent or asymptomatic coronary heart disease, angina, myocardial infarction, myocardial fibrosis and sudden death. Coronary artery disease often develops above the age of 40, affecting more men than women, especially brain workers.

In Chinese medicine, this condition falls under the category of "chest *qi* impediment," "chest pain" or "cardiac pain." The main contributing factors include kidney *qi* deficiency due to aging, impairment of the spleen and stomach due to overingestion of sweet fatty food, *qi* stagnation and blood stasis due to emotional disturbance, and blockage of chest yang following contraction of cold.

Failure of the spleen and stomach to transport and transform may produce internal phlegm dampness to block the heart collaterals. Kidney yang (*qi*) deficiency may also cause heart yang deficiency, and coupled with contraction of cold may obstruct the circulation of heart blood. Emotional disturbance may cause liver *qi* stagnation and subsequent blood stasis.

Clinical manifestations

The main symptoms of coronary artery disease are chest tightness, chest pain and palpitations. In mild cases, patients may experience only a suffocating sensation with unsmooth breathing. In severe cases, patients may experience cardiac pain radiating to the back with profuse sweating. The pain is often located behind the sternum or in the left chest, possibly radiating to the left shoulder, arm, neck and gastric region. Each episode lasts a couple of minutes to dozens of minutes. Palpitations are often present along with chest tightness and chest pain.

Pattern identification and treatment

Cold retention in the heart vessels

Signs and symptoms

Chest pain that can be aggravated by cold, palpitations, shortness of breath, cold limbs and pallor; in severe cases, cardiac pain radiating to the back or vice versa may be present.

Tongue: pale, with a thin white coating
Pulse: wiry and tense

Treatment principle

Unblock yang, warm the meridians and dissipate cold.

Formula

Modified *Dāng Guī Sì Nì Tāng* (当归四逆汤, "Chinese Angelica Frigid Extremities Decoction").

当归	*dāng guī*	9 g	*Radix Angelicae Sinensis*
桂枝	*guì zhī*	9 g	*Ramulus Cinnamomi*
细辛	*xì xīn*	3 g	*Radix et Rhizoma Asari*
炙甘草	*zhì gān cǎo*	9 g	*Radix et Rhizoma Glycyrrhizae Praeparata cum Melle*
通草	*tōng cǎo*	9 g	*Medulla Tetrapanacis*
枳壳	*zhǐ qiào*	9 g	*Fructus Aurantii*
薤白	*xiè bái*	9 g	*Bulbus Allii Macrostemi*

Modifications

- For a severe chest pain, combine with *zhì chuān wū* (制川乌, *Radix Aconiti Praeparata*) 9 g and *chì shí zhī* (赤石脂, *Halloysitum Rubrum*) 12 g (decoct first).
- For nausea and vomiting, combine with *wú zhū yú* (吴茱萸, *Fructus Evodiae*) 6 g, *bàn xià* (半夏, *Rhizoma Pinelliae*) 9 g and *chén pí* (陈皮, *Pericarpium Citri Reticulatae*) 9 g.
- For cold intolerance and cold limbs, combine with *páo fù zǐ* (炮附子, *Radix Aconiti Lateralis Praeparata*) 6 g (decoct first) and *ròu guì* (肉桂, *Cortex Cinnamomi*) 4.5 g (decoct later).

Liver qi stagnation

Signs and symptoms

Chest fullness with migratory pain that can radiate to the shoulder and chest (the pain can be aggravated by emotions or anger) shortness of breath, fatigue and frequent sighing.

Tongue: pale, with a thin white coating

Pulse: wiry and tense

Treatment principle

Formula

Modified *Chái Hú Shū Gān Săn* (柴胡疏肝散, "Bupleurum Liver-Soothing Powder").

柴胡	*chái hú*	9 g	*Radix Bupleuri*
白芍	*bái sháo*	9 g	*Radix Paeoniae Alba*
陈皮	*chén pí*	9 g	*Pericarpium Citri Reticulatae*
川芎	*chuān xiōng*	12 g	*Rhizoma Chuanxiong*
甘草	*gān cǎo*	6 g	*Radix et Rhizoma Glycyrrhizae*
枳壳	*zhǐ qiào*	9 g	*Fructus Aurantii*
香附	*xiāng fù*	9 g	*Rhizoma Cyperi*
郁金	*yù jīn*	9 g	*Radix Curcumae*

Modifications

- For a severe chest pain, combine with *yán hú suǒ* (延胡索, *Rhizoma Corydalis*) 9 g and *chuān liàn zǐ* (川楝子, *Fructus Toosendan*) 9 g.
- For a tongue with ecchymosis, combine with *yán hú suǒ* (延胡索, *Rhizoma Corydalis*) 9 g and *chuān liàn zǐ* (川楝子, *Fructus Toosendan*) 9 g.
- For chest tightness and a greasy tongue coating, combine with *cāng zhú* (苍术, *Rhizoma Atractylodis*) 9 g and *hòu pò* (厚朴, *Cortex Magnoliae Officinalis*) 9 g.
- For a dry mouth with a bitter taste, combine with *huáng lián* (黄连, *Rhizoma Coptidis*) 3 g and *shān zhī* (山栀, *Fructus Gardeniae*) 9 g.

Heart blood stasis

Signs and symptoms

A stabbing chest pain in a fixed position (especially at night), palpitations, restlessness, insomnia and a dark complexion.

Tongue: dark, purple or with ecchymosis
Pulse: wiry and hesitant

Treatment principle

Invigorate blood, resolve stasis, unblock collaterals and relieve pain.

Formula

Modified *Xuè Fŭ Zhú Yū Tāng* (血府逐瘀汤, "Blood Stasis–Expelling Decoction").

柴胡	*chái hú*	9 g	*Radix Bupleuri*
赤芍	*chì sháo*	9 g	*Radix Paeoniae Rubra*
枳壳	*zhǐ qiào*	9 g	*Fructus Aurantii*
当归	*dāng guī*	9 g	*Radix Angelicae Sinensis*
川芎	*chuān xiōng*	9 g	*Rhizoma Chuanxiong*
桃仁	*táo rén*	9 g	*Semen Persicae*
红花	*hóng huā*	9 g	*Flos Carthami*
甘草	*gān cǎo*	9 g	*Radix et Rhizoma Glycyrrhizae*
丹参	*dān shēn*	15 g	*Radix et Rhizoma Salviae Miltiorrhizae*
桔梗	*Jié gěng*	6 g	*Radix Platycodonis*

Modifications

- For intense chest pain, combine with *rŭ xiāng* (乳香, *Olibanum*) 6 g, *mò yào* (水蛭, *Myrrha*) 6 g and *shuĭ zhì* (水蛭, *Hirudo*) 6 g.
- For distension in the hypochondriac regions, combine with *xiāng fù* (香附, *Rhizoma Cyperi*) 9 g and *chuān liàn zǐ* (川楝子, *Fructus Toosendan*) 9 g.
- For a dry mouth with a bitter taste, combine with *huáng lián* (黄连, *Rhizoma Coptidis*) 3 g and *shān zhī* (山栀, *Fructus Gardeniae*) 9 g.
- For constipation, combine with *má rén* (麻仁, *Fructus Cannabis*) 9 g and *yù lĭ rén* (郁李仁, *Semen Pruni*) 9 g.

Phlegm turbidity blocking chest yang

Signs and symptoms

Chest tightness and pain, obesity, a general heavy sensation, fatigue, panting, shortness of breath, profuse sticky sputum, nausea and a poor appetite.
Tongue coating: thick, greasy or turbid
Pulse: wiry and slippery

Treatment principle

Resolve phlegm, discharge turbidity and unblock yang.

Formula

Modified *Guā Lóu Xiè Bái Bái Jiǔ Tāng* (瓜蒌薤白白酒汤, "Trichosanthes, Chinese Chives and White Wine Decoction").

瓜蒌	*guā lóu*	15 g	*Fructus Trichosanthis*
薤白	*xiè bái*	9 g	*Bulbus Allii Macrostemi*
茯苓	*fú líng*	9 g	*Poria*
半夏	*bàn xià*	9 g	*Rhizoma Pinelliae*
陈皮	*chén pí*	9 g	*Pericarpium Citri Reticulatae*
厚朴	*hòu pò*	9 g	*Cortex Magnoliae Officinalis*
石菖蒲	*shí chāng pú*	9 g	*Rhizoma Acori Tatarinowii*

Modifications

- For epigastric fullness with a sense of *qi* ascending, combine with *zhǐ shí* (枳实, *Fructus Aurantii Immaturus*) 9 g and *guì zhī* (桂枝, *Ramulus Cinnamomi*) 9 g.
- For yellow sticky sputum, combine with *chuān bèi mǔ* (川贝母, *Bulbus Fritillariae Cirrhosae*) 9 g, *zhú rú* (竹茹, *Caulis Bambusae in Taenia*) 9 g and *huáng lián* (黄连, *Rhizoma Coptidis*) 3 g.
- For severe chest tightness and pain due to an impediment to chest yang, combine with one pill of *Sū Hé Xiāng Wán* (苏合香丸, "Storax Pill") (swallow).

Deficiency of qi and yin

Signs and symptoms

Intermittent dull or burning chest pain, mild or severe palpitations, shortness of breath, fatigue, restlessness, poor sleep, a dry mouth, night sweats and spontaneous sweating.

Tongue: red, with no or a scanty coating
Pulse: wiry, thready and possibly rapid

Treatment principle

Supplement *qi*, nourish yin and tonify heart vessels.

Formula

Modified *Shēng Mài Sǎn* (生脉散, "Pulse-Engendering Powder").

太子参	*tài zǐ shēn*	12 g	*Radix Pseudostellariae*
麦冬	*mài dōng*	15 g	*Radix Ophiopogonis*
五味子	*wǔ wèi zǐ*	9 g	*Fructus Schisandrae Chinensis*
生地	*Shēng dì*	15 g	*Radix Rehmanniae*
炙甘草	*zhì gān cǎo*	9 g	*Radix et Rhizoma Glycyrrhizae Praeparata cum Melle*
桂枝	*guì zhī*	9 g	*Ramulus Cinnamomi*
白芍	*bái sháo*	9 g	*Radix Paeoniae Alba*

Modifications

- For severe palpitations, combine with *suān zǎo rén* (酸枣仁, *Semen Ziziphi Spinosae*) 9 g and *bǎi zǐ rén* (柏子仁, *Semen Platycladi*) 9 g.
- For severe chest pain, combine with *yù jīn* (郁金, *Radix Curcumae*) 9 g and *chén xiāng* (沉香, *Lignum Aquilariae Resinatum*) 3 g.
- For a dry mouth and constipation, combine with *yù zhú* (玉竹, *Rhizoma Polygonati Odorati*) 9 g and *má rén* (麻仁, *Fructus Cannabis*) 9 g.
- For restlessness with severe insomnia, combine with *zhī mǔ* (知母, *Rhizoma Anemarrhenae*) 9 g and *lián zǐ xīn* (莲子心, *Plumula Nelumbinis*) 9 g.

Kidney yang deficiency

Signs and symptoms

Cardiac pain, shortness of breath, mental fatigue, pallor, cold limbs, soreness and weakness of the low back and knee joints, and clear profuse urine.

Tongue: pale, with a white coating
Pulse: deep, thready and weak

Treatment principle

Warm kidney yang and invigorate heart blood.

Formula

Modified *Jīn Guì Shèn Qì Wán* (金匮肾气丸, "Golden Cabinet's Kidney *Qi* Pill").

制附子	*zhì fù zǐ*	9 g	*Radix Aconiti Lateralis Praeparata* (decoct first)
肉桂	*ròu guì,*	6 g	*Cortex Cinnamomi* (decoct later)
山茱萸	*shān zhū yú*	9 g	*Fructus Corni*
熟地黄	*shú dì huáng*	9 g	*Radix Rehmanniae Praeparata*
山药	*shān yào*	15 g	*Rhizoma Dioscoreae*
牡丹皮	*mǔ dān pí*	9 g	*Cortex Moutan*
茯苓	*fú líng*	9 g	*Poria*
杜仲	*dù zhòng*	9 g	*Cortex Eucommiae*

Modifications

- For severe chest pain, combine with *zhì chuān wū* (制川乌, *Radix Aconiti Praeparata*) 9 g and *gāo liáng jiāng* (高良姜, *Rhizoma Alpiniae Officinarum*) 9 g.
- For severe palpitations and insomnia, combine with *lóng gǔ* (龙骨, *Os Draconis*) 30 g (decoct first) and *mǔ lì* (牡蛎, *Concha Ostreae*) 30 g (decoct first).

- For impotence and premature ejaculations, combine with *xiān máo* (仙茅, *Rhizoma Curculiginis*) 9 g and *xiān líng pí* (仙灵脾, *Herba Epimedii*) 9 g.
- For facial puffiness and edema in the eyelids, combine with *chē qián zǐ* (车前子, *Semen Plantaginis*) 30 g and *zhū líng* (猪苓, *Polyporus*) 15 g.

Collapse of yang–qi

Signs and symptoms

Chest pain, profuse sweating, cold limbs, pallor and apathy or mental confusion.

Tongue: pale, with a white coating
Pulse: thready and faint

Treatment principle

Resuscitate yang and supplement *qi*.

Formula

Modified *Shēn Fù Lóng Mǔ Tāng* (参附龙牡汤, "Ginseng, Aconite *Os Draconis* and *Concha Ostreae* Decoction").

人参	*rén shēn*	9 g	*Radix et Rhizoma Ginseng* (decoct separately)
制附子	*zhì fù zǐ*	9 g	*Radix Aconiti Lateralis Praeparata* (decoct first)
龙骨	*lóng gǔ*	30 g	*Os Draconis* (decoct first)
牡蛎	*mǔ lì*	30 g	*Concha Ostreae* (decoct first)
炙甘草	*zhì gān cǎo*	9 g	*Radix et Rhizoma Glycyrrhizae Praeparata cum Melle*
黄芪	*huáng qí*	30 g	*Radix Astragali*
五味子	*wǔ wèi zǐ*	9 g	*Fructus Schisandrae Chinensis*
肉桂	*ròu guì,*	4.5 g	*Cortex Cinnamomi* (decoct later)

Modifications

- For a bluish-purple complexion with difficulty in breathing, combine with *chén xiāng* (沉香, *Lignum Aquilariae Resinatum*) 3 g and *Hēi Xī Dān* (黑锡丹, *Galenite Elixir*) 6 g (swallow).
- For a severe chest pain, combine with *yán hú suō* (延胡索, *Rhizoma Corydalis*) 9 g and *dān shēn* (丹参, *Radix et Rhizoma Salviae Miltiorrhizae*) 9 g.

QUESTIONS

1. Describe the common complications of coronary artery disease.
2. List the pattern identifications and treatment methods of coronary artery disease in Chinese medicine.
3. *Case study.* Try to make a pattern identification and give a prescription for the following case:

Mr. Zhang, 65, suffered from chest tightness and pain for 20 years and was diagnosed with coronary artery disease. Three days prior to treatment following a cold attack, he experienced chest pain radiating to the back, shortness of breath, fatigue, palpitations and cold limbs. The tongue was pale, with a thin white coating. The pulse was wiry and tense.

Viral Myocarditis

Overview

Viral myocarditis is inflammation of the heart muscle (myocardium) following viral infections, most commonly by the viruses that can cause intestinal and upper respiratory tract infections. This condition can develop at any age, but more commonly in young adults, and more men than women suffer from it.

In Chinese medicine, viral myocarditis falls under the category of "palpitations." The main contributing factors include deficiency of antipathogenic *qi*, contraction of external damp–heat and toxins affecting the heart.

Clinical manifestations

The main symptoms of viral myocarditis are palpitations, chest tightness, chest pain and arrhythmias. However, the signs and symptoms may vary greatly, from an absence of symptoms to sudden death, depending on the severity and area. Most patients have a history of symptoms consistent with a recent viral infection, including chills, fever, general discomfort, a sore throat, coughing, abdominal pain and diarrhea. After this, palpitations, chest tightness, shortness of breath, fatigue, dull chest pain, dizziness, nausea and arrhythmias may be present. In rare cases, syncope or Adams–Strokes syndrome may be present. In some cases, the condition may develop rapidly, leading to heart failure, cardiogenic shock or even sudden death.

Pattern identification and treatment

Wind–cold attacking the heart

Signs and symptoms

Fever, chills, headache, nasal congestion, coughing with scanty sputum, pain of the bones and limbs, chest tightness and discomfort, palpitations and shortness of breath.

Tongue: a thin white or slightly yellow coating
Pulse: floating and regularly/irregularly intermittent

Treatment principle

Expel wind, dissipate cold and calm the mind.

Formula

Modified *Jīng Fáng Bài Dú Sǎn* (荆防败毒散, "Schizonepeta and Saposhnikovia Toxin–Resolving Powder").

荆芥	*jīng jiè*	9 g	*Herba Schizonepetae*
防风	*fáng fēng*	9 g	*Radix Saposhnikoviae*
羌活	*qiāng huó*	9 g	*Rhizoma et Radix Notopterygii*
独活	*Dú huó*	9 g	*Radix Angelicae Pubescentis*

茯神	*Fú shén*	9 g	*Sclerotium Poriae Pararadicis*
前胡	*qián hú*	9 g	*Radix Peucedani*
枳壳	*zhǐ qiào*	9 g	*Fructus Aurantii*
桔梗	*Jié gěng*	6 g	*Radix Platycodonis*
丹参	*dān shēn*	15 g	*Radix et Rhizoma Salviae Miltiorrhizae*
甘草	*gān cǎo*	9 g	*Radix et Rhizoma Glycyrrhizae*

Modifications

- For headache with pain of the bones, combine with *guì zhī* (桂枝, *Ramulus Cinnamomi*) 6 g and *bái zhǐ* (白芷, *Radix Angelicae Dahuricae*) 9 g.
- For a dry mouth with a bitter taste, combine with *jīn yín huā* (金银花, *Flos Lonicerae Japonicae*) 9 g and *lián qiào* (连翘, *Fructus Forsythiae*) 9 g.
- For severe coughing, combine with *chuān bèi mǔ* (川贝母, *Bulbus Fritillariae Cirrhosae*) 9 g and *zǐ wǎn* (紫菀, *Radix et Rhizoma Asteris*) 9 g.
- For severe palpitations, combine with *suān zǎo rén* (酸枣仁, *Semen Ziziphi Spinosae*) 9 g and *yuǎn zhì* (远志, *Radix Polygalae*) 9 g.

Wind–heat attacking the heart

Signs and symptoms

Fever with or without sweating, headache, coughing, a dry mouth with a sore throat, palpitations and chest tightness.

Tongue: red, with a thin yellow coating
Pulse: floating, rapid and regularly/irregularly intermittent

Treatment principle

Clear heat, expel wind and calm the mind.

Formula

Modified *Yín Qiào Sǎn* (银翘散, "Lonicera and Forsythia Powder").

金银花	jīn yín huā	9 g	Flos Lonicerae Japonicae
连翘	lián qiào	9 g	Fructus Forsythiae
黄连	huáng lián	3 g	Rhizoma Coptidis
黄芩	huáng qín	9 g	Radix Scutellariae
牛蒡子	niú bàng zǐ	9 g	Fructus Arctii
桑叶	sāng yè	9 g	Folium Mori
山栀	shān zhī	9 g	Fructus Gardeniae
丹参	dān shēn	15 g	Radix et Rhizoma Salviae Miltiorrhizae
麦冬	mài dōng	9 g	Radix Ophiopogonis
柏子仁	bǎi zǐ rén	9 g	Semen Platycladi

Modifications

- For constipation, combine with *dà huáng* (大黄, *Radix et Rhizoma Rhei*) 9 g (decoct later) and *máng xiāo* (芒硝, *Natrii Sulfas*) 9 g.
- For severe palpitations, combine with *suān zǎo rén* (酸枣仁, *Semen Ziziphi Spinosae*) 9 g and *yè jiāo téng* (夜交藤, *Caulis Polygoni Multiflori*) 15 g.
- For a severe sore throat, combine with *shè gān* (射干, (*Rhizoma Belamcandae*) 6 g and *jié gěng* (桔梗, *Radix Platycodonis*) 6 g.
- For a dry mouth with a desire to drink water, combine with *shēng dì* (生地, *Radix Rehmanniae*) 12 g and *shí hú* (石斛, *Caulis Dendrobii*) 9 g.

Toxic cold retention in the heart

Signs and symptoms

Chills, fever, absence of sweating, general pain, ache of the bones and joints, a clear nasal discharge, coughing with white sputum, chest tightness and pain, palpitations and panting.

Tongue: pale, with a thin white coating
Pulse: floating, slow and regularly/irregularly intermittent

Treatment principle

Dissipate cold and warm the heart.

Formula

Modified *Má Huáng Fù Zǐ Xì Xīn Tāng* (麻黄附子细辛汤, "Ephedra, Aconite and Asarum Decoction").

麻黄	*má huáng*	9 g	Herba Ephedrae
炮附子	*páo fù zǐ*	9 g	Radix Aconiti Lateralis Praeparata (decoct first)
细辛	*xì xīn*	3 g	Radix et Rhizoma Asari
桂枝	*guì zhī*	9 g	Ramulus Cinnamomi
丹参	*dān shēn*	15 g	Radix et Rhizoma Salviae Miltiorrhizae
瓜蒌	*guā lóu*	15 g	Fructus Trichosanthis

Modifications

- For severe chest tightness and pain, combine with *yù jīn* (郁金, *Radix Curcumae*) 9 g and *xiè bái* (薤白, *Bulbus Allii Macrostemi*) 9 g.
- For coughing with profuse sputum, combine with *jiāng bàn xià* (姜半夏, *Rhizoma Pinelliae Praeparatum*) 9 g and *jiāng zhú rú* (姜竹茹, *Caulis Bambusae in Taenia Praeparatum*) 9 g.
- For severe palpitations, combine with *suān zǎo rén* (酸枣仁, *Semen Ziziphi Spinosae*) 9 g and *bǎi zǐ rén* (柏子仁, *Semen Platycladi*) 9 g.
- For a significant general pain, combine with *qiāng huó* (羌活, *Rhizoma et Radix Notopterygii*) 9 g and *dú huó* (独活, *Radix Angelicae Pubescentis*) 9 g.

Phlegm dampness obstructing the heart

Signs and symptoms

Chest tightness, shortness of breath, palpitations, a general heavy sensation, fatigue, dizziness, a poor appetite, gastric and abdominal fullness, and loose stools.

Tongue: pale and swollen, with a white, slippery or greasy coating
Pulse: slippery and regularly/irregularly intermittent

Treatment principle

Resolve phlegm, remove dampness and unblock heart collaterals.

Formula

Modified *Wēn Dǎn Tāng* (温胆汤, "Gallbladder-Warming Decoction").

半夏	*bàn xià*	9 g	*Rhizoma Pinelliae*
陈皮	*chén pí*	9 g	*Pericarpium Citri Reticulatae*
枳壳	*zhǐ qiào*	9 g	*Fructus Aurantii*
竹茹	*zhú rú*	9 g	*Caulis Bambusae in Taenia*
茯神	*fú shén*	9 g	*Sclerotium Poriae Pararadicis*
苍术	*cāng zhú*	12 g	*Rhizoma Atractylodis*
川朴	*chuān pò*	9 g	*Cortex Magnoliae Officinalis*
丹参	*dān shēn*	15 g	*Radix et Rhizoma Salviae Miltiorrhizae*

Modifications

- For severe chest tightness due to dampness, combine with *zǐ sū gěng* (紫苏梗, *Caulis Perillae*) 9 g and *huò xiāng* (藿香, *Herba Agastachis*) 9 g.
- For a severe poor appetite, combine with *jī nèi jīn* (鸡内金, *Endothelium Corneum Gigeriae Galli*) 9 g and *mài yá* (麦芽, *Fructus Hordei Germinatus*) 12 g.
- For severe palpitations, combine with *yuǎn zhì* (远志, *Radix Polygalae*) 9 g and *lóng gǔ* (龙骨, *Os Draconis*) 15 g (decoct first).
- For fatigue and loose stools, combine with *shān yào* (山药, *Rhizoma Dioscoreae*) 9 g and *bái zhú* (白术, *Rhizoma Atractylodis Macrocephalae*) 9 g.

Qi stagnation and blood stasis

Signs and symptoms

Chest tightness, palpitations, dull or colic chest pain, shortness of breath, fatigue and dark-purple lips.

Tongue: dark-red, with ecchymosis
Pulse: wiry, thready and regularly/irregularly intermittent

Treatment principle

Invigorate blood, regulate *qi*, unblock collaterals and nourish the heart.

Formula

Modified *Dān Shēn Yǐn* (丹参饮, "Salvia Beverage").

丹参	*dān shēn*	15 g	*Radix et Rhizoma Salviae Miltiorrhizae*
檀香	*tán xiāng*	3 g	*Lignum Santali Albi*
川芎	*chuān xiōng*	9 g	*Rhizoma Chuanxiong*
赤芍	*chì sháo*	9 g	*Radix Paeoniae Rubra*
蒲黄	*pú huáng*	15 g	*Pollen Typhae* (wrapped)
五灵脂	*wǔ líng zhī*	9 g	*Faeces Trogopterori* (wrapped)
延胡索	*yán hú suǒ*	9 g	*Rhizoma Corydalis*
酸枣仁	*suān zǎo rén*	9 g	*Semen Ziziphi Spinosae*

Modifications

- For a severe stabbing pain in the chest, combine with *rǔ xiāng* (乳香, *Olibanum*) 6 g and *mò yào* (没药, *Myrrha*) 6 g.
- For chest tightness and fullness, combine with *yù jīn* (郁金, *Radix Curcumae*) 9 g and *lù lù tōng* (路路通, *Fructus Liquidambaris*) 9 g.
- For severe palpitations, combine with *bǎi zǐ rén* (柏子仁, *Semen Platycladi*) 9 g and *zhēn zhū mǔ* (珍珠母, *Concha Margaritiferae Usta*) 15 g (decoct first) and.
- For a severe dry mouth, combine with *shēng dì* (生地, *Radix Rehmanniae*) 15 g and *mài dōng* (麦冬, *Radix Ophiopogonis*) 9 g.

Deficiency of qi and yin

Signs and symptoms

Palpitations, shortness of breath, chest tightness and pain, mental fatigue, restlessness, poor sleep and a dry mouth and throat.

Tongue: dry and red
Pulse: thready and regularly/irregularly intermittent

Treatment principle

Supplement *qi*, nourish yin and calm the mind.

Formula

Supplemented *Shēng Mài Sǎn* (生脉散, "Pulse-Engendering Powder").

太子参	*tài zǐ shēn*	15 g	*Radix Pseudostellariae*
麦冬	*mài dōng*	9 g	*Radix Ophiopogonis*
五味子	*wǔ wèi zǐ*	9 g	*Fructus Schisandrae Chinensis*
生地	*shēng dì*	12 g	*Radix Rehmanniae*
百合	*bǎi hé*	12 g	*Bulbus Lilii*
丹参	*dān shēn*	15 g	*Radix et Rhizoma Salviae Miltiorrhizae*
琥珀	*hǔ pò*	2 g	*Succinum* (powder)

Modifications

- For restlessness and irritability, combine with *zhú yè* (竹叶, *Folium Phyllostachydis Henonis*) 9 g and *huáng lián* (黄连, *Rhizoma Coptidis*) 4.5 g.
- For palpitations and severe insomnia, combine with *suān zǎo rén* (酸枣仁, *Semen Ziziphi Spinosae*) 9 g *bǎi zǐ rén* (柏子仁, *Semen Platycladi*) 9 g.

Collapse of yang-qi

Signs and symptoms

Palpitations, shortness of breath, an inability to lie flat, profuse sweating, cold limbs and pallor.

Tongue: pale, with a thin coating
Pulse: thready, faint and regularly/irregularly intermittent

Treatment principle

Resuscitate yang, supplement and calm the heart.

Formula

Modified *Shēn Fù Lóng Mǔ Tāng* (参附龙牡汤, "Ginseng, Aconite *Os Draconis* and *Concha Ostreae* Decoction")

人参	*rén shēn*	9 g	*Radix et Rhizoma Ginseng* (decoct separately)
制附子	*zhì fù zǐ*	9 g	*Radix Aconiti Lateralis Praeparata* (decoct first)
龙骨	*lóng gǔ*	30 g	*Os Draconis* (decoct first)
牡蛎	*mǔ lì*	30 g	*Concha Ostreae* (decoct first)
炙甘草	*zhì gān cǎo*	9 g	*Radix et Rhizoma Glycyrrhizae Praeparata cum Melle*
五味子	*wǔ wèi zǐ*	9 g	*Fructus Schisandrae Chinensis*
麦冬	*mài dōng*	9 g	*Radix Ophiopogonis*

Modifications

- For unconsciousness, combine with a pill of *Sū Hé Xiāng Wán* (苏合香丸, "Storax Pill") (swallow).
- For a severe chest pain, combine with *dān shēn* (丹参, *Radix et Rhizoma Salviae Miltiorrhizae*) 12 g and *tán xiāng* (檀香, *Lignum Santali Albi*) 3 g.
- For hemiplegia, combine with *táo rén* (桃仁, *Semen Persicae*) 9 g, *hóng huā* (红花, *Flos Carthami*) 9 g and *dì lóng* (地龙, *Pheretima*) 9 g.
- For persistent sweating, combine with *huáng qí* (黄芪, *Radix Astragali*) 15 g and *bái zhú* (白术, *Rhizoma Atractylodis Macrocephalae*) 9 g.

QUESTIONS

1. Describe the common complications of viral myocarditis.
2. List the pattern identifications and treatment methods of viral myocarditis in Chinese medicine.
3. *Case study.* Try to make a pattern identification and give a prescription for the following case:

Ms. Li, 35, suffered from a common cold two weeks prior to treatment. The day prior to treatment, she experienced palpitations, chest tightness, a stabbing chest pain, distension in the hypochondriac regions, a poor appetite and unsmooth bowel movements. The tongue was dark-red, with ecchymosis. The pulse was wiry, thready and regularly/irregularly intermittent.

COMMON URINARY SYSTEM CONDITIONS

Chronic Glomerulonephritis

Overview

Chronic glomerulonephritis, also known as chronic nephritis, is the advanced stage of a group of kidney disorders, resulting in inflammation and gradual, progressive destruction of the glomeruli (internal kidney structures). This may eventually cause irreversible damage to the kidneys and subsequent kidney failure.

In Chinese medicine, chronic nephritis falls under the category of "edema," "chronic deficiency and consumption" or "low back pain." The main contributing factors include contraction of external pathogens and deficiency of the zang–fu organs.

Pathogenic wind–cold may impair the dispersing and descending of lung *qi* and result in water retention. Long-term living in humid places may also play a role. An improper diet may impair the transportation and transformation of the spleen and stomach, resulting in internal water–dampness. Dysfunctions of the lungs, spleen and kidneys may compromise the *qi* transformation and cause disordered water distribution. Over time, the kidney conditions may affect the liver, leading to yin deficiency of the liver and kidneys and subsequent hyperactivity of liver yang. Eventually, deficiency of yin and yang may be present.

Clinical manifestations

The main symptoms of chronic nephritis are proteinuria, hematuria, cylindruria, edema, hypertension and kidney insufficiency. Proteinuria is the most common symptom. Edema is often seen in the eyelids and face in the morning and in the lower limbs in the afternoon. General edema may also be present in acute conditions. The hypertension can be persistent or intermittent, especially involving elevated diastolic pressure. The kidney insufficiency mainly manifests as elevated nonprotein nitrogen, urea and creatinine. Chronic nephritis is characterized by a long duration (over a year) with slow progress.

Pattern identification and treatment

Failure of the lungs to disperse and descend

Signs and symptoms

Sudden aggravation of facial puffiness, chills, fever, headache, a sore throat, coughing with panting and white sticky sputum.
Tongue: pale, with a thin white coating
Pulse: floating

Treatment principle

Formula

Modified *Yuè Bì Jiā Zhú Tāng* (越婢加术汤, "Maidservant from Yue Decoction Plus *Atractylodis Macrocephalae*").

麻黄	*má huáng*	9 g	*Herba Ephedrae*
石膏	*shí gāo*	30 g	*Gypsum Fibrosum* (ground, and decoct first)
白术	*bái zhú*	9 g	*Rhizoma Atractylodis Macrocephalae*
甘草	*gān cǎo*	9 g	*Radix et Rhizoma Glycyrrhizae*
浮萍	*fú píng*	9 g	*Herba Spirodelae*
猪苓	*zhū líng*	9 g	*Polyporus*
桑白皮	*sāng bái pí*	9 g	*Cortex Mori*
茯苓	*fú líng*	9 g	*Poria*

Modifications

- For a severe sore throat, combine with *jīn yín huā* (金银花, *Flos Lonicerae Japonicae*) 9 g and *jié gěng* (桔梗, *Radix Platycodonis*) 6 g.
- For severe coughing, combine with *xìng rén* (杏仁, *Semen Armeniacae Amarum*) 9 g and *zǐ wǎn* (紫菀, *Radix et Rhizoma Asteris*) 9 g.
- For severe headache with chills, combine with *bái zhǐ* (白芷, *Radix Angelicae Dahuricae*) 9 g and *jīng jiè* (荆芥, *Herba Schizonepetae*) 9 g.
- For visible edema, combine with *chē qián zǐ* (车前子, *Semen Plantaginis*) 30 g (wrapped) and *chē qián cǎo* (车前草, *Herba Plantaginis*) 30 g.

Spleen qi deficiency

Signs and symptoms

Persistent edema in the eyelids, a poor appetite, nausea, mental fatigue, a lusterless complexion and loose stools.

Tongue: pale, with a thin greasy coating
Pulse: soft and thready

Treatment principle

Strengthen the spleen, supplement *qi*, promote urination and resolve edema.

Formula

Modified *Huáng Qí Bǔ Zhōng Tāng* (黄芪补中汤, "Astragalus *Qi*-Supplementing Decoction").

黄芪	*huáng qí*	30 g	*Radix Astragali*
党参	*dǎng shēn*	9 g	*Radix Codonopsis*
白术	*bái zhú*	9 g	*Rhizoma Atractylodis Macrocephalae*
陈皮	*chén pí*	9 g	*Pericarpium Citri Reticulatae*
茯苓	*fú líng*	9 g	*Poria*
猪苓	*zhū líng*	9 g	*Polyporus*
炙甘草	*zhì gān cǎo*	9 g	*Radix et Rhizoma Glycyrrhizae Praeparata cum Melle*

Modifications

- For severe edema, combine with *chē qián zǐ* (车前子, *Semen Plantaginis*) 15 g (wrapped) and *zé xiè* (泽泻, *Rhizoma Alismatis*) 9 g.
- For mental fatigue and severe loose stools, combine with *shān yào* (山药, *Rhizoma Dioscoreae*) 9 g and *bái biǎn dòu* (白扁豆, *Semen Lablab Album*) 9 g.
- For a poor appetite, combine with *mài yá* (麦芽, *Fructus Hordei Germinatus*) 9 g and *jī nèi jīn* (鸡内金, *Endothelium Corneum Gigeriae Galli*) 9 g.

- For chest tightness and fullness, combine with *mù xiāng* (木香, *Radix Aucklandiae*) 9 g and *hòu pò* (厚朴, *Cortex Magnoliae Officinalis*) 9 g.

Yang deficiency of the spleen and kidneys

Signs and symptoms

General edema, hydrothorax or ascites, bloating, scanty urine, a poor appetite, nausea, pallor, mental fatigue, and soreness and weakness of the low back and knee joints.

Tongue: pale, with a thin white coating
Pulse: thready and weak

Treatment principle

Warm and tonify the spleen and kidneys, transform *qi* and promote urination.

Formula

Modified *Zhēn Wǔ Tāng* (真武汤, "True Warrior Decoction") and *Wǔ Líng Sǎn* (五苓散, "Five Substances Powder with Poria").

炮附子	*páo fù zǐ*	9 g	*Radix Aconiti Lateralis Praeparata* (decoct first)
干姜	*gān jiāng*	6 g	*Rhizoma Zingiberis*
白术	*bái zhú*	9 g	*Rhizoma Atractylodis Macrocephalae*
猪苓	*zhū líng*	9 g	*Polyporus*
大腹皮	*dà fù pí*	9 g	*Pericarpium Arecae*
肉桂	*ròu guì*	3 g	*Cortex Cinnamomi* (decoct later)
车前子	*chē qián zǐ*	30 g	*Semen Plantaginis* (wrapped)
泽泻	*zé xiè*	15 g	*Rhizoma Alismatis*

Modifications

- For severe bloating, combine with *mù xiāng* (木香, *Radix Aucklandiae*) 9 g and *hòu pò* (厚朴, *Cortex Magnoliae Officinalis*) 9 g.

- For dyspnea with an inability to lie flat, combine with *sāng bái pí* (桑白皮, *Cortex Mori*) 12 g and *huā jiāo* (花椒, *Pericarpium Zanthoxyli*) 9 g.
- For nausea and vomiting, combine with *jiāng bàn xià* (姜半夏, *Rhizoma Pinelliae Praeparatum*) 9 g and *chén pí* (陈皮, *Pericarpium Citri Reticulatae*) 9 g.
- For ascites with scanty urine, combine with *hú lú* (葫芦, *Fructus Lagenariae*) 15 g and *chē qián cǎo* (车前草, *Herba Plantaginis*) 30 g.

Deficiency of the spleen and kidneys

Signs and symptoms

Edema in the eyelids, fatigue, a lusterless complexion, a poor appetite, dizziness, tinnitus, soreness and weakness of the low back and knee joints, and loose stools.

Tongue: pale, with a thin coating
Pulse: soft and thready

Treatment principle

Strengthen the spleen, tonify the kidneys, supplement *qi* and nourish blood.

Formula

Modified *Dà Bǔ Yuán Jiān* (大补元煎, "Major *Yuan*-Supplementing Decoction").

黄芪	huáng qí	30 g	Radix Astragali
党参	dǎng shēn	9 g	Radix Codonopsis
白术	bái zhú	9 g	Rhizoma Atractylodis Macrocephalae
茯苓	fú líng	9 g	Poria
枸杞子	gǒu qǐ zǐ	9 g	Fructus Lycii
杜仲	dù zhòng	9 g	Cortex Eucommiae
当归	dāng guī	9 g	Radix Angelicae Sinensis

熟地黄	shú dì huáng	9 g	Radix Rehmanniae Praeparata
猪苓	zhū líng	9 g	Polyporus
炙甘草	zhì gān cǎo	9 g	Radix et Rhizoma Glycyrrhizae Praeparata cum Melle

Modifications

- For loose stools, combine with *shān yào* (山药, *Rhizoma Dioscoreae*) 9 g and *bái biǎn dòu* (白扁豆, *Semen Lablab Album*) 9 g.
- For edema in the eyelids, combine with *chē qián zǐ* (车前子, *Semen Plantaginis*) 15 g (wrapped) and *zé xiè* (泽泻, *Rhizoma Alismatis*) 9 g.
- For severe soreness and weakness of the low back and knee joints, combine with *chuān xù duàn* (川续断, *Radix Dipsaci*) 9 g and *gǒu jǐ* (狗脊, *Rhizoma Cibotii*) 15 g.
- For chest tightness and a poor appetite, combine with *fó shǒu* (佛手, *Fructus Citri Sarcodactylis*) 9 g and *shā rén* (砂仁, *Fructus Amomi*) 6 g (decoct later).

Yin deficiency of the liver and kidneys

Signs and symptoms

Rosy cheeks, tidal fever, a dry throat, thirst, dizziness, headache, palpitations, insomnia, soreness and weakness of the low back and knee joints, nocturnal emissions, premature ejaculations and slight edema in the lower extremities.

Tongue: red, with no or a scanty coating
Pulse: thready and rapid

Treatment principle

Nourish the liver and kidneys, soothe the liver and suppress yang.

Formula

Modified *Dì Huáng Yǐn Zǐ* (地黄饮子, "Rehmannia Drink").

生地	shēng dì	9 g	Radix Rehmanniae
天冬	tiān dōng	9 g	Radix Asparagi
麦冬	mài dōng	9 g	Radix Ophiopogonis
石斛	shí hú	9 g	Caulis Dendrobii
杜仲	dù zhòng	9 g	Cortex Eucommiae
枸杞子	gǒu qǐ zǐ	9 g	Fructus Lycii
山茱萸	shān zhū yú	9 g	Fructus Corni
牡蛎	mǔ lì	30 g	Concha Ostreae
石决明	shí jué míng	30 g	Concha Haliotidis
龟板	guī bǎn	15 g	Plastrum Testudinis (decoct first)

Modifications

- For severe vertigo, combine with *lü dòu yī* (绿豆衣, *Testa Glycinis*) 12 g and *gōu téng* (钩藤, *Ramulus Uncariae Cum Uncis*) 9 g (decoct later).

- For visible edema, combine with *chē qián zǐ* (车前子, *Semen Plantaginis*) 15 g and *zhū líng* (猪苓, *Polyporus*) 15 g.

- For restlessness with insomnia, combine with *zhēn zhū mǔ* (珍珠母, *Concha Margaritiferae Usta*) 15 g and *suān zǎo rén* (酸枣仁, *Semen Ziziphi Spinosae*) 9 g.

- For severe nocturnal emissions, combine with *jīn yīng zǐ* (金樱子, *Fructus Rosae Laevigatae*) 9 g and *qiàn shí* (芡实, *Semen Euryales*) 15 g.

Deficiency of the spleen and kidneys

Signs and symptoms

A dark-gray complexion with facial puffiness, a low spirit, weight loss, chest tightness, bloating, a poor appetite, nausea, vomiting, clear profuse or scanty urine and diarrhea or constipation; restlessness, coma and convulsions may also be present.

Tongue: pale and swollen, with a white greasy or yellow greasy coating
Pulse: deep–thready or wiry–thready

Treatment principle

Tonify the spleen and kidneys, and downregulate turbidity.

Formula

Modified *Wēn Pí Tāng* (温脾汤, "Spleen-Warming Decoction").

炮附子	*páo fù zǐ*	9 g	Radix Aconiti Lateralis Praeparata (decoct first)
人参	*rén shēn*	9 g	Radix et Rhizoma Ginseng (decoct separately)
大黄	*dà huáng*	9 g	Radix et Rhizoma Rhei (decoct later)
半夏	*bàn xià*	9 g	Rhizoma Pinelliae
生姜	*shēng jiāng*	4.5 g	Rhizoma Zingiberis Recens
陈皮	*chén pí*	9 g	Pericarpium Citri Reticulatae
茯苓	*fú líng*	9 g	Poria
竹茹	*zhú rú*	9 g	Caulis Bambusae in Taenia
厚朴	*hòu pò*	9 g	Cortex Magnoliae Officinalis

Modifications

- For a bitter taste and a yellow greasy tongue coating, combine with *huáng lián* (黄连, *Rhizoma Coptidis*) 3 g and *cāng zhú* (苍术, *Rhizoma Atractylodis*) 9 g.
- For scanty urine, combine with *bái chǒu* (白丑, *Semen Pharbitidis*) 6 g.
- For convulsions, combine with *lóng gǔ* (龙骨, *Os Draconis*) 30 g (decoct first) and *mǔ lì* (牡蛎, *Concha Ostreae*) 30 g (decoct first).
- For coma, combine with one pill of *Sū Hé Xiāng Wán* (苏合香丸, "Storax Pill") (swallow).

QUESTIONS

1. Describe the common complications of chronic nephritis.
2. List the pattern identifications and treatment methods of chronic nephritis in Chinese medicine.
3. *Case study.* Try to make a pattern identification and give a prescription for the following case:

Mr. Huang, age 50, suffered from proteinuria, edema and hypertension for over 10 years and was diagnosed with chronic nephritis, which has responded well

> to integrative Chinese and Western therapies. However, he started to experience the following symptoms at the time of treatment: visible pitting edema in the lower extremities, bloating, scanty urine, nausea, a poor appetite, a low spirit, fatigue, soreness and weakness of the low back and knee joints, and pallor. The tongue was pale, with a thin coating. The pulse was deep and thready.

Pyelonephritis

Overview

Pyelonephritis is an ascending urinary tract infection that has reached the *pyelum* of the kidney. According to the duration and symptoms, it can be either acute or chronic. Acute pyelonephritis can develop at any age, but more commonly in young women. In rare cases, persistent infections, extended duration and repeated attacks may result in chronic pyelonephritis and subsequent kidney insufficiency.

In Chinese medicine, this condition falls under the category of "micturition disorders" or "low back pain." Damp–heat accumulating in the urinary bladder is considered the major contributing factor.

Contraction of damp–heat or internal damp–heat due to overingestion of sweet fatty food coupled with excessive consumption of alcohol may impair the *qi* transformation of the urinary bladder, leading to this condition.

Clinical manifestations

The main symptoms of pyelonephritis are dysuria, low back pain and bacteriuria. In acute conditions, patients may present with frequent urgent painful voiding of urine and bacteriuria, followed by dull pain or ache in the low back. Some patients may experience abdominal colic radiating to the urinary bladder along the ureter, accompanied by a high-grade fever and chills. In chronic conditions, patients may have asymptomatic bacteriuria. Other common symptoms include fatigue, a low-grade fever, a poor appetite, lumbar soreness and pain, as well as frequent urgent painful urination.

Pattern identification and treatment

Damp–heat in the urinary bladder

Signs and symptoms

Cold intolerance, fever, frequent urgent painful urination with a burning sensation, dark-yellow urine, abdominal pain, tenderness and distending pain in the lower abdomen.

Tongue: a yellow greasy coating
Pulse: soft–rapid or slippery–rapid

Treatment principle

Clear heat, resolve dampness and promote urination.

Formula

Modified *Bā Zhèng Sǎn* (八正散, "Eight Corrections Powder").

瞿麦	*qú mài*	9 g	Herba Dianthi
萹蓄	*biǎn xù*	9 g	Herba Polygoni Avicularis
川木通	*chuān mù tōng*	6 g	Caulis Clematidis Armandii
山栀	*shān zhī*	9 g	Fructus Gardeniae
滑石	*huá shí*	15 g	Talcum (decoct first)
金银花	*jīn yín huā*	9 g	Flos Lonicerae Japonicae
连翘	*lián qiào*	9 g	Fructus Forsythiae
车前子	*chē qián zǐ*	30 g	Semen Plantaginis (wrapped)
甘草梢	*gān cǎo shāo*	6 g	Radix Tenuis Glycyrrhizae

Modifications

- For constipation, combine with *dà huáng* (大黄, *Radix et Rhizoma Rhei*) 9 g (decoct later) and *máng xiāo* (芒硝, *Natrii Sulfas*) 9 g.
- For severe distending pain in the lower abdomen, combine with *wū yào* (乌药, *Radix Linderae*) 9 g and *zhǐ qiào* (枳壳, *Fructus Aurantii*) 9 g.

- For chest tightness and a poor appetite, combine with *shā rén* (砂仁, *Fructus Amomi*) 6 g (decoct later) and *bái dòu kòu* (白豆蔻, *Fructus Amomi Kravanh*) 6 g (decoct later).
- For chills and fever, combine with *jīng jiè* (荆芥, *Herba Schizonepetae*) 9 g and *dòu chī* (豆豉, *Semen Sojae Praeparatum*) 9 g.

Heat accumulating in the liver and gallbladder

Signs and symptoms

Frequent urgent painful urination with a burning sensation, dark-yellow urine, low back pain, bloating, alternating fever and chills, restlessness, nausea and a bitter taste with a dry throat.

Tongue: a yellow–white thin greasy coating
Pulse: wiry and rapid

Treatment principle

Clear heat in the liver and gallbladder, and regulate water passage.

Formula

Modified *Lóng Dǎn Xiè Gān Tāng* (龙胆泻肝汤, "Gentian Liver-Draining Decoction").

龙胆草	*lóng dǎn cǎo*	9 g	*Radix et Rhizoma Gentianae*
黄芩	*huáng qín*	9 g	*Radix Scutellariae*
山栀	*shān zhī*	9 g	*Fructus Gardeniae*
柴胡	*chái hú*	9 g	*Radix Bupleuri*
生地	*shēng dì*	12 g	*Radix Rehmanniae*
川楝子	*chuān liàn zǐ*	9 g	*Fructus Toosendan*
延胡索	*yán hú suǒ*	9 g	*Rhizoma Corydalis*
川木通	*chuān mù tōng*	6 g	*Caulis Clematidis Armandii*
车前子	*chē qián zǐ*	30 g	*Semen Plantaginis* (wrapped)
甘草梢	*gān cǎo shāo*	6 g	*Radix Tenuis Glycyrrhizae*

Modifications

- For abdominal fullness with constipation, combine with *dà huáng* (大黄, *Radix et Rhizoma Rhei*) 9 g (decoct later) and *zhǐ shí* (枳实, *Fructus Aurantii Immaturus*) 9 g.
- For a poor appetite and nausea, combine with *jiāng bàn xià* (姜半夏, *Rhizoma Pinelliae Praeparatum*) 9 g and *jiāng zhú rú* (姜竹茹, *Caulis Bambusae in Taenia Praeparatum*) 9 g.
- For headache and a sore throat, combine with *sāng yè* (桑叶, *Folium Mori*) 9 g and *niú bàng zǐ* (牛蒡子, *Fructus Arctii*) 9 g.
- For thirst with a desire to drink water, combine with *lú gēn* (芦根, *Rhizoma Phragmitis*) 30 g and *shí hú* (石斛, *Caulis Dendrobii*) 9 g.

Excessive heat in the stomach and intestine

Signs and symptoms

Frequent urgent painful urination, abdominal pain, tenderness, a persistent strong fever, sweating, a foul breath, thirst with a desire to drink water, abdominal pain and constipation.

Tongue: a yellow greasy coating
Pulse: wiry and rapid

Treatment principle

Clear heat, remove toxins and unblock the stomach and intestine.

Formula

Modified *Dǎo Chì Chéng Qì Tāng* (导赤承气汤, "Red Guiding Purgative Decoction").

生地	*shēng dì*	12 g	*Radix Rehmanniae*
黄连	*huáng lián*	3 g	*Rhizoma Coptidis*
大黄	*dà huáng*	9 g	*Radix et Rhizoma Rhei* (decoct later)
黄柏	*huáng bǎi*	9 g	*Cortex Phellodendri Chinensis*
川木通	*chuān mù tōng*	6 g	*Caulis Clematidis Armandii*
甘草梢	*gān cǎo shāo*	6 g	*Radix Tenuis Glycyrrhizae*
车前子	*chē qián zǐ*	15 g	*Semen Plantaginis* (wrapped)

Modifications

- For constipation, combine with *máng xiāo* (芒硝, *Natrii Sulfas*) 9 g and *má rén* (麻仁, *Fructus Cannabis*) 9 g.
- For severe abdominal pain, combine with *zhǐ shí* (枳实, *Fructus Aurantii Immaturus*) 9 g and *hòu pò* (厚朴, *Cortex Magnoliae Officinalis*) 9 g.
- For a high-grade fever, combine with *shí gāo* (石膏, *Gypsum Fibrosum*) 30 g (decoct first) and *shān zhī* (山栀, *Fructus Gardeniae*) 9 g.
- For thirst, combine with *tiān huā fěn* (天花粉, *Radix Trichosanthis*) 15 g and *lú gēn* (芦根, *Rhizoma Phragmitis*) 30 g.

Kidney yin deficiency

Signs and symptoms

Frequent scanty painful urination, dizziness, tinnitus, dry throat and lips, soreness and weakness of the low back and knee joints; a low-grade fever and feverish sensations of the palms, soles and chest may also be present.

Tongue: red, with a thin or scanty coating
Pulse: wiry, thready and rapid

Treatment principle

Nourish yin, benefit the kidneys and clear heat.

Formula

Modified *Zhī Bǎi Dì Huáng Wán* (知柏地黄丸, "Anemarrhena, Phellodendron and Rehmannia Pill").

生地	*shēng dì*	12 g	*Radix Rehmanniae*
山茱萸	*shān zhū yú*	9 g	*Fructus Corni*
山药	*shān yào*	15 g	*Rhizoma Dioscoreae*
猪苓	*zhū líng*	9 g	*Polyporus*
牡丹皮	*mǔ dān pí*	9 g	*Cortex Moutan*
泽泻	*zé xiè*	9 g	*Rhizoma Alismatis*
知母	*zhī mǔ*	9 g	*Rhizoma Anemarrhenae*
黄柏	*huáng bǎi*	9 g	*Cortex Phellodendri Chinensis*
金樱子	*jīn yīng zǐ*	9 g	*Fructus Rosae Laevigatae*

Modifications

- For urination with a burning sensation, combine with *huáng lián* (黄连, *Rhizoma Coptidis*) 3 g and *chuān mù tōng* (川木通, *Caulis Clematidis Armandii*).
- For lower abdominal distension and pain, combine with *zhǐ qiào* (枳壳, *Fructus Aurantii*) 9 g and *chuān liàn zǐ* (川楝子, *Fructus Toosendan*) 9 g.
- For a dry mouth with a desire to drink water, combine with *shí hú* (石斛, *Caulis Dendrobii*) 9 g and *yù zhú* (玉竹, *Rhizoma Polygonati Odorati*) 9 g.
- For severe dizziness, combine with *jú huā* (菊花, *Flos Chrysanthemi*) 9 g and *bái jí lí* (白蒺藜, *Fructus Tribuli*) 9 g.

Yang deficiency of the spleen and kidneys

Signs and symptoms

Frequent dribbling urination, facial puffiness, edema in the lower extremities, a poor appetite, bloating, mental fatigue, soreness and weakness of the low back and knee joints, and loose stools.

Tongue: pale, with a thin white coating
Pulse: deep and thready

Treatment principle

Strengthen the spleen, benefit the kidneys and resolve dampness.

Formula

Shēn Líng Bái Zhú Sǎn (参苓白术散, "Ginseng, Poria and *Atractylodes Macrocephalae* Powder") and *Èr Xiān Tāng* (二仙汤, "*Chong* and *Ren*-Regulating Decoction").

党参	*dǎng shēn*	9 g	*Radix Codonopsis*
茯苓	*fú líng*	9 g	*Poria*
白术	*bái zhú*	9 g	*Rhizoma Atractylodis Macrocephalae*
白扁豆	*bái biǎn dòu*	9 g	*Semen Lablab Album*
山药	*shān yào*	15 g	*Rhizoma Dioscoreae*

薏苡仁	*yì yǐ rén*	9 g	Semen Coicis
仙茅	*xiān máo*	9 g	Rhizoma Curculiginis
仙灵脾	*xiān líng pí*	15 g	Herba Epimedii
知母	*zhī mǔ*	9 g	Rhizoma Anemarrhenae
黄柏	*huáng bǎi*	9 g	Cortex Phellodendri Chinensis

Modifications

- For severe lower abdominal fullness and distension, combine with *hòu pò* (厚朴, *Cortex Magnoliae Officinalis*) 9 g and *wū yào* (乌药, *Radix Linderae*) 9 g.
- For dribbling urination, combine with *guì zhī* (桂枝, *Ramulus Cinnamomi*) 6 g and *chē qián zǐ* (车前子, *Semen Plantaginis*) 15 g (wrapped).
- For severe lumbar soreness, combine with *xù duàn* (续断, *Radix Dipsaci*) 9 g and *dù zhòng* (杜仲, *Cortex Eucommiae*) 9 g.
- For a poor appetite and nausea, combine with *bàn xià* (半夏, *Rhizoma Pinelliae*) 9 g and *shén qū* (神曲, *Massa Medicata Fermentata*) 9 g.

QUESTIONS

1. Describe the common complications of pyelonephritis.
2. List the pattern identifications and treatment methods of pyelonephritis in Chinese medicine.
3. *Case study.* Try to make a pattern identification and give a prescription for the following case:

Ms. Ye, 25, experienced sudden frequent urgent painful urination three days prior to treatment. Other symptoms included a burning sensation in the urethra, low back pain on the right side, chills, fever, a poor appetite, chest fullness and a dry mouth with a desire to drink water. The tongue coating was yellow and greasy. The pulse was slippery and rapid.

Urinary System Stones

Overview

Urinary system stones, also known as urinary calculi, are solid particles in the urinary system. According to the positions of the stones, urinary calculi can be categorized into four patterns: kidney stones, urethral stones, bladder stones and urerthal stones. Urinary calculi are associated with the environment, systemic conditions and urinary system disease. They may obstruct the urethra, cause secondary infection and damage the urethral mucosa. In rare cases, they may impair the kidney functions.

In Chinese medicine, urinary calculi fall under the category of "stony stranguria," "sandy stranguria," "bloody stranguria" or "low back pain." The main contributing factors include damp–heat accumulating in the lower *jiao* and fire–*qi* affecting the lower *jiao*.

External damp–heat or internal damp–heat (due to overingestion of sweet fatty food or excessive consumption of alcohol) may accumulate in the lower *jiao*, consume fluids and form stones. Emotional disturbance may cause liver *qi* stagnation, which later transforms into fire to affect the lower *jiao*.

Clinical manifestations

The main symptoms of urinary calculi are painful urination, bloody urine, dysuria or passing of urine containing stones. The pain is often located in the lower back and abdomen. It may also radiate to other areas. The pain can be distending, dull, sore or colic. Local tenderness or sensitivity to percussion may be present. Patients may experience alternating mild and severe recurrent pain. Bloody urine often follows pain, exercise or fatigue. The color of the blood can be pink, fresh red or purple–brown. Blood clots may sometimes be present. In addition, patients may suffer from frequent painful dribbling urination, coupled with lower abdominal cramp (which may radiate to the low back and the entire abdomen). Sometimes, interrupted urination or passing of stones may be present.

Pattern identification and treatment

Accumulation of damp–heat

Signs and symptoms

Passing of stones in the urine, painful or interrupted urination, intolerable low back pain or abdominal colic and bloody urine.

Tongue: red, with a thin yellow coating
Pulse: wiry and rapid

Treatment principle

Clear heat, resolve dampness, promote urination and resolve stones.

Formula

Supplemented *Shí Wéi Sǎn* (石韦散, *"Folium Pyrrosiae Powder"*).

石苇	*shí wéi*	30 g	*Folium Pyrrosiae*
冬葵子	*dōng kuí zǐ*	15 g	*Fructus Malvae*
海金沙	*hǎi jīn shā*	15 g	*Spora Lygodii* (wrapped)
鸡内金	*jī nèi jīn*	9 g	*Endothelium Corneum Gigeriae Galli*
车前子	*chē qián zǐ*	30 g	*Semen Plantaginis* (wrapped)
滑石	*huá shí*	15 g	*Talcum* (decoct first)
瞿麦	*qú mài*	9 g	*Herba Dianthi*

Modifications

- For visible bloody urine, combine with *dà jì* (大蓟, *Herba Cirsii Japonici*) 12 g, *xiǎo jì* (小蓟, *Herba Cirsii*) 9 g and *bái máo gēn* (白茅根, *Rhizoma Imperatae*) 15 g.
- For severe pain, combine with *bái sháo* (白芍, *Radix Paeoniae Alba*) 9 g and *gān cǎo* (甘草, *Radix et Rhizoma Glycyrrhizae*) 6 g.
- For urination with a severe burning sensation, combine with *pú gōng yīng* (蒲公英, *Herba Taraxaci*) 30 g and *biǎn xù* (萹蓄, *Herba Polygoni Avicularis*) 9 g.
- For a yellow greasy tongue coating, combine with *cāng zhú* (苍术, *Rhizoma Atractylodis*) 9 g and *huáng bǎi* (黄柏, *Cortex Phellodendri Chinensis*) 9 g.

Liver qi stagnation

Signs and symptoms

Distending pain in the low back and hypochondriac regions, chest tightness, painful dribbling urination (the low back pain can radiate to the lower abdomen), interrupted urination and bloating.

Tongue: a thin yellow or thin white coating
Pulse: wiry and slippery

Treatment principle

Soothe the liver, regulate *qi*, promote urination and resolve stones.

Formula

Modified *Chái Hú Shū Gān Sǎn* (柴胡疏肝散, "Bupleurum Liver-Soothing Powder").

柴胡	*chái hú*	9 g	*Radix Bupleuri*
枳壳	*zhǐ qiào*	9 g	*Fructus Aurantii*
赤芍	*chì sháo*	9 g	*Radix Paeoniae Rubra*
白芍	*bái sháo*	9 g	*Radix Paeoniae Alba*
当归	*dāng guī*	9 g	*Radix Angelicae Sinensis*
陈皮	*chén pí*	9 g	*Pericarpium Citri Reticulatae*
石苇	*shí wéi*	30 g	*Folium Pyrrosiae*
冬葵子	*dōng kuí zǐ*	15 g	*Fructus Malvae*
王不留行	*wáng bù liú xíng*	9 g	*Semen Vaccariae*
金钱草	*jīn qián cǎo*	30 g	*Herba Lysimachiae*
川木通	*chuān mù tōng*	6 g	*Caulis Clematidis Armandii*
海金沙	*hǎi jīn shā*	15 g	*Spora Lygodii* (wrapped)

Modifications

- For severe low back and abdominal pain, combine with *yán hú suǒ* (延胡索, *Rhizoma Corydalis*) 9 g, *chuān liàn zǐ* (川楝子, *Fructus Toosendan*) 9 g and *wū yào* (乌药, *Radix Linderae*) 9 g.
- For severe bloody urine, combine with *bái máo gēn* (白茅根, *Rhizoma Imperatae*) 30 g, *ǒu jié* (藕节, *Nodus Nelumbinis Rhizomatis*) 9 g and *pú huáng* (蒲黄, *Pollen Typhae*) 9 g (wrapped).

- For blocked urination, combine with *dà huáng* (大黄, *Radix et Rhizoma Rhei*) 9 g , *hǔ zhàng* (虎杖, *Rhizoma Polygoni Cuspidati*) 15 g and *Zī Shèn Tōng Guān Wán* (滋肾通关丸, "Kidney-Nourishing and Gate-Unblocking Pill").
- For a yellow tongue coating due to excessive heat, combine with *huáng bǎi* (黄柏, *Cortex Phellodendri Chinensis*) 9 g, *shān zhī* (山栀, *Fructus Gardeniae*) 9 g and *qú mài* (瞿麦, *Herba Dianthi*) 9 g.

Blood stasis

Signs and symptoms

Low back and abdominal pain in a fixed position, palpable masses, tenderness, repeated dark-purple bloody urine or with blood clots, painful urination and lower abdominal distension and fullness.

Tongue: dark-purple or with ecchymosis
Pulse: wiry and hesitant

Treatment principle

Invigorate blood, resolve stasis, promote urination and resolve stones.

Formula

Modified *Shào Fǔ Zhú Yū Tāng* (少腹逐瘀汤, "Lower Abdominal Stasis–Expelling Decoction").

当归	*dāng guī*	9 g	Radix Angelicae Sinensis
川芎	*chuān xiōng*	9 g	Rhizoma Chuanxiong
赤芍	*chì sháo*	9 g	Radix Paeoniae Rubra
王不留行	*wáng bù liú xíng*	9 g	Semen Vaccariae
枳壳	*zhǐ qiào*	9 g	Fructus Aurantii
乌药	*wū yào*	9 g	Radix Linderae
石苇	*shí wéi*	30 g	Folium Pyrrosiae
冬葵子	*dōng kuí zǐ*	15 g	Fructus Malvae
蒲黄	*pú huáng*	9 g	Pollen Typhae (wrapped)
海金沙	*hǎi jīn shā*	15 g	Spora Lygodii (wrapped)

Modifications

- For unresolved masses, combine with *sān léng* (三棱, *Rhizoma Sparganii*) 9 g, *é zhú* (莪术, *Rhizoma Curcumae*) 9 g and *chuān shān jiǎ* (穿山甲, *Squama Manitis*) 9 g (decoct first).
- For frequent urgent painful urination, combine with *pú gōng yīng* (蒲公英, *Herba Taraxaci*) 30 g, *hǔ zhàng* (虎杖, *Rhizoma Polygoni Cuspidati*) 15 g and *jīn qián cǎo* (金钱草, *Herba Lysimachiae*) 30 g.
- For severe bloating, combine with *hòu pò* (厚朴, *Cortex Magnoliae Officinalis*) 9 g, *wū yào* (乌药, *Radix Linderae*) 9 g and *bīng láng* (槟榔, *Semen Arecae*) 9 g.
- For constipation, combine with *dà huáng* (大黄, *Radix et Rhizoma Rhei*) 9 g (decoct later) and *máng xiāo* (芒硝, *Natrii Sulfas*) 9 g.

Deficiency of the spleen and kidneys

Signs and symptoms

Persistent unresolved stones, painful urination, dull pain in the low back and abdomen, pallor, a low spirit and fatigue.

Tongue: pale, with tooth marks
Pulse: soft and thready

Treatment principle

Strengthen the spleen, benefit the kidneys, promote urination and resolve stones.

Formula

Modified *Wú Bǐ Shān Yào Wán* (无比山药丸, "Incomparable Dioscoreae Pill").

熟地黄	shú dì huáng	9 g	*Radix Rehmanniae Praeparata*
山茱萸	shān zhū yú	9 g	*Fructus Corni*
山药	shān yào	15 g	*Rhizoma Dioscoreae*
巴戟天	bā jǐ tiān	9 g	*Radix Morindae Officinalis*
杜仲	dù zhòng	9 g	*Cortex Eucommiae*

续断	xù duàn	9 g	Radix Dipsaci
泽泻	zé xiè	9 g	Rhizoma Alismatis
海金沙	hǎi jīn shā	15 g	Spora Lygodii (wrapped)
滑石	huá shí	15 g	Talcum (decoct first)
黄芪	huáng qí	30 g	Radix Astragali

Modifications

- For unsmooth dribbling urination, combine with *jī nèi jīn* (鸡内金, Endothelium Corneum Gigeriae Galli) 9 g, *chē qián zǐ* (车前子, Semen Plantaginis) 15 g (wrapped) and *hǔ zhàng* (虎杖, Rhizoma Polygoni Cuspidati) 15 g.
- For severe lower abdominal fullness and distension, combine with *hòu pò* (厚朴, Cortex Magnoliae Officinalis) 9 g, *wū yào* (乌药, Radix Linderae) 9 g and *zhǐ shí* (枳实, Fructus Aurantii Immaturus) 9 g.
- For feverish sensations of the palms and soles, and a red tongue with a scanty coating, combine with *gǒu qǐ zǐ* (枸杞子, Fructus Lycii) 9 g, *hàn lián cǎo* (旱莲草, Herba Ecliptae) 9 g and *nǔ zhēn zǐ* (女贞子, Fructus Ligustri Lucidi) 9 g.
- For a greasy tongue coating and a general heavy sensation, combine with *cāng zhú* (苍术, Rhizoma Atractylodis) 9 g, *jiāng bàn xià* (姜半夏, Rhizoma Pinelliae Praeparatum) 9 g and *chén pí* (陈皮, Pericarpium Citri Reticulatae) 9 g.

Deficiency of qi *and yin*

Signs and symptoms

Persistent unresolved stones, painful urination, dizziness, tinnitus, a dry mouth and throat, restlessness, insomnia, feverish sensations of the palms and soles, and dull lingering low back pain.

Tongue: red, with a scanty coating
Pulse: wiry, thready and rapid

Treatment principle

Supplement *qi*, nourish yin, promote urination and resolve stones.

Formula

Modified *Shēng Mài Sǎn* (生脉散, "Pulse-Engendering Powder").

太子参	*tài zǐ shēn*	15 g	*Radix Pseudostellariae*
麦冬	*mài dōng*	9 g	*Radix Ophiopogonis*
五味子	*wǔ wèi zǐ*	9 g	*Fructus Schisandrae Chinensis*
生地	*shēng dì*	12 g	*Radix Rehmanniae*
山茱萸	*shān zhū yú*	9 g	*Fructus Corni*
牡丹皮	*mǔ dān pí*	9 g	*Cortex Moutan*
车前子	*chē qián zǐ*	30 g	*Semen Plantaginis* (wrapped)
海金沙	*hǎi jīn shā*	15 g	*Spora Lygodii* (wrapped)
枸杞子	*gǒu qǐ zǐ*	15 g	*Fructus Lycii*
石苇	*shí wéi*	30 g	*Folium Pyrrosiae*

Modifications

- For a dry mouth with a desire to drink water, combine with *yù zhú* (玉竹, *Rhizoma Polygonati Odorati*) 9 g, *shí hú* (石斛, *Caulis Dendrobii*) 9 g and *shā shēn* (沙参, *Radix Adenophorae seu Glehniae*) 9 g.
- For visible bloody urine, combine with *bái máo gēn* (白茅根, *Rhizoma Imperatae*) 30 g, *hàn lián cǎo* (旱莲草, *Herba Ecliptae*) 9 g and *ē jiāo* (阿胶, *Colla Corii Asini*) 12 g (melted).
- For severe low back pain, combine with *gǒu jǐ* (狗脊, *Rhizoma Cibotii*) 15 g, *chuān xù duàn* (川续断, *Radix Dipsaci*) 9 g and *dù zhòng* (杜仲, *Cortex Eucommiae*) 9 g.
- For restlessness with severe insomnia, combine with *suān zǎo rén* (酸枣仁, *Semen Ziziphi Spinosae*) 9 g, *bǎi zǐ rén* (柏子仁, *Semen Platycladi*) 9 g and *yè jiāo téng* (夜交藤, *Caulis Polygoni Multiflori*) 15 g.

COMMON HEMATOPOIETIC SYSTEM CONDITIONS

Aplastic Anemia

Overview

Aplastic anemia is a condition where the bone marrow does not produce sufficient new cells to replenish blood cells. It can result in lower counts of all three blood cell types (red blood cells, white blood cells and platelets), termed "pancytopenia." This condition can be either acute or chronic. Aplastic anemia can develop at any age; however, chronic aplastic anemia is more common in the elderly (slightly more males than females).

In Chinese medicine, aplastic anemia falls under the category of "chronic deficiency" and "bleeding syndrome." The main contributing factors include overexertion, contraction of pathogens or toxins damaging *qi* and blood.

Failure of the spleen to control blood within vessels, failure of the heart to dominate blood, failure of the liver to store blood and failure of the kidney to store essence can all result in susceptibility to external contraction. Among the five *zang* organs, aplastic anemia is especially associated with the spleen and kidneys.

Clinical manifestations

The main symptoms of aplastic anemia are anemia, bleeding, infection and pancytopenia. The anemia is often progressive. Depending on the severity and duration, patients may present with a sallow complexion, pallor, fatigue, dizziness, blurred vision, palpitations and shortness of breath. The bleeding often involves the nostrils, gums, menstruation and skin. In severe cases, patients may experience hematemesis, black stools, bloody urine and hemoptysis. The infection often causes fever. Localized infections can be seen in the oral mucosa, gums, tonsils and throat, leading to ulcerations or necrosis.

Pattern identification and treatment

Weakness of the spleen with blood deficiency

Signs and symptoms

A sallow complexion, mental fatigue, palpitations, shortness of breath, dizziness, lumbar soreness, dream-disturbed sleep, a poor appetite, bleeding at the gums and from the nostrils, and menorrhagia.

Tongue: pale, with a thin white coating
Pulse: soft and thready

Treatment principle

Strengthen the spleen and nourish blood.

Formula

Modified *Guī Pí Tāng* (归脾汤, "Spleen-Restoring Decoction").

党参	*dǎng shēn*	9 g	*Radix Codonopsis*
黄芪	*huáng qí*	30 g	*Radix Astragali*
白术	*bái zhú*	9 g	*Rhizoma Atractylodis Macrocephalae*
白芍	*bái sháo*	9 g	*Radix Paeoniae Alba*
山药	*shān yào*	15 g	*Rhizoma Dioscoreae*
何首乌	*hé shǒu wū*	15 g	*Radix Polygoni Multiflori*
酸枣仁	*suān zǎo rén*	9 g	*Semen Ziziphi Spinosae*
仙鹤草	*xiān hè cǎo*	15 g	*Herba Agrimoniae*
大枣	*dà zǎo*	10 p	*Fructus Jujubae*
炙甘草	*zhì gān cǎo*	9 g	*Radix et Rhizoma Glycyrrhizae Praeparata cum Melle*

Modifications

- For severe mental fatigue, combine with *shēng shài shēn* (生晒参, *Radix et Rhizoma Ginseng Cruda*) 6 g (decoct separately).
- For rough scaly skin, combine with *dān shēn* (丹参, *Radix et Rhizoma Salviae Miltiorrhizae*) 15 g and *shú dì huáng* (熟地黄, *Radix Rehmanniae Praeparata*) 12 g.
- For severe bleeding, combine with *huā ruǐ shí* (花蕊石, *Ophicalcitum*) 30 g, *chén zōng tàn* (陈棕炭, *Petiolus Trachycarpi Carbonisatus*) and *pú huáng tàn* (蒲黄炭, *Pollen Typhae Carbonisatus*) 9 g (wrapped).
- For abdominal distension with loose stools, combine with *bàn xià* (半夏, *Rhizoma Pinelliae*) 9 g, *chén pí* (陈皮, *Pericarpium Citri Reticulatae*) 9 g and *shā rén* (砂仁, *Fructus Amomi*) 6 g (decoct later).

Kidney yin deficiency

Signs and symptoms

Dizziness, blurred vision, palpitations, tinnitus, restlessness, irritability, feverish sensations of the soles and palms, a low-grade fever, night sweats, a dry mouth and throat, soreness and weakness of the low back and knee joints, nocturnal emissions, bleeding from the nostrils and at the gums, and subcutaneous purpura.

Tongue: red, with a thin or scanty coating
Pulse: thready and rapid

Treatment principle

Nourish yin and fill essence.

Formula

Modified *Dà Bǔ Yuán Jiān* (大补元煎, "Major *Yuan*–Supplementing Decoction").

太子参	*tài zǐ shēn*	9 g	*Radix Pseudostellariae*
生地	*shēng dì*	12 g	*Radix Rehmanniae*
熟地黄	*shú dì huáng*	9 g	*Radix Rehmanniae Praeparata*
山茱萸	*shān zhū yú*	9 g	*Fructus Corni*
枸杞子	*gǒu qǐ zǐ*	9 g	*Fructus Lycii*
杜仲	*dù zhòng*	9 g	*Cortex Eucommiae*
当归	*dāng guī*	9 g	*Radix Angelicae Sinensis*
何首乌	*hé shǒu wū*	15 g	*Radix Polygoni Multiflori*
龟板	*guī bǎn*	15 g	*Plastrum Testudinis* (decoct first)
阿胶	*ē jiāo*	9 g	*Colla Corii Asini* (melted)

Modifications

- For severe purpura, combine with *hàn lián cǎo* (旱莲草, *Herba Ecliptae*) 9 g and *xiān hè cǎo* (仙鹤草, *Herba Agrimoniae*) 30 g.
- For severe bleeding from the nostril and at the gums, combine with *bái máo gēn* (白茅根, *Rhizoma Imperatae*) 30 g and *cè bǎi yè* (侧柏叶, *Cacumen Platycladi*) 12 g.
- For a severe fever, combine with *qīng hāo* (青蒿, *Herba Artemisiae Annuae*) 9 g and *dì gū pí* (地骨皮, *Cortex Lycii*) 9 g.
- For a severe dry mouth, combine with *yù zhú* (玉竹, *Rhizoma Polygonati Odorati*) 9 g and *shí hú* (石斛, *Caulis Dendrobii*) 9 g.

Kidney yang insufficiency

Signs and symptoms

Pallor, cold intolerance, cold limbs, edema in the eyelids, fatigue, shortness of breath, a poor appetite, loose stools, clear profuse urine at night, bleeding from the nostrils and at the gums, and skin purpura.

Tongue: pale, with a thin white coating
Pulse: deep and thready

Treatment principle

Warm the kidneys and benefit the marrow.

Formula

Modified *Jīn Guì Shèn Qì Wán* (金匮肾气丸, "Golden Cabinet's Kidney *Qi* Pill").

制附子	*zhì fù zǐ*	9 g	*Radix Aconiti Lateralis Praeparata* (decoct first)
肉桂	*ròu guì,*	4.5 g	*Cortex Cinnamomi* (decoct later)
熟地黄	*shú dì huáng*	9 g	*Radix Rehmanniae Praeparata*
山茱萸	*shān zhū yú*	15 g	*Fructus Corni*
山药	*shān yào*	15 g	*Rhizoma Dioscoreae*
茯苓	*fú líng*	9 g	*Poria*
泽泻	*zé xiè*	9 g	*Rhizoma Alismatis*
鹿角	*lù jiǎo*	9 g	*Cornu Cervi*
菟丝子	*tù sī zǐ*	9 g	*Semen Cuscutae*

Modifications

- For severe cold intolerance and cold limbs, combine with *xiān máo* (仙茅, *Rhizoma Curculiginis*) 9 g and *xiān líng pí* (仙灵脾, *Herba Epimedii*) 9 g.
- For severe bleeding, combine with *chén zōng tàn* (陈棕炭, *Petiolus Trachycarpi Carbonisatus*) and *lián fáng tàn* (莲房炭, *Receptaculum Nelumbinis Carbonisatus*) 9 g.

- For a severe poor appetite with loose stools, combine with *shā rén* (砂仁, *Fructus Amomi*) 6 g (decoct later) and *gān jiāng* (干姜, *Rhizoma Zingiberis*) 6 g.
- For severe edema, combine with *chē qián zǐ* (车前子, *Semen Plantaginis*) 15 g (wrapped) and *zhū líng* (猪苓, *Polyporus*) 15 g.

Deficiency of yin and yang

Signs and symptoms

Cold intolerance, cold limbs, mental fatigue, feverish sensations of the palms and soles, night sweats, spontaneous sweating, soreness and weakness of the low back and knee joints, pallor and bleeding from the nostrils and at the gums.

Tongue: pale, with a scanty coating
Pulse: thready and weak

Treatment principle

Tonify yin and yang.

Formula

Modified *Qī Bǎo Měi Rán Dān* (七宝美髯丹, "Seven Treasures Beard-Blackening Elixir").

何首乌	*hé shǒu wū*	15 g	Radix Polygoni Multiflori
茯苓	*fú líng*	9 g	Poria
当归	*dāng guī*	9 g	Radix Angelicae Sinensis
枸杞子	*gǒu qǐ zǐ*	9 g	Fructus Lycii
菟丝子	*tù sī zǐ*	9 g	Semen Cuscutae
补骨脂	*bǔ gǔ zhī*	9 g	Fructus Psoraleae
巴戟天	*bā jǐ tiān*	9 g	Radix Morindae Officinalis
黄精	*huáng jīng*	9 g	Rhizoma Polygonati
女贞子	*nǚ zhēn zǐ*	9 g	Fructus Ligustri Lucidi

Modifications

- For severe bleeding tendency, combine with *huā ruǐ shí* (花蕊石, *Ophicalcitum*) 30 g and *zōng lǚ tàn* (棕榈炭, *Petiolus Trachycarpi Carbonisatus*) 9 g.

- For a poor appetite with loose stools, combine with *shān yào* (山药, *Rhizoma Dioscoreae*) 9 g and *bái biǎn dòu* (白扁豆, *Semen Lablab Album*) 9 g.
- For severe cold intolerance, combine with *páo fù zǐ* (炮附子, *Radix Aconiti Lateralis Praeparata*) 6 g (decoct first) and *ròu guì* (肉桂, *Cortex Cinnamomi*) 4.5 g (decoct later).
- For severe feverish sensations of the palms, soles and chest, combine with *shēng dì* (生地, *Radix Rehmanniae*) 15 g and *mài dōng* (麦冬, *Radix Ophiopogonis*) 9 g.

Toxic heat entering the ying and blood

Signs and symptoms

Dizziness, headache, a persistent strong fever, hematemesis, subcutaneous bruises, a dry mouth with a sore throat, ulcerations at the gums, palpitations and shortness of breath.

Tongue: dry and red, with a yellow coating
Pulse: deficient, big and rapid

Treatment principle

Remove toxins and cool blood.

Formula

Modified *Xī Jiǎo Dì Huáng Tāng* (犀角地黄汤, "Rhinoceros Horn and Rehmannia Decoction").

水牛角	*shuǐ niú jiǎo*	30 g	*Cornu Bubali* (decoct first)
生地	*shēng dì*	15 g	*Radix Rehmanniae*
玄参	*xuán shēn*	9 g	*Radix Scrophulariae*
牡丹皮	*mǔ dān pí*	9 g	*Cortex Moutan*
赤芍	*chì sháo*	9 g	*Radix Paeoniae Rubra*
山栀	*shān zhī*	9 g	*Fructus Gardeniae*
麦冬	*mài dōng*	9 g	*Radix Ophiopogonis*
白茅根	*bái máo gēn*	30 g	*Rhizoma Imperatae*

Modifications

- For severe bleeding, combine with *Shí Huī Wán* (十灰丸, *Ten Charred Substances Pill*) 6 g (swallow with water), *dà jì* (大蓟, *Herba Cirsii Japonici*) 9 g and *xiǎo jì* (小蓟, *Herba Cirsii*) 9 g.
- For coma and delirium, combine with one pill of *Ān Gōng Niú Huáng Wán* (安宫牛黄丸, "Peaceful Palace Bovine Bezoar Pill").
- For a severe fever, combine with *Zǐ Xu Dān* (紫雪丹, "Purple Snow Elixir") 6 g.

Kidney deficiency with blood stasis

Signs and symptoms

A dark-gray complexion, rough scaly skin, soreness and weakness of the low back and knee joints, clear profuse urine, impotence, spermatorrhea, mental fatigue, palpitations, shortness of breath, and bleeding from the nostrils, and at the gums.

Tongue: purple, with ecchymosis
Pulse: thready and hesitant

Treatment principle

Warm the kidneys and resolve phlegm.

Formula

Modified *Yòu Guī Wán* (右归丸, "Right-Restoring Pill") and *Táo Hóng Sì Wù Tāng* (桃红四物汤, "Peach Kernel and Carthamus Four Substances Decoction").

熟地黄	shú dì huáng	9 g	Radix Rehmanniae Praeparata
制附子	zhì fù zǐ	9 g	Radix Aconiti Lateralis Praeparata (decoct first)
肉桂	ròu guì,	3 g	Cortex Cinnamomi (decoct later)
山茱萸	shān zhū yú	9 g	Fructus Corni
山药	shān yào	15 g	Rhizoma Dioscoreae

桃仁	*táo rén*	9 g	*Semen Persicae*
红花	*hóng huā*	9 g	*Flos Carthami*
当归	*dāng guī*	9 g	*Radix Angelicae Sinensis*
川芎	*chuān xiōng*	9 g	*Rhizoma Chuanxiong*
补骨脂	*bǔ gǔ zhī*	9 g	*Fructus Psoraleae*
肉苁蓉	*ròu cōng róng*	9 g	*Herba Cistanches*

Modifications

- For severe cold intolerance and cold limbs, combine with *xiān máo* (仙茅, *Rhizoma Curculiginis*) 9 g and *xiān líng pí* (仙灵脾, *Herba Epimedii*) 9 g.

- For impotence and spermatorrhea, combine with *wǔ wèi zǐ* (五味子, *Fructus Schisandrae Chinensis*) 9 g and *fù pén zǐ* (覆盆子, *Fructus Rubi*) 9 g.

- For a dark-purple tongue due to severe blood stasis, combine with *sān léng* (三棱, *Rhizoma Sparganii*) 9 g and *é zhú* (莪术, *Rhizoma Curcumae*) 9 g.

- For fatigue and loose stools, combine with *dǎng shēn* (党参, *Radix Codonopsis*) 9 g and *bái zhú* (白术, *Rhizoma Atractylodis Macrocephalae*) 9 g.

QUESTIONS

1. Describe the common symptoms of aplastic anemia.
2. List the pattern identifications and treatment methods of aplastic anemia in Chinese medicine.
3. *Case study.* Try to make a pattern identification and give a prescription for the following case:

Ms. Lin, 40, suffered from the following symptoms for one month: mental fatigue, palpitations, shortness of breath, dream-disturbed sleep, a poor appetite, dizziness, tinnitus, bleeding from the nostrils and at the gums, and heavy lingering menstruation. She was diagnosed with aplastic anema. The tongue was pale, with a thin coating. The pulse was soft and thready.

Idiopathic Thrombocytopenic Purpura

Overview

Idiopathic thrombocytopenic purpura (ITP), also known as autoimmune thrombocytopenic purpura, is the condition of having a low platelet count of no known cause. Most causes appear to be related to IgG antibodies against platelets. Clinically, ITP can be either acute or chronic. Acute ITP is often primary and is more commonly seen in children, while chronic ITP is more commonly seen in young females, with a slim probability of durable remission.

In Chinese medicine, ITP falls under the category of "bleeding syndrome" or "chronic deficiency or consumption." The main contributing factors include toxic heat retention in the *ying* and blood and deficiency of *qi* and blood of the *zang–fu* organs.

Retention of toxic heat in the *ying* and blood or exuberance of stomach heat may accelerate the flow of blood, leading to purpura. Failure of (spleen) *qi* to control blood within the vessels may cause blood to leak. Kidney yin deficiency may cause internal stirring of deficient fire to disturb the *ying* and blood. Kidney yang deficiency may produce internal yin cold, resulting in ascending of the rootless fire to impair the normal circulation of blood.

Clinical manifestations

The symptoms of ITP include bleeding, fever and an absolute drop in platelet counts. The bleeding can be persistent or recurrent, typically manifesting as bruises or petechiae. The petechiae can be as small as a pillet in a bright-red or dark-red color. The bruises are especially seen on the lower extremities. Bleeding from the nostrils, bleeding at the gums, bloody stools and urine, and menorrhagia may also be present. Severe bleeding may occur in acute ITP. In severe cases, patients may present with headache, vomiting, coma or even life-threatening signs due to intracranial bleeding.

Pattern identification and treatment

Retention of toxic heat

Signs and symptoms

Fever, subcutaneous purple petechiae or bruises (especially on the lower extremities), bleeding from the nostrils, bleeding at the gums, bloody urine and stools, a dry mouth, restlessness, dark-yellow urine and constipation.

Tongue: red, with a yellow coating
Pulse: wiry and rapid

Treatment principle

Clear heat, remove toxins, cool blood and relieve bruises.

Formula

Modified *Huà Bān Tāng* (化斑汤, "Stasis Resolving Decoction").

水牛角	*shuǐ niú jiǎo*	30 g	*Cornu Bubali* (decoct first)
生地	*shēng dì*	15 g	*Radix Rehmanniae*
玄参	*xuán shēn*	9 g	*Radix Scrophulariae*
竹叶	*zhú yè*	4 g	*Folium Phyllostachydis Henonis*
金银花	*jīn yín huā*	9 g	*Flos Lonicerae Japonicae*
连翘	*lián qiào*	12 g	*Fructus Forsythiae*
牡丹皮	*mǔ dān pí*	9 g	*Cortex Moutan*
紫草	*zǐ cǎo*	9 g	*Radix Arnebiae*
白茅根	*bái máo gēn*	30 g	*Rhizoma Imperatae*

Modifications

- For a severe fever, combine with *shí gāo* (石膏, Gypsum Fibrosum) 30 g (decoct first), *lóng dǎn cǎo* (龙胆草, *Radix et Rhizoma Gentianae*) 9 g and *Zǐ Xuě Dān* (紫雪丹, "Purple Snow Elixir") 6 g.
- For severe bleeding, combine with *zōng lǘ tàn* (棕榈炭, *Petiolus Trachycarpi Carbonisatus*) 9 g, *cè bǎi tàn* (侧柏炭, *Cacumen Platycladi*

Carbonisatus) 9 g and *dì yú tàn* (地榆炭, *Radix Sanguisorbae Carbonisatus*) 9 g.

- For constipation, combine with *dà huáng* (大黄, *Radix et Rhizoma Rhei*) 9 g (decoct later) and *máng xiāo* (芒硝, *Natrii Sulfas*) 9 g.
- For a thirst with a desire to drink water, combine with *yù zhú* (玉竹, *Rhizoma Polygonati Odorati*) 9 g, *mài dōng* (麦冬, *Radix Ophiopogonis*) 9 g and *shí hú* (石斛, *Caulis Dendrobii*) 9 g.

Hyperactivity of fire due to yin deficiency

Signs and symptoms

Alternating mild and severe red or purple–red subcutaneous petechiae or bruises (especially on the lower extremities), bleeding from the nostrils, bleeding at the gums, heavy menstruation, restlessness, insomnia, a dry throat, feverish sensations of the palms and soles, tidal fever and night sweats

Tongue: red, with a scanty coating
Pulse: thready and rapid

Treatment principle

Nourish yin, reduce fire, calm the collaterals and arrest bleeding.

Formula

Modified *Qiàn Gēn Sàn* (茜根散, "Rubiae Powder").

茜草	qiàn cǎo	15 g	Radix et Rhizoma Rubiae
黄芩	huáng qín	9 g	Radix Scutellariae
阿胶	ē jiāo	9 g	Colla Corii Asini (melted)
侧柏炭	cè bǎi tàn	9 g	Cacumen Platycladi Carbonisatus
生地	shēng dì	15 g	Radix Rehmanniae
甘草	gān cǎo	6 g	Radix et Rhizoma Glycyrrhizae
麦冬	mài dōng	9 g	Radix Ophiopogonis
知母	zhī mǔ	9 g	Rhizoma Anemarrhenae

Modifications

- For restlessness and irritability, combine with *huáng lián* (黄连, *Rhizoma Coptidis*) 4.5 g and *lián zǐ xīn* (莲子心, *Plumula Nelumbinis*) 9 g.
- For bleeding, combine with *hàn lián cǎo* (旱莲草, *Herba Ecliptae*) 9 g, *dà jì* (大蓟, *Herba Cirsii Japonici*) 9 g and *xiǎo jì* (小蓟, *Herba Cirsii*) 9 g.
- For a dry mouth with a desire to drink water, combine with *yù zhú* (玉竹, *Rhizoma Polygonati Odorati*) 9 g, *shí hú* (石斛, *Caulis Dendrobii*) 9 g and *tiān huā fěn* (天花粉, *Radix Trichosanthis*) 9 g.
- For severe insomnia, combine with *wū wèi zǐ* (五味子, *Fructus Schisandrae Chinensis*) 9 g, *suān zǎo rén* (酸枣仁, *Semen Ziziphi Spinosae*) 9 g and *bǎi zǐ rén* (柏子仁, *Semen Platycladi*) 9 g.

Spleen qi *deficiency*

Signs and symptoms

Pale hidden intermittent subcutaneous bruises that can be aggravated by fatigue, a sallow complexion, a low spirit, dizziness, fatigue, a poor appetite and heavy menstruation.

Tongue: pale and swollen, with a thin coating
Pulse: soft and moderate

Treatment principle

Supplement *qi* to control blood and strengthen the spleen to nourish blood.

Formula

Modified *Guī Pí Tāng* (归脾汤, "Spleen-Restoring Decoction").

黄芪	huáng qí	15 g	Radix Astragali
党参	dǎng shēn	9 g	Radix Codonopsis
当归	dāng guī	9 g	Radix Angelicae Sinensis
白术	bái zhú	9 g	Rhizoma Atractylodis Macrocephalae

白芍	*bái sháo*	9 g	Radix Paeoniae Alba
木香	*mù xiāng*	6 g	Radix Aucklandiae
远志	*yuǎn zhì*	9 g	Radix Polygalae
酸枣仁	*suān zǎo rén*	9 g	Semen Ziziphi Spinosae
龙眼肉	*lóng yǎn ròu*	9 g	Arillus Longan
仙鹤草	*xiān hè cǎo*	15 g	Herba Agrimoniae
蒲黄	*pú huáng*	9 g	Pollen Typhae (wrapped)
甘草	*gān cǎo*	6 g	Radix et Rhizoma Glycyrrhizae

Modifications

- For severe bleeding, combine with *dì yú* (地榆, *Radix Sanguisorbae*) 9 g and *zōng lǚ tàn* (棕榈炭, *Petiolus Trachycarpi Carbonisatus*) 9 g.
- For a severe poor appetite, combine with *shā rén* (砂仁, *Fructus Amomi*) 6 g (decoct later) and *shén qū* (神曲, *Massa Medicata Fermentata*) 9 g.
- For soreness and weakness of the low back and knee joints, combine with *xù duàn* (续断, *Radix Dipsaci*) 9 g and *dù zhòng* (杜仲, *Cortex Eucommiae*) 9 g.
- For chest tightness and discomfort, combine with *zhǐ qiào* (枳壳, *Fructus Aurantii*) 9 g and *chén pí* (陈皮, *Pericarpium Citri Reticulatae*) 9 g.

Yang deficiency of the spleen and kidneys

Signs and symptoms

Recurrent subcutaneous bruises in a pale color, bleeding from the nostrils, bleeding at the gums, fatigue, cold intolerance, cold limbs, pallor, soreness and weakness of the low back and knee joints, and heavy menstruation.

Tongue: pale, with a thin white coating
Pulse: deep and thready

Treatment principle

Warm and tonify the spleen and kidneys, nourish blood and arrest bleeding.

Formula

Modified *Jīn Guì Shèn Qì Wán* (金匮肾气丸, "Golden Cabinet's Kidney *Qi* Pill").

制附子	*zhì fù zǐ*	9 g	*Radix Aconiti Lateralis Praeparata* (decoct first)
肉桂	*ròu guì,*	4.5 g	*Cortex Cinnamomi* (decoct later)
熟地黄	*shú dì huáng*	15 g	*Radix Rehmanniae Praeparata*
山药	*shān yào*	15 g	*Rhizoma Dioscoreae*
山茱萸	*shān zhū yú*	9 g	*Fructus Corni*
茯苓	*fú líng*	9 g	*Poria*
灶心土	*zào xīn tǔ*	30 g	*Terra Flava Usta* (wrapped)

Modifications

- For severe cold intolerance and cold limbs, combine with *xiān máo* (仙茅, *Rhizoma Curculiginis*) 9 g and *xiān líng pí* (仙灵脾, *Herba Epimedii*) 9 g.
- For severe fatigue, combine with *dǎng shēn* (党参, *Radix Codonopsis*) 9 g and *huáng qí* (黄芪, *Radix Astragali*) 15 g.
- For severe soreness and weakness of the low back and knee joints, combine with *dù zhòng* (杜仲, *Cortex Eucommiae*) 9 g and *tù sī zǐ* (菟丝子, *Semen Cuscutae*).
- For severe bleeding tendency, combine with *sān qī* (三七, *Radix et Rhizoma Notoginseng*) 9 g and *ǒu jié tàn* (藕节炭, *Nodus Nelumbinis Rhizomatis Carbonisatus*) 9 g.

Retention of internal blood stasis

Signs and symptoms

Subcutaneous bruises or dark petechiae, masses in the hypochondrium, low back pain, bleeding at the gums or vomiting up dark-purple blood.

Tongue: dark, with ecchymosis
Pulse: wiry and hesitant

Treatment principle

Circulate *qi*, invigorate blood, resolve stasis and arrest bleeding.

Formula

Modified *Xuè Fǔ Zhú Yū Tāng* (血府逐瘀汤, "Blood Stasis–Expelling Decoction").

当归	*dāng guī*	9 g	*Radix Angelicae Sinensis*
赤芍	*chì sháo*	9 g	*Radix Paeoniae Rubra*
川芎	*chuān xiōng*	9 g	*Rhizoma Chuanxiong*
桃仁	*táo rén*	9 g	*Semen Persicae*
红花	*hóng huā*	9 g	*Flos Carthami*
柴胡	*chái hú*	9 g	*Radix Bupleuri*
枳壳	*zhǐ qiào*	9 g	*Fructus Aurantii*
牛膝	*niú xī*	9 g	*Radix Achyranthis Bidentatae*
甘草	*gān cǎo*	9 g	*Radix et Rhizoma Glycyrrhizae*

Modifications

- For distending pain in the hepatic and hypochondriac regions, combine with *yán hú suǒ* (延胡索, *Rhizoma Corydalis*) 9 g and *chuān liàn zǐ* (川楝子, *Fructus Toosendan*) 9 g.
- For masses in the hypochondrium, combine with *wǔ líng zhī* (五灵脂, *Faeces Trogopterori*) 9 g (wrapped) and *pú huáng* (蒲黄, *Pollen Typhae*) 9 g (wrapped).
- For bleeding, combine with *sān qī* (三七, *Radix et Rhizoma Notoginseng*) 9 g (mix with water and swallow).
- For constipation, combine with *dà huáng* (大黄, *Radix et Rhizoma Rhei*) 9 g (decoct later) and *má rén* (麻仁, *Fructus Cannabis*) 9 g.

QUESTIONS

1. Describe the common symptoms of idiopathic thrombocytopenic purpura.
2. List the pattern identifications and treatment methods of idiopathic thrombocytopenic purpura in Chinese medicine.
3. *Case study.* Try to make a pattern identification and give a prescription for the following case:

Ms. Zhang, 25, suffered from sudden recent subcutaneous red bruises on the thigh with no pain or itching. Other symptoms included bleeding from the nostrils, a dry mouth with a desire to drink water, restlessness, irritability, dark-yellow urine and constipation. The tongue was red, with a dry yellow coating. The pulse was wiry and rapid.

COMMON NERVOUS SYSTEM CONDITIONS

Migraine

Overview

Migraine is a medical condition characterized by recurrent attacks of moderate-to-severe headaches. Although much about the cause of migraine is not understood, genetics seems to play a role. Approximately 50% of patients with migraine have a family history. The condition more commonly affects women, and this is often associated with menstruation. Mental stress, overexertion, a sudden change of weather, light stimulus, sunlight and hypoglycemia may trigger attacks of migraine. In addition, vasodilators or reserpine, ingestion of chocolate, cheese and oranges or tangerines, and drinking alcoholic beverages may also induce migraine. Currently, this condition can be categorized into five patterns migraine without an aura, migraine with an aura, retinal migraine, childhood periodic syndromes and persistent migraine.

In Chinese medicine, migraine falls under the category of "headache" or "head wind." It is closely associated with the liver, spleen and kidneys. The causative factors include hyperactivity of liver yang due to liver yin deficiency, liver *qi* stagnation transforming into fire, deficiency of *qi* and blood (due to spleen deficiency) and internal cold or hyperactive wind yang (due to kidney deficiency). Persistent headache with a stabbing sensation is often caused by blood stasis in the collaterals.

Clinical manifestations

Migraine is characterized by intense headache. The typical migraine headache is unilateral; however, the entire head and nape may also be affected. The pain is pulsating, with a distending and burning sensation. In severe cases, the pain can be splitting. The migraine headache often occurs in the morning, lasting from hours to 1–2 days. The pain can be relieved by bed rest. Migraines during daytime can be periodic but irregular. Migraines during the night are often regular, lasting from dozens of minutes to 1–2 h and requiring an extended remission stage. Other symptoms may include nausea, vomiting, dizziness, palpitations, sweating and photophobia.

Pattern identification and treatment

Migraine due to hyperactivity of liver yang

Signs and symptoms

Pulsating or splitting headache with a sense of distension (the pain can involve the eyes and nape), restlessness, irritability, red face and eyes, a dry mouth with a bitter taste and distending pain or discomfort in the hypochondriac regions.

Tongue: red, with a thin yellow coating
Pulse: wiry and rapid

Treatment principle

Soothe the liver and suppress yang.

Formula

Modified *Tiān Má Gōu Téng Yǐn* (天麻钩藤饮, "Gastrodia and Uncaria Beverage").

天麻	*tiān má*	9 g	*Rhizoma Gastrodiae*
钩藤	*gōu téng*	12 g	*Ramulus Uncariae Cum Uncis* (decoct later)
石决明	*shí jué míng*	30 g	*Concha Haliotidis*
山栀	*shān zhī*	9 g	*Fructus Gardeniae*
茯神	*fú shén*	9 g	*Sclerotium Poriae Pararadicis*
牛膝	*niú xī*	9 g	*Radix Achyranthis Bidentatae*
生地	*shēng dì*	15 g	*Radix Rehmanniae*

Modifications

- For severe headache, combine with *zhēn zhū mǔ* (珍珠母, *Concha Margaritiferae Usta*) 30 g (decoct first) and *lóng dǎn cǎo* (龙胆草, *Radix et Rhizoma Gentianae*) 9 g.
- For tinnitus and weakness of the knee joints, combine with *gǒu qǐzǐ* (枸杞子, *Fructus Lycii*) 9 g and *nǚ zhēn zǐ* (女贞子, *Fructus Ligustri Lucidi*) 9 g.
- For a dry mouth with a desire to drink water, combine with *yù zhú* (玉竹, *Rhizoma Polygonati Odorati*) 9 g and *shí hú* (石斛, *Caulis Dendrobii*) 9 g.
- For constipation, combine with *dà huáng* (大黄, *Radix et Rhizoma Rhei*) 9 g (decoct later) and *máng xiāo* (芒硝, *Natrii Sulfas*) 9 g.

Migraine due to phlegm turbidity

Signs and symptoms

Headache with mental cloudiness, chest or gastric fullness, nausea, vomiting, a poor appetite and a dry mouth with no desire to drink water.

Tongue: a white greasy coating
Pulse: wiry and slippery

Treatment principle

Resolve phlegm and downregulate *qi*.

Formula

Modified *Bàn Xià Bái Zhú Tiān Má Tāng* (半夏白术天麻汤, "Pinellia, *Atractylodes Macrocephala* and Gastrodia Decoction").

半夏	*bàn xià*	9 g	*Rhizoma Pinelliae*
白术	*bái zhú*	9 g	*Rhizoma Atractylodis Macrocephalae*
天麻	*tiān má*	9 g	*Rhizoma Gastrodiae*
茯苓	*fú líng*	9 g	*Poria*
陈皮	*chén pí*	9 g	*Pericarpium Citri Reticulatae*
蔓荆子	*màn jīng zǐ*	9 g	*Fructus Viticis*
制南星	*zhì nán xīng*	9 g	*Rhizoma Arisaematis praeparatum*
竹茹	*zhú rú*	9 g	*Caulis Bambusae in Taenia*

Modifications

- For severe chest fullness, combine with *hòu pò* (厚朴, *Cortex Magnoliae Officinalis*) 9 g and *zhǐ qiào* (枳壳, *Fructus Aurantii*) 9 g.
- For a severe bitter taste, combine with *huáng lián* (黄连, *Rhizoma Coptidis*) 4.5 g and *huáng qín* (黄芩, *Radix Scutellariae*) 9 g.
- For severe headache, combine with *bái zhǐ* (白芷, *Radix Angelicae Dahuricae*) 9 g and *qiāng huó* (羌活, *Rhizoma et Radix Notopterygii*) 9 g.
- For a poor appetitle or loss of appetite, combine with *cāng zhú* (苍术, *Rhizoma Atractylodis*) 9 g and *shén qū* (神曲, *Massa Medicata Fermentata*) 9 g.

Migraine due to blood stasis

Signs and symptoms

Persistent severe headache with a stabbing sensation in a fixed position and a dark-gray complexion.

Tongue: dark-purple or with ecchymosis or petechia
Pulse: thready and hesitant

Treatment principle

Invigorate blood and resolve stasis.

Formula

Modified *Tōng Qiào Huó Xuè Tāng* (通窍活血汤, "Orifice-Unblocking and Blood-Invigorating Decoction").

桃仁	táo rén	9 g	Semen Persicae
红花	hóng huā	9 g	Flos Carthami
川芎	chuān xiōng	12 g	Rhizoma Chuanxiong
赤芍	chì sháo	9 g	Radix Paeoniae Rubra
麝香	shè xiāng	0.1 g	Moschus
当归	dāng guī	9 g	Radix Angelicae Sinensis
葱白	cōng bái	2 p	Bulbus Allii Fistulosi

Modifications

- For severe headache, combine with *quán xiē* (全蝎, *Scorpio*) 3 g and *wú gōng* (蜈蚣, *Scolopendra*) 3 g.
- For cold intolerance, combine with *guì zhī* (桂枝, *Ramulus Cinnamomi*) 6 g and *xì xīn* (细辛, *Radix et Rhizoma Asari*) 4.5 g.
- For chest tightness and discomfort, combine with *hòu pò* (厚朴, *Cortex Magnoliae Officinalis*) 9 g and *chuān liàn zǐ* (川楝子, *Fructus Toosendan*) 9 g.
- For poor sleep, combine with *suān zǎo rén* (酸枣仁, *Semen Ziziphi Spinosae*) 9 g and *cí shí* (磁石, *Magnetitum*) 30 g.

Migraine due to qi deficiency

Signs and symptoms

Dull lingering intermittent headache that can be worsened by fatigue, lassitude, cold intolerance, lack of energy, tastelessness and a poor appetite.

Tongue: pale, with a thin coating
Pulse: soft and thready

Treatment principle

Supplement *qi* and lift clean *qi*.

Formula

Modified *Shùn Qì Hé Zhōng Tāng* (顺气和中汤, "*Qi*-Balancing and Middle *Jiao*–Harmonizing Decoction").

党参	*dǎng shēn*	9 g	*Radix Codonopsis*
黄芪	*huáng qí*	30 g	*Radix Astragali*
白术	*bái zhú*	9 g	*Rhizoma Atractylodis Macrocephalae*
甘草	*gān cǎo*	9 g	*Radix et Rhizoma Glycyrrhizae*
当归	*dāng guī*	9 g	*Radix Angelicae Sinensis*
白芍	*bái sháo*	9 g	*Radix Paeoniae Alba*

陈皮	*chén pí*	9 g	*Pericarpium Citri Reticulatae*
升麻	*shēng má*	9 g	*Rhizoma Cimicifugae*
蔓荆子	*màn jīng zǐ*	9 g	*Fructus Viticis*
白芷	*bái zhǐ*	9 g	*Radix Angelicae Dahuricae*
川芎	*chuān xiōng*	12 g	*Rhizoma Chuanxiong*

Modifications

- For severe headache and vertigo, combine with *xì xīn* (细辛, *Radix et Rhizoma Asari*) 4.5 g and *bái jí lí* (白蒺藜, *Fructus Tribuli*) 9 g.
- For soreness and weakness of the low back and knee joints, combine with *xù duàn* (续断, *Radix Dipsaci*) 9 g and *dù zhòng* (杜仲, *Cortex Eucommiae*) 9 g.
- For feverish sensations of the palms, soles and chest, combine with *hàn lián cǎo* (旱莲草, *Herba Ecliptae*) 9 g and *gǒu qǐzǐ* (枸杞子, *Fructus Lycii*) 9 g.
- For chest tightness and discomfort, combine with *zhǐ qiào* (枳壳, *Fructus Aurantii*) 9 g and *lù lù tōng* (路路通, *Fructus Liquidambaris*) 9 g.

Migraine due to blood deficiency

Signs and symptoms

Headache, vertigo, a lusterless complexion, mild or severe palpitations, a low spirit and fatigue.

Tongue: pale, with a thin coating
Pulse: thready

Treatment principle

Nourish blood and relieve pain.

Formula

Supplemented *Sì Wù Tāng* (四物汤, "Four Substances Decoction").

熟地黄	*shú dì huáng*	15 g	*Radix Rehmanniae Praeparata*
当归	*dāng guī*	9 g	*Radix Angelicae Sinensis*
赤芍	*chì sháo*	9 g	*Radix Paeoniae Rubra*
白芍	*bái sháo*	9 g	*Radix Paeoniae Alba*
川芎	*chuān xiōng*	12 g	*Rhizoma Chuanxiong*
蔓荆子	*màn jīng zǐ*	9 g	*Fructus Viticis*
菊花	*jú huā*	9 g	*Flos Chrysanthemi*
桑椹	*sāng shèn*	9 g	*Fructus Mori*

Modifications

- For tinnitus and insomnia, combine with *suān zǎo rén* (酸枣仁, *Semen Ziziphi Spinosae*) 9 g and *cí shí* (磁石, *Magnetitum*) 30 g.
- For soreness and weakness of the low back and knee joints, combine with *huáng jīng* (黄精, *Rhizoma Polygonati*) 15 g and *nǚ zhēn zǐ* (女贞子, *Fructus Ligustri Lucidi*) 15 g.
- For feverish sensations of the palms, soles and chest, combine with *gǒu qǐzǐ* (枸杞子, Fructus Lycii) 9 g and *zhī mǔ* (知母, *Rhizoma Anemarrhenae*) 9 g.
- For headache with a sense of distension, combine with *shí jué míng* (石决明, *Concha Haliotidis*) 30 g (decoct first) and *mǔ lì* (牡蛎, *Concha Ostreae*) 30 g (decoct first).

Migraine due to kidney deficiency

Signs and symptoms

Headache with a hollow sensation, dizziness, blurred vision, tinnitus, insomnia, cold intolerance, cold limbs, soreness and weakness of the low back and knee joints, nocturnal emissions and leukorrhea.

Tongue: pale, with a thin coating
Pulse: deep, thready and weak

Treatment principle

Tonify the kidneys and fill essence.

Formula

Modified *Dà Bǔ Yuán Jiān* (大补元煎, "Major *Yuan*–Supplementing Decoction")

熟地黄	*shú dì huáng*	15 g	Radix Rehmanniae Praeparata
山药	*shān yào*	15 g	Rhizoma Dioscoreae
山茱萸	*shān zhū yú*	9 g	Fructus Corni
枸杞子	*gǒu qǐ zǐ*	9 g	Fructus Lycii
当归	*dāng guī*	9 g	Radix Angelicae Sinensis
杜仲	*dù zhòng*	9 g	Cortex Eucommiae
党参	*dǎng shēn*	12 g	Radix Codonopsis

Modifications

- For severe headache, combine with *chuān xiōng* (川芎, *Rhizoma Chuanxiong*) 12 g and *bái zhǐ* (白芷, *Radix Angelicae Dahuricae*) 9 g.
- For frequent nocturnal emissions, combine with *jīn yīng zǐ* (金樱子, *Fructus Rosae Laevigatae*) 9 g and *qiàn shí* (芡实, *Semen Euryales*) 15 g.
- For severe leukorrhea, combine with *hǎi piāo xiāo* (海螵蛸, *Endoconcha Sepiae*) 9 g and *chūn gēn pí* (椿根皮, *Cortex Ailanthi*) 9 g.
- For severe cold intolerance, combine with *ròu cōng róng* (肉苁蓉, *Herba Cistanches*) 9 g and *lù jiǎo* (鹿角, *Cornu Cervi*) 9 g (decoct first).

QUESTIONS

1. Describe the main clinical symptoms of migraine.
2. List the possible contributing or triggering factors of migraine.
3. *Case study*. Try to make a pattern identification and give a prescription for the following case:

Ms. Zhuang, 40, suffered for 20 years from migraines that were associated with menstruation, weather changes, emotions and fatigue. Two days prior to treatment, she experienced headache with a distending sensation in the temporal regions, chest tightness, nausea, a poor appetite and loose stools. The tongue coating was white and greasy. The pulse was soft.

Acute Cerebrovascular Disease

Overview

Acute cerebrovascular disease, also known as a cerebrovascular accident (CVA) or a stroke, is the rapidly developing loss of brain functions due to disturbance in the blood supply to the brain. This can be due to ischemia (lack of blood flow) caused by blockages (thrombosis, arterial embolism) or a hemorrhage (leakage of blood). As a result, the affected area of the brain is unable to function, leading to a sudden collapse, deviation of the mouth and eyes, inability to move one or more limbs on one side of the body, and inability to understand or formulate speech.

This condition is marked by a sudden onset, rapid progression, high mortality and a substantial sequela. Its incidence increases exponentially from 40 years of age. The elderly with hypertension are the most common risk group. Ischemic strokes are those that are caused by interruption of the blood supply, including transient ischemic attack (TIA), atherosclerotic infarct of the brain and brain embolism; while hemorrhagic strokes are the ones which result from rupture of a blood vessel or an abnormal vascular structure, including hypertensive cerebral hemorrhage or subarachnoid hemorrhage.

In Chinese medicine, acute cerebrovascular disease is known as "windstroke" or "apoplexy." The main contributing factors include emotional disturbance, overingestion of fatty food and overexertion.

Emotional disturbance may cause a sudden hyperactivity of liver yang and subsequent disorder of *qi* and blood, which in turn may ascend to affect the mind. Excessive ingestion of fatty food may impair the spleen and stomach, leading to internal phlegm dampness. Over time, the phlegm dampness may transform into fire and stir liver wind to affect the brain. Overexertion may consume yin blood and result in hyperactivity of deficient fire to affect the brain.

Clinical manifestations

Typical symptoms of acute cerebrovascular disease are sudden collapse, unconsciousness, deviation of the eyes and mouth, hemiplegia and slurred speech. Patients with the ischemic type can remain conscious. However, some patients may stay conscious at first but gradually became confused. In severe cases, patients may experience immediate mental confusion. In most cases, patients may experience an inability to move one side of the body and some may become totally paralyzed after hours or 2–3 days. The hemorrhagic type can be fatal. In mild cases, patients may remain conscious but still develop hemiplegia.

Pattern identification and treatment

Sudden hyperactivity of liver yang

Signs and symptoms

Hemiplegia, numbness on one side of the body, deviation of the mouth and eyes, tongue stiffness, slurred speech or an inability to formulate speech, dizziness, blurred vision, headache with a sense of distension, red face and eyes, a dry throat with a bitter taste, restlessness, irritability, dark-yellow urine and constipation

Tongue: red or dark-red, with a thin yellow coating
Pulse: wiry

Treatment principle

Soothe the liver and reduce fire.

Formula

Modified *Tiān Má Gōu Téng Yǐn* (天麻钩藤饮, "Gastrodia and Uncaria Beverage").

天麻	*tiān má*	9 g	Rhizoma Gastrodiae
钩藤	*gōu téng*	12 g	Ramulus Uncariae Cum Uncis (decoct later)
石决明	*shí jué míng*	30 g	Concha Haliotidis
黄芩	*huáng qín*	9 g	Radix Scutellariae
山栀	*shān zhī*	9 g	Fructus Gardeniae
牡丹皮	*mǔ dān pí*	9 g	Cortex Moutan
赤芍	*chì sháo*	9 g	Radix Paeoniae Rubra
夏枯草	*xià kū cǎo*	9 g	Spica Prunellae

Modifications

- For severe headache with red eyes, combine with *lóng dǎn cǎo* (龙胆草, *Radix et Rhizoma Gentianae*) 9 g and *jué míng zǐ* (决明子, *Semen Cassiae*) 30 g.
- For constipation, combine with *dà huáng* (大黄, *Radix et Rhizoma Rhei*) 9 g (decoct later) and *máng xiāo* (芒硝, *Natrii Sulfas*) 9 g.
- For restlessness and insomnia, combine with *zhēn zhū mǔ* (珍珠母, *Concha Margaritiferae Usta*) 30 g and *suān zǎo rén* (酸枣仁, *Semen Ziziphi Spinosae*) 9 g.
- For thirst with a desire to drink water, combine with *shēng dì* (生地, *Radix Rehmanniae*) 15 g and *shí hú* (石斛, *Caulis Dendrobii*) 9 g.

Wind phlegm with bloods stasis

Signs and symptoms

Hemiplegia, deviation of the mouth and eyes, tongue stiffness, slurred speech or an inability to formulate speech, numbness on one side of the body, dizziness, blurred vision and chest tightness.

Tongue: gray–pale, with a thin white or white greasy coating
Pulse: wiry and slippery

Treatment principle

Expel wind and resolve phlegm.

Formula

Modified *Bàn Xià Bái Zhú Tiān Má Tāng* (半夏白术天麻汤, "Pinellia, Atractylodes Macrocephala and Gastrodia Decoction").

半夏	*bàn xià*	9 g	*Rhizoma Pinelliae*
白术	*bái zhú*	9 g	*Rhizoma Atractylodis Macrocephalae*
天麻	*tiān má*	9 g	*Rhizoma Gastrodiae*
胆南星	*dǎn nán xīng*	9 g	*Arisaema cum Bile*
丹参	*dān shēn*	15 g	*Radix et Rhizoma Salviae Miltiorrhizae*
制大黄	*zhì dà huáng*	9 g	*Radix et Rhizoma Rhei Praeparata* (decoct later)
香附	*xiāng fù*	9 g	*Rhizoma Cyperi*

Modifications

- For a bitter taste and a red tongue, combine with *huáng qín* (黄芩, *Radix Scutellariae*) 9 g and *shān zhī* (山栀, *Fructus Gardeniae*) 9 g.
- For headache with a sense of distension, combine with *shí jué míng* (石决明, *Concha Haliotidis*) 15 g (decoct first) and *jú huā* (菊花, *Flos Chrysanthemi*) 9 g.
- For profuse sputum, combine with *guā lóu* (瓜蒌, *Fructus Trichosanthis*) 15 g and *zhú rú* (竹茹, *Caulis Bambusae in Taenia*) 9 g.
- For severe chest fullness or tightness, combine with *hòu pò* (厚朴, *Cortex Magnoliae Officinalis*) 9 g and *zhǐ shí* (枳实, *Fructus Aurantii Immaturus*) 9 g.

Retention of phlegm heat

Signs and symptoms

Hemiplegia, deviation of the mouth and eyes, tongue stiffness or slurred speech, numbness on one side of the body, dizziness, blurred vision, profuse sputum, gastric or abdominal fullness and distension, dark-yellow urine and constipation.

Tongue: dark-red or gray–pale, with a yellow or yellow greasy coating
Pulse: wiry and slippery

Treatment principle

Clear heat and resolve phlegm.

Formula

Modified *Dà Chéng Qì Tāng* (大承气汤, "Major Purgative Decoction") and *Dǎo Tán Tāng* (导痰汤, "Phlegm-Expelling Decoction").

大黄	*dà huáng*	9 g	*Radix et Rhizoma Rhei* (decoct later)
芒硝	*máng xiāo*	6 g	*Natrii Sulfas*
枳实	*zhǐ shí*	9 g	*Fructus Aurantii Immaturus*
厚朴	*hòu pò*	9 g	*Cortex Magnoliae Officinalis*

半夏	*bàn xià*	9 g	*Rhizoma Pinelliae*
胆南星	*dǎn nán xīng*	9 g	*Arisaema cum Bile*
瓜蒌	*guā lóu*	15 g	*Fructus Trichosanthis*
黄连	*huáng lián*	3 g	*Rhizoma Coptidis*

Modifications

- For yellow sticky sputum, combine with *tiān zhú huáng* (天竺黄, *Concretio Silicea Bambusae*) 9 g and *zhú rú* (竹茹, *Caulis Bambusae in Taenia*) 9 g.

- For a dry mouth and throat, combine with *lú gēn* (芦根, *Rhizoma Phragmitis*) 15 g and *tiān huā fēn* (天花粉, *Radix Trichosanthis*) 9 g.

- For severe headache and dizziness, combine with *zhēn zhū mǔ* (珍珠母, *Concha Margaritiferae Usta*) 30 g and *gōu téng* (钩藤, *Ramulus Uncariae Cum Uncis*) 12 g (decoct later).

- For gastric and abdominal fullness and distension, combine with *dà fù pí* (大腹皮, *Pericarpium Arecae*) 9 g and *lù lù tōng* (路路通, *Fructus Liquidambaris*) 9 g.

Qi deficiency with blood stasis

Signs and symptoms

Hemiplegia, deviation of the mouth and eyes, slurred speech or an inability to formulate speech, numbness on one side of the body, pallor, fatigue, palpitations, shortness of breath, salivation, spontaneous sweating and loose stools.

Tongue: gray–pale, with a thin white or thin greasy coating
Pulse: wiry and thready

Treatment principle

Supplement *qi* and invigorate blood.

Formula

Modified *Bǔ Yáng Huán Wǔ Tāng* (补阳还五汤, "Yang-Supplementing and Five-Returning Decoction").

黄芪	huáng qí	15 g	Radix Astragali
桃仁	táo rén	9 g	Semen Persicae
红花	hóng huā	9 g	Flos Carthami
当归	dāng guī	9 g	Radix Angelicae Sinensis
川芎	chuān xiōng	9 g	Rhizoma Chuanxiong
赤芍	chì sháo	9 g	Radix Paeoniae Rubra
地龙	dì lóng	9 g	Pheretima
丹参	dān shēn	15 g	Radix et Rhizoma Salviae Miltiorrhizae

Modifications

- For severe fatigue, combine with *dǎng shēn* (党参, *Radix Codonopsis*) 9 g and *xiān hè cǎo* (仙鹤草, *Herba Agrimoniae*) 30 g.
- For loose stools, combine with *shān yào* (山药, *Rhizoma Dioscoreae*) 9 g and *bái biǎn dòu* (白扁豆, *Semen Lablab Album*) 9 g.
- For a greasy tongue coating, combine with *cāng zhú* (苍术, *Rhizoma Atractylodis*) 9 g and *bái zhú* (白术, *Rhizoma Atractylodis Macrocephalae*) 9 g.
- For a dark-purple tongue, combine with *sān léng* (三棱, *Rhizoma Sparganii*) 9 g and *tū biē chóng* (土鳖虫, *Eupolyphaga seu Steleophaga*) 6 g.

Wind stirring due to yin deficiency

Signs and symptoms

Hemiplegia, deviation of the mouth and eyes, tongue stiffness, slurred speech, numbness on one side of the body, restlessness, palpitations, insomnia, dizziness, tinnitus, feverish sensations of the palms and soles.

Tongue: dark-red, with no or a scanty coating
Pulse: wiry, thready and rapid

Treatment principle

Nourish yin and expel wind.

Formula

Modified *Zhèn Gān Xī Fēng Tāng* (镇肝息风汤, "Liver-Sedating and Wind-Extinguishing Decoction").

生地	*shēng dì*	15 g	*Radix Rehmanniae*
玄参	*xuán shēn*	9 g	*Radix Scrophulariae*
女贞子	*nǚ zhēn zǐ*	9 g	*Fructus Ligustri Lucidi*
钩藤	*gōu téng*	12 g	*Ramulus Uncariae Cum Uncis* (decoct later)
白芍	*bái sháo*	9 g	*Radix Paeoniae Alba*
丹参	*dān shēn*	15 g	*Radix et Rhizoma Salviae Miltiorrhizae*
龙骨	*lóng gǔ*	30 g	*Os Draconis* (decoct first)

Modifications

- For dizziness and tinnitus, combine with *mǔ lì* (牡蛎, *Concha Ostreae*) 30 g (decoct first) and *zhēn zhū mǔ* (珍珠母, *Concha Margaritiferae Usta*) 30 g.
- For restlessness and insomnia, combine with *lián zǐ xīn* (莲子心, *Plumula Nelumbinis*) 9 g and *suān zǎo rén* (酸枣仁, *Semen Ziziphi Spinosae*) 9 g.
- For constipation, combine with *má rén* (麻仁, *Fructus Cannabis*) 9 g and *yù lǐ rén* (郁李仁, *Semen Pruni*) 9 g.
- For a dry dark-red tongue with no coating, combine with *shí hú* (石斛, *Caulis Dendrobii*) 9 g and *guī bǎn* (龟板, *Plastrum Testudinis*) 15 g (decoct first).

Wind–fire disturbing the mind

Signs and symptoms

Mental confusion or unconsciousness, hemiplegia, stiffness and contracture of the limbs, and constipation.

Tongue: dark-red, with a dry yellow coating
Pulse: wiry, slippery and rapid

Treatment principle

Clear heat, expel wind and refresh the mind.

Formula

Modified *Líng Jiǎo Gōu Téng Yǐn* (羚角钩藤饮, "Antelope Horn and Uncaria Beverage")

羚羊角	*líng yáng jiǎo*	0.6 g	*Cornu Saigae Tataricae*
天麻	*tiān má*	9 g	*Rhizoma Gastrodiae*
钩藤	*gōu téng*	12 g	*Ramulus Uncariae Cum Uncis* (decoct later)
石决明	*shí jué míng*	30 g	*Concha Haliotidis*
黄芩	*huáng qín*	9 g	*Radix Scutellariae*
山栀	*shān zhī*	9 g	*Fructus Gardeniae*
大黄	*dà huáng*	9 g	*Radix et Rhizoma Rhei* (decoct later)
牡蛎	*mǔ lì*	30 g	*Concha Ostreae*

Modifications

- For a greasy coating due to phlegm dampness, combine with *shí chāng pú* (石菖蒲, *Rhizoma Acori Tatarinowii*) 15 g and *cāng zhú* (苍术, *Rhizoma Atractylodis*) 9 g.
- For a red face and eyes, combine with *lóng dǎn cǎo* (龙胆草, *Radix et Rhizoma Gentianae*) 9 g and *xià kū cǎo* (夏枯草, *Spica Prunellae*) 9 g.
- For severe convulsions, combine with *lóng gǔ* (龙骨, *Os Draconis*) 30 g (decoct first) and *quán xiē* (全蝎, *Scorpio*) 3 g.
- For a severe dry tongue, combine with *shēng dì* (生地, *Radix Rehmanniae*) 15 g and *mài dōng* (麦冬, *Radix Ophiopogonis*) 9 g.

Phlegm misting the mind

Signs and symptoms

Unconsciousness, hemiplegia, cold, loosened limbs, pallor, dark lips and profuse salivation.

Tongue: gray–pale with a white greasy coating
Pulse: deep and slippery

Treatment principle

Dry dampness, resolve phlegm and refresh the mind.

Formula

Modified *Dí Tán Tāng* (涤痰汤, "Phlegm-Flushing Decoction").

半夏	*bàn xià*	9 g	*Rhizoma Pinelliae*
陈皮	*chén pí*	9 g	*Pericarpium Citri Reticulatae*
枳实	*zhǐ shí*	9 g	*Fructus Aurantii Immaturus*
胆南星	*dǎn nán xīng*	9 g	*Arisaema cum Bile*
石菖蒲	*shí chāng pú*	9 g	*Rhizoma Acori Tatarinowii*
竹茹	*zhú rú*	9 g	*Caulis Bambusae in Taenia*
远志	*yuǎn zhì*	9 g	*Radix Polygalae*
苏合香丸	*Sū Hé Xiāng Wán*	1 pill	*"Storax Pill"*

Modifications

- For severe cold limbs, combine with *páo fù zǐ* (炮附子, *Radix Aconiti Lateralis Praeparata*) 6 g (decoct first) and *guì zhī* (桂枝, *Ramulus Cinnamomi*) 6 g.
- For severe convulsions, combine with *quán xiē* (全蝎, *Scorpio*) 3 g and *wú gōng* (蜈蚣, *Scolopendra*) 3 g.
- For a yellow greasy tongue coating, combine with *tiān zhú huáng* (天竺黄, *Concretio Silicea Bambusae*) 9 g and *xià kū cǎo* (夏枯草, *Spica Prunellae*) 9 g.

Phlegm heat blocking the mind

Signs and symptoms

Unconsciousness, hemiplegia, a phlegm sound in the throat, stiffness and contracture of the limbs, feverish sensations of the body and restlessness.

Tongue: dark-red, with a dry yellow greasy coating
Pulse: wiry, slippery and rapid

Treatment principle

Clear heat, resolve phlegm and open the orifice.

Formula

Modified *Qīng Qì Huà Tán Wán* (清气化痰丸, "*Qi*-Clearing and Phlegm-Transforming Pill").

胆南星	*dǎn nán xīng*	9 g	*Arisaema cum Bile*
半夏	*bàn xià*	9 g	*Rhizoma Pinelliae*
枳实	*zhǐ shí*	9 g	*Fructus Aurantii Immaturus*
黄芩	*huáng qín*	9 g	*Radix Scutellariae*
瓜蒌	*guā lóu*	15 g	*Fructus Trichosanthis*
陈皮	*chén pí*	9 g	*Pericarpium Citri Reticulatae*
天竺黄	*tiān zhú huáng*	9 g	*Concretio Silicea Bambusae*
石菖蒲	*shí chāng pú*	9 g	*Rhizoma Acori Tatarinowii*
安宫牛黄丸	*Ān Gōng Niú Huáng Wán*	1 pill	*"Peaceful Palace Bovine Bezoar Pill"*

Modifications

- For severe convulsions, combine with a powder of *líng yáng jiǎo* (羚羊角, *Cornu Saigae Tataricae*) 0.6 g and *shuǐ niú jiǎo* (水牛角, *Cornu Bubali*) 30 g (decoct first).
- For a severe feverish sensation of the body, combine with *huáng qín* (黄芩, *Radix Scutellariae*) 9 g and *shān zhī* (山栀, *Fructus Gardeniae*) 9 g.
- For constipation, combine with *dà huáng* (大黄, *Radix et Rhizoma Rhei*) 9 g (decoct later) and *máng xiāo* (芒硝, *Natrii Sulfas*) 9 g.
- For severe restlessness, combine with *lián zǐ xīn* (莲子心, *Plumula Nelumbinis*) 9 g and *mài dōng* (麦冬, *Radix Ophiopogonis*) 9 g.

Collapse of yuan primordial qi

Signs and symptoms

Unconsciousness, paralysis of the limbs, cold limbs, profuse cold sweating, and urinary and fecal incontinence.

Tongue: dark-purple, with a white greasy coating
Pulse: deep and faint

Treatment principle

Tonify *yuan* primordial *qi* and resuscitate yang.

Formula

Modified *Shēn Fù Tāng* (参附汤, "Ginseng and Aconite Decoction").

人参	*rén shēn*	15 g	Radix et Rhizoma Ginseng
制附子	*zhì fù zǐ*	9 g	Radix Aconiti Lateralis Praeparata (decoct first)
石菖蒲	*shí chāng pú*	9 g	Rhizoma Acori Tatarinowii
五味子	*wǔ wèi zǐ*	9 g	Fructus Schisandrae Chinensis
炙甘草	*zhì gān cǎo*	9 g	Radix et Rhizoma Glycyrrhizae Praeparata cum Melle

Modifications

- For extreme sweating, combine with *lóng gǔ* (龙骨, Os Draconis) 30 g (decoct first) and *mǔ lì* (牡蛎, Concha Ostreae) 30 g (decoct first).
- For a red tongue, combine with *xī yáng shēn* (西洋参, *Radix Panacis Quinquefolii*) 6 g (separately) and *guī bǎn* (龟板, *Plastrum Testudinis*) 15 g (decoct first).

QUESTIONS

1. Describe the main types of acute cerebrovascular disease.
2. Describe the clinical manifestations of acute cerebrovascular disease.
3. *Case study.* Try to make a pattern identification and give a prescription for the following case:

Mr. Lin, 60, suffered from hypertension for 20 years. On the day of treatment, he experienced sudden dizziness and collapse after getting up in the morning, followed by an inability to move the left-sided limb, deviation of the mouth and eyes, tongue stiffness and slurred speech. Other symptoms included a red face and eyes, restlessness, a dry mouth with a bitter taste and constipation. The tongue was red, with a thin yellow coating. The pulse was wiry and tense.

COMMON METABOLIC CONDITIONS

Diabetes Mellitus

Overview

Diabetes mellitus, often simply referred to as diabetes, is a common metabolic endocrine condition. Most cases are primary and genetic, because the body does not produce enough insulin, resulting in metabolic disorders of glucose, protein, fat, water and electrolyte. In severe cases, acid–base imbalance may be present. It is characterized by high blood sugar, glycosuria, decreased glucose tolerance and an abnormal insulin releasing test. Symptoms may develop slowly and may be subtle or absent at the early stages. However, over time, the patient may experience the classical symptoms of polyuria (frequent urination), polydipsia (increased thirst) and polyphagia (increased hunger), weight loss and fatigue. Common complications in the later stages are diabetic cardiovascular disease, nephropathy, ophthalmopathy and neuropathy. In severe cases, diabetic ketoacidosis, nonketotic hyperosmolar coma and lactic acidosis may be present. Additionally, pyogenic infection, urinary tract infection and pulmonary tuberculosis may also be present.

The incidence of diabetes increases with age, especially from the age of 45 to 60. Clinically, diabetes can be categorized into two patterns: insulin-dependent type and non-insulin-dependent type. The former can affect anyone but more commonly affects children and teenagers. The latter often develops more slowly in adults and the elderly. In rare cases, it can also be seen in children.

In Chinese medicine, diabetes falls under the category of "thirsting and wasting," "diaphragm wasting," "lung wasting" or "wasting of the middle *jiao*." The main contributing factors include an improper diet, emotional disturbance, sex indulgence, congenital deficiency, and an overdose of warm and dry-property medications.

Overingestion of hot, spicy, sweet or fatty food may damage the spleen and stomach, leading to internal heat consuming fluids. Long-term depressed anger may impair the liver, leading to liver *qi* stagnation, which may in turn transform into fire. The fire–heat may further consume stomach fluid and kidney essence. Congenital deficiency of the five *zang* organs may eventually result in consumption of essence and fluid.

Clinical manifestations

The classical symptoms of diabetes are polyuria, polydipsia and polyphagia, as well as weight loss and fatigue. For polyuria, patients may have frequent urination of more than 20 time a day, amounting to 2–3 or even 10 L. For polydipsia, patients may drink 5, 10 or 20 L of water a day. For polyphagia, patients can have 5–6 meals with fast hunger. In addition, patients may present with a rapid weight loss and fatigue. Other symptoms may include soreness and weakness of the four limbs, lumbar soreness, reduced libido, impotence, vision changes, irregular menstruation and itchy skin rashes. In severe cases, ketoacidosis, shock or acute renal failure may be present.

Pattern identification and treatment

Dry heat in the lungs and stomach

Signs and symptoms

A dry mouth and tongue, thirst with a desire to drink water, fast hunger with an increased appetite, frequent urination with profuse yellow urine, weight loss and fatigue.

Tongue: red, with a scanty coating
Pulse: slippery and rapid

Treatment principle

Clear heat, moisten the lungs, promote regeneration of fluids and relieve thirst.

Formula

Modified *Xiāo Kě Fāng* (消渴方, "Diabetes-Relieving Formula").

天花粉	*tiān huā fěn*	15 g	*Radix Trichosanthis*
黄连	*huáng lián*	3 g	*Rhizoma Coptidis*
知母	*zhī mǔ*	15 g	*Rhizoma Anemarrhenae*
生地	*shēng dì*	15 g	*Radix Rehmanniae*
葛根	*gé gēn*	9 g	*Radix Puerariae Lobatae*
甘草	*gān cǎo*	9 g	*Radix et Rhizoma Glycyrrhizae*

Modifications

- For a bitter taste, combine with *huáng qín* (黄芩, *Radix Scutellariae*) 9 g, *zhú yè* (竹叶, *Folium Phyllostachydis Henonis*) 9 g and *lián zǐ xīn* (莲子心, *Plumula Nelumbinis*) 9 g.
- For dry stools, combine with *dà huáng* (大黄, *Radix et Rhizoma Rhei*) 9 g (decoct later) and *zhǐ shí* (枳实, *Fructus Aurantii Immaturus*) 9 g.
- For a gastric upset, combine with *shí gāo* (石膏, *Gypsum Fibrosum*) 30 g (ground, and decoct first) and *jīng mī* (粳米, *Oryza Sativa L.*) 9 g.
- For rosy cheeks due to a tidal fever, combine with *mài dōng* (麦冬, *Radix Ophiopogonis*) 9 g and *shā shēn* (沙参, *Radix Adenophorae seu Glehniae*) 9 g.

Exuberance of stomach heat

Signs and symptoms

Fast hunger with an increased appetite, thirst with a desire to drink water and dry stools or constipation.

Tongue: dry and red, with a yellow coating
Pulse: slippery, excessive and powerful

Treatment principle

Clear stomach fire and promote regeneration of fluids.

Formula

Modified *Zēng Yè Chéng Qì Tāng* (增液承气汤, "Humor-Increasing Purgative Decoction").

大黄	*dà huáng*	9 g	*Radix et Rhizoma Rhei* (decoct later)
芒硝	*máng xiāo*	6 g	*Natrii Sulfas*
枳实	*zhǐ shí*	9 g	*Fructus Aurantii Immaturus*
生地	*shēng dì*	15 g	*Radix Rehmanniae*
玄参	*xuán shēn*	9 g	*Radix Scrophulariae*
麦冬	*mài dōng*	9 g	*Radix Ophiopogonis*

Modifications

- For chest tightness and a greasy tongue coating, combine with *cāng zhú* (苍术, *Rhizoma Atractylodis*) 9 g, *cǎo dòu kòu* (草豆蔻, *Semen Alpiniae Katsumadai*) 6 g and *shā rén* (砂仁, *Fructus Amomi*) 6 g (decoct later).
- For severe damage to fluids, combine with *tiān huā fěn* (天花粉, *Radix Trichosanthis*) 9 g and *shí hú* (石斛, *Caulis Dendrobii*) 9 g.
- For a gastric upset with heartburn, combine with *shí gāo* (石膏, *Gypsum Fibrosum*) 30 g (ground, and decoct first) and *zhī mǔ* (知母, *Rhizoma Anemarrhenae*) 12 g.
- For a bitter taste due to exuberant heat, combine with *huáng lián* (黄连, *Rhizoma Coptidis*) 3 g and *huáng bǎi* (黄柏, *Cortex Phellodendri Chinensis*) 9 g.

Deficiency of qi *and* yin

Signs and symptoms

Lack of energy, fatigue, worsened lassitude after physical exertion, spontaneous sweating, night sweats, a dry mouth with a desire to drink water, feverish sensations of the palms, soles and chest, mild or severe palpitations and frequent urination.

Tongue: red, with no or a scanty coating
Pulse: thready and rapid

Treatment principle

Supplement *qi* and nourish yin.

Formula

Modified *Shēng Mài Sǎn* (生脉散, "Pulse-Engendering Powder").

太子参	*tài zǐ shēn*	12 g	Radix Pseudostellariae
麦冬	*mài dōng*	15 g	Radix Ophiopogonis
五味子	*wǔ wèi zǐ*	9 g	Fructus Schisandrae Chinensis
黄芪	*huáng qí*	15 g	Radix Astragali
生地	*shēng dì*	12 g	Radix Rehmanniae
煅牡蛎	*duàn mǔ lì*	30 g	Concha Ostreae Praeparatum

Modifications

- For a severe dry mouth, combine with *tiān huā fěn* (天花粉, *Radix Trichosanthis*) 9 g and *wū méi* (乌梅, *Fructus Mume*) 9 g.
- For severe feverish sensations of the soles, palms and chest, combine with *dì gǔ pí* (地骨皮, *Cortex Lycii*) 9 g and *lián zǐ xīn* (莲子心, *Plumula Nelumbinis*) 9 g.
- For mild and severe palpitations, combine with *suān zǎo rén* (酸枣仁, *Semen Ziziphi Spinosae*) 9 g and *bǎi zǐ rén* (柏子仁, *Semen Platycladi*) 9 g.
- For a gastric upset and heartburn, combine with *shí gāo* (石膏, *Gypsum Fibrosum*) 30 g (ground, and decoct first) and *zhī mǔ* (知母, *Rhizoma Anemarrhenae*) 12 g.

Yin deficiency of the liver and kidneys

Signs and symptoms

Frequent urination with profuse turbid urine, soreness and weakness of the low back and knee joints, fatigue, a dry mouth, dizziness, blurred vision, tinnitus, poor sleep, nocturnal emissions, premature ejaculation, dry skin and general itching.

Tongue: red, with a scanty coating
Pulse: thready and rapid

Treatment principle

Nourish the liver and kidneys, fill essence and moisten dryness.

Formula

Modified *Liù Wèi Dì Huáng Wán* (六味地黄丸, "Six Ingredient Rehmannia Pill").

熟地黄	*shú dì huáng*	15 g	*Radix Rehmanniae Praeparata*
山茱萸	*shān zhū yú*	9 g	*Fructus Corni*
山药	*shān yào*	15 g	*Rhizoma Dioscoreae*
牡丹皮	*mǔ dān pí*	9 g	*Cortex Moutan*
泽泻	*zé xiè*	9 g	*Rhizoma Alismatis*
何首乌	*hé shǒu wū*	15 g	*Radix Polygoni Multiflori*
天花粉	*tiān huā fěn*	15 g	*Radix Trichosanthis*

Modifications

- For blurred vision, combine with *jué míng zǐ* (决明子, *Semen Cassiae*) 30 g and *gǒu qǐzǐ* (枸杞子, *Fructus Lycii*) 9 g.
- For bone steam tidal fever, combine with *zhī mǔ* (知母, *Rhizoma Anemarrhenae*) 12 g and *huáng bǎi* (黄柏, *Cortex Phellodendri Chinensis*) 9 g.
- For general skin itching, combine with *dāng guī* (当归, *Radix Angelicae Sinensis*) 9 g and *bái jí lí* (白蒺藜, *Fructus Tribuli*) 12 g.
- For frequent turbid urine, combine with *sāng piāo xiāo* (桑螵蛸, *Oötheca Mantidis*) 9 g and *yì zhì rén* (益智仁, *Fructus Alpiniae Oxyphyllae*) 9 g.

Deficiency of yin and yang

Signs and symptoms

Clear profuse urine, a withered complexion, cold intolerance, cold limbs, soreness and weakness of the low back and knee joints, cold hands and feet, dizziness, tinnitus and a dry mouth and throat.

Tongue: pale, with a thin coating
Pulse: deep, thready and weak

Treatment principle

Warm yang, nourish yin and tonify the kidneys.

Formula

Modified *Jīn Guì Shèn Qì Wán* (金匮肾气丸, "Golden Cabinet's Kidney *Qi* Pill").

肉桂	*ròu guì,*	4.5 g	*Cortex Cinnamomi* (decoct later)
制附子	*zhì fù zǐ*	9 g	*Radix Aconiti Lateralis Praeparata* (decoct first)
熟地黄	*shú dì huáng*	15 g	*Radix Rehmanniae Praeparata*
山茱萸	*shān zhū yú*	9 g	*Fructus Corni*
泽泻	*zé xiè*	9 g	*Rhizoma Alismatis*
牡丹皮	*mm dān pí*	9 g	*Cortex Moutan*
茯苓	*fú líng*	9 g	*Poria*
杜仲	*dù zhòng*	9 g	*Cortex Eucommiae*
牛膝	*niú xī*	9 g	*Radix Achyranthis Bidentatae*

Modifications

- For loose stools, combine with *ròu dòu kòu* (肉豆蔻, *Semen Myristicae*) and *bǔ gǔ zhī* (补骨脂, *Fructus Psoraleae*) 9 g.
- For edema in the limbs, combine with *zhū líng* (猪苓, *Polyporus*) 15 g and *fáng jǐ* (防己, *Radix Stephaniae Tetrandrae*) 9 g.
- For frequent urination, combine with *sāng piāo xiāo* (桑螵蛸, *Oötheca Mantidis*) 9 g and *yì zhì rén* (益智仁, *Fructus Alpiniae Oxyphyllae*) 9 g.
- For a dark-purple tongue, combine with *chì sháo* (赤芍, *Radix Paeoniae Rubra*) 9 g, *táo rén* (桃仁, *Semen Persicae*) 9 g and *dān shēn* (丹参, *Radix et Rhizoma Salviae Miltiorrhizae*) 9 g.

Deficiency of the spleen and stomach

Signs and symptoms

Thirst with excessive drinking, fast hunger with an increased appetite, loose stools, a low spirit and fatigue.

Tongue: pale and swollen, with a dry white coating
Pulse: thready and weak

Treatment principle

Strengthen the spleen, supplement *qi*, promote regeneration of fluids and relieve thirst.

Formula

Modified *Qī Wèi Bái Zhú Sàn* (七味白术散, "Seven-Ingredient *Atractylodis Macrocephalae* Powder").

党参	*dǎng shēn*	12 g	*Radix Codonopsis*
白术	*bái zhú*	9 g	*Rhizoma Atractylodis Macrocephalae*
茯苓	*fú líng*	9 g	*Poria*
葛根	*gé gēn*	9 g	*Radix Puerariae Lobatae*
木香	*mù xiāng*	6 g	*Radix Aucklandiae*
山药	*shān yào*	15 g	*Rhizoma Dioscoreae*
砂仁	*shā rén*	3 g	*Fructus Amomi* (decoct later)
炙甘草	*zhì gān cǎo*	9 g	*Radix et Rhizoma Glycyrrhizae Praeparata cum Melle*

Modifications

- For gastric or abdominal distension after eating food, combine with *shén qū* (神曲, *Massa Medicata Fermentata*) 9 g and *shān zhā* (山楂, *Fructus Crataegi*) 9 g.
- For severe fatigue, combine with *huáng qí* (黄芪, *Radix Astragali*) 15 g and *bái biǎn dòu* (白扁豆, *Semen Lablab Album*) 9 g.
- For frequent diarrhea, combine with *páo fù zǐ* (炮附子, *Radix Aconiti Lateralis Praeparata*) 6 g (decoct first) and *gān jiāng* (干姜, *Rhizoma Zingiberis*) 6 g.
- For severe lumbar soreness, combine with *ròu dòu kòu* (肉豆蔻, *Semen Myristicae*) and *bǔ gǔ zhī* (补骨脂, *Fructus Psoraleae*) 9 g.

Stagnant blood obstructing the collaterals

Signs and symptoms

A dark or dark-gray complexion, a dry mouth with no desire to drink water, fast hunger with an increased appetite, stabbing pain in the chest, numbness of the extremities, dizziness, blurred vision, palpitations and poor memory.

Tongue: dark-purple or with ecchymosis and a thin coating
Pulse: hesitant

Treatment principle

Invigorate blood and resolve stasis.

Formula

Modified *Táo Hóng Sì Wù Tāng* (桃红四物汤, "Peach Kernel and Carthamus Four Substances Decoction").

桃仁	táo rén	9 g	Semen Persicae
红花	hóng huā	9 g	Flos Carthami
赤芍	chì sháo	9 g	Radix Paeoniae Rubra
川芎	chuān xiōng	9 g	Rhizoma Chuanxiong
当归	dāng guī	9 g	Radix Angelicae Sinensis
丹参	dān shēn	15 g	Radix et Rhizoma Salviae Miltiorrhizae
葛根	gé gēn	9 g	Radix Puerariae Lobatae
益母草	yì mǔ cǎo	30 g	Herba Leonuri

Modifications

- For chest pain, combine with *yù jīn* (郁金, *Radix Curcumae*) 9 g, *sān qī* (三七, *Radix et Rhizoma Notoginseng*) 9 g and *yán hú suǒ* (延胡索, *Rhizoma Corydalis*) 9 g.
- For hemiplegia, combine with *dì lóng* (地龙, *Pheretima*) 9 g, *guì zhī* (桂枝, *Ramulus Cinnamomi*) 6 g and *jī xuè téng* (鸡血藤, *Caulis Spatholobi*) 15 g.
- For thirst with a desire to drink water, combine with *shēng dì* (生地, *Radix Rehmanniae*) 15 g, *shí hú* (石斛, *Caulis Dendrobii*) 9 g and *mài dōng* (麦冬, *Radix Ophiopogonis*) 9 g.
- For feverish sensations of the soles, palms and chest, combine with *lián zǐ xīn* (莲子心, *Plumula Nelumbinis*) 9 g and *lóng chǐ* (龙齿, *Dens Draconis*) 15 g (decoct first).

QUESTIONS

1. Describe the main clinical symptoms of diabetes mellitus.
2. Describe the severe complications of diabetes mellitus.
3. *Case study.* Try to make a pattern identification and give a prescription for the following case:

Mr. Lin, 60, suffered from non-insulin-dependent diabetes for five years. Recently he experienced a low spirit, fatigue and a dry mouth with a desire to drink water. Other symptoms included spontaneous sweating, night sweats, feverish sensations of the palms and soles, restlessness, palpitations, insomnia and frequent urination. The tongue was red, with a scanty coating. The pulse was thready and rapid.

Gout

Overview

Gout is a medical condition caused by purine metabolism disorder. It is clinically characterized by elevated levels of uric acid in the blood (hyperuricemia), repeated bouts of acute gouty arthritis, gouty deposition, chronic arthritis due to gouty deposition and joint deformity. This condition can often affect the kidneys, resulting in chronic interstitial nephritis and uric acid kidney stones. It can be primary or secondary. Except for lack of enzymes, causes of primary gouts are still unknown. However, it is considered as a genetic disease often accompanied by hyperlipidemia, obesity, diabetes, hypertension, atherosclerosis and coronary artery disease. Secondary gout can be attributed to kidney conditions, hematologic diseases and medications. The incidence of gout increases with age. Men are more likely to develop gout (male–female ratio of incidence: approximately 20:1). Gout can occur all year round, particularly in spring and autumn.

In Chinese medicine, gout falls under the category of "*qi* impediment syndrome" or "joint pain." The main contributing factors include deficiency of the spleen and stomach, an improper diet and contraction of external pathogens.

Failure of the spleen and stomach to transport and transform may cause internal damp–heat to affect the meridians. Overingestion of sweet and fatty food may impair the spleen and stomach, leading to phlegm dampness blocking the collaterals. Contraction of external damp–heat may also contribute to joint pain.

Clinical manifestations

Common symptoms of gout are red tender hot swollen joints, presence of gouty nodules, urinary stones and hyperuricemia. For inflammatory arthritis, the metatarsal–phalangeal joint at the base of the big toe is the most commonly affected. It may also be present at the ankle, knee, finger, wrist and elbow joints. With a sudden onset, gout often occurs during night sleep, causing visible redness, swelling and intense pain of the joints and surrounding soft tissue. Patients may experience restricted movement. The symptoms may resolve after a couple of days or weeks. Initially, a single joint can be affected. However, repeated bouts may involve multiple joints, eventually resulting in joint stiffness and deformity. Gouty nodules are often seen in the helix, extensor aspect of the forearms, toes, fingers and elbows. A longer duration causes increased gouty nodules. In addition, uric acid stones can be present in 20%–25% of the patients, causing renal colic, hematuria and urinary infections.

Pattern identification and treatment

Retention of wind–damp–heat

Signs and symptoms

Red swollen hot painful joints (particularly at night; the pain can be relieved by cold compression), dark-yellow urine and constipation; fever may also be present.

Tongue: red, with a thin yellow coating
Pulse: wiry and rapid

Treatment principle

Expel wind, clear heat, resolve dampness and unblock collaterals.

Formula

Modified *Sì Miào Wán* (四妙丸, "Wonderfully Effective Four Pill").

苍术	*cāng zhú*	12 g	Rhizoma Atractylodis
黄柏	*huáng bǎi*	9 g	Cortex Phellodendri Chinensis
牛膝	*niú xī*	9 g	Radix Achyranthis Bidentatae
薏苡仁	*yì yǐ rén*	9 g	Semen Coicis
忍冬藤	*rěn dōng téng*	15 g	Caulis Lonicerae Japonicae
金银花	*jīn yín huā*	9 g	Flos Lonicerae Japonicae
海桐皮	*hǎi tóng pí*	15 g	Cortex Erythrinae
蚕沙	*cán shā*	9 g	Faeces Bombycis
木瓜	*mù guā*	9 g	Fructus Chaenomelis

Modifications

- For severe fever, combine with *shí gāo* (石膏, *Gypsum Fibrosum*) 30 g (ground, and decoct first), *zhī mǔ* (知母, *Rhizoma Anemarrhenae*) 12 g and *shān zhī* (山栀, *Fructus Gardeniae*) 9 g.
- For a greasy tongue coating due to dampness, combine with *hàn fáng jǐ* (汉防己, *Radix Stephaniae Tetrandrae*) 9 g and *chē qián zǐ* (车前子, *Semen Plantaginis*) 15 g (wrapped).
- For intense joint pain, combine with *yán hú suǒ* (延胡索, *Rhizoma Corydalis*) 9 g, *rǔ xiāng* (乳香, *Olibanum*) 6 g and *mò yào* (没药, *Myrrha*) 6 g.
- For severe constipation, combine with *dà huáng* (大黄, *Radix et Rhizoma Rhei*) 9 g (decoct later) and *máng xiāo* (芒硝, *Natrii Sulfas*) 9 g.

Retention of wind–cold–damp

Signs and symptoms

Sore and painful joints with an absence of redness, restricted movement, cold intolerance and cold limbs; the pain can be relieved by warmth.

Tongue: pale, with a thin white coating
Pulse: wiry and thready

Treatment principle

Expel wind, dissipate cold, resolve dampness and unblock collaterals.

Formula

Modified *Dà Wū Tóu Jiān* (大乌头煎, "Aconiti Decoction").

麻黄	*má huáng*	9 g	Herba Ephedrae
桂枝	*guì zhī*	9 g	Ramulus Cinnamomi
制川乌	*zhì chuān wū*	9 g	Radix Aconiti Praeparata (decoct first)
制草乌	*zhì cǎo wū*	9 g	Radix Aconiti Kusnezoffii Praeparata (decoct first)
白芍	*bái sháo*	9 g	Radix Paeoniae Alba
白术	*bái zhú*	9 g	Rhizoma Atractylodis Macrocephalae
防风	*fáng fēng*	12 g	Radix Saposhnikoviae
露蜂房	*lù fēng fáng*	9 g	Nidus Vespae

Modifications

- For intense pain, combine with *wēi líng xiān* (威灵仙, *Radix et Rhizoma Clematidis*) 9 g and *xú cháng qīng* (徐长卿, *Radix et Rhizoma Cynanchi Paniculati*) 9 g.
- For severe joint swelling, combine with *shān cí gū* (山慈菇, *Pseudobulbus Cremastrae seu Pleiones*) 9 g and *tǔ fú líng* (土茯苓, *Rhizoma Smilacis Glabrae*) 30 g.
- For severe fatigue, combine with *dǎng shēn* (党参, *Radix Codonopsis*) 9 g and *huáng qí* (黄芪, *Radix Astragali*) 15 g.
- For gastric discomfort, combine with *bàn xià* (半夏, *Rhizoma Pinelliae*) 9 g and *chén pí* (陈皮, *Pericarpium Citri Reticulatae*) 9 g.

Retention of phlegm stasis

Signs and symptoms

Joint deformity, swelling and pain with restricted movement.

Tongue: dark or with ecchymosis and a thin white coating
Pulse: wiry and thready

Treatment principle

Resolve phlegm stasis, remove masses and unblock collaterals.

Formula

Modified *Shēn Tòng Zhú Yū Tāng* (身痛逐瘀汤, "Generalized Pain Stasis–Expelling Decoction").

牡蛎	*mǔ lì*	30 g	Concha Ostreae
当归	*dāng guī*	9 g	Radix Angelicae Sinensis
川芎	*chuān xiōng*	9 g	Rhizoma Chuanxiong
桃仁	*táo rén*	9 g	Semen Persicae
红花	*hóng huā*	9 g	Flos Carthami
五灵脂	*wǔ líng zhī*	9 g	Faeces Trogopterori (wrapped)
香附	*xiāng fù*	9 g	Rhizoma Cyperi
地龙	*dì lóng*	9 g	Pheretima
秦艽	*qín jiāo*	9 g	Radix Gentianae Macrophyllae
豨莶草	*xī xiān cǎo*	15 g	Herba Siegesbeckiae
牛膝	*niú xī*	9 g	Radix Achyranthis Bidentatae
杜仲	*dù zhòng*	9 g	Cortex Eucommiae

Modifications

- For severe cold intolerance, combine with *lù jiǎo* (鹿角, *Cornu Cervi*) 9 g (decoct first) and *má huáng* (麻黄, *Herba Ephedrae*) 9 g.
- For intolerable pain, combine with *zhì cǎo wū* (制草乌, *Radix Aconiti Kusnezoffii Praeparata*) 9 g (decoct first) and *zhì chuān wū* (制川乌, *Radix Aconiti Praeparata*) 9 g (decoct first).
- For severe fatigue, combine with *dǎng shēn* (党参, *Radix Codonopsis*) 9 g and *huáng qí* (黄芪, *Radix Astragali*) 15 g.
- For a severe dark-purple tongue, combine with *sān léng* (三棱, *Rhizoma Sparganii*) 9 g and *é zhú* (莪术, *Rhizoma Curcumae*) 9 g.

Damp–heat in the urinary bladder

Signs and symptoms

Intense lower back pain, difficult urination mixed with stones, frequent and urgent urination, a burning pain in the urethra and bloody urine.

Tongue: red, with a yellow greasy coating
Pulse: wiry and rapid

Treatment principle

Clear heat, resolve dampness and promote urination.

Formula

Modified *Bā Zhèng Sǎn* (八正散, "Eight Corrections Powder").

瞿麦	*qú mài*	9 g	*Herba Dianthi*
萹蓄	*biǎn xù*	9 g	*Herba Polygoni Avicularis*
石韦	*shí wéi*	15 g	*Folium Pyrrosiae*
黄柏	*huáng bǎi*	9 g	*Cortex Phellodendri Chinensis*
海金沙	*hǎi jīn shā*	15 g	*Spora Lygodii* (wrapped)
金钱草	*jīn qián cǎo*	30 g	*Herba Lysimachiae*
鸡内金	*jī nèi jīn*	9 g	*Endothelium Corneum Gigeriae Galli*
枳壳	*zhǐ qiào*	9 g	*Fructus Aurantii*

Modifications

- For severe low back pain, combine with *yán hú suǒ* (延胡索, *Rhizoma Corydalis*) 9 g and *bái sháo* (白芍, *Radix Paeoniae Alba*) 9 g.
- For hematuria, combine with *bái máo gēn* (白茅根, *Rhizoma Imperatae*) 30 g and *dà jì* (大蓟, *Herba Cirsii Japonici*) 9 g.
- For a greasy tongue coating, combine with *cāng zhú* (苍术, *Rhizoma Atractylodis*) 9 g and *hòu pò* (厚朴, *Cortex Magnoliae Officinalis*) 9 g.
- For constipation, combine with *dà huáng* (大黄, *Radix et Rhizoma Rhei*) 9 g (decoct later) and *máng xiāo* (芒硝, *Natrii Sulfas*) 9 g.

Yang deficiency of the spleen and kidneys

Signs and symptoms

Mental fatigue, lassitude, cold intolerance, cold limbs, soreness and weakness of the low back and knee joints, edema in the lower limbs, deformed painful joints and restricted movement.

Tongue: pale, with a thin white coating
Pulse: deep, thready and weak

Treatment principle

Supplement *qi*, strengthen the spleen, warm the kidneys and unblock collaterals.

Formula

Modified *Fù Zǐ Tāng* (附子汤, "Aconite Decoction").

炮附子	*páo fù zǐ*	9 g	*Radix Aconiti Lateralis Praeparata* (decoct first)
党参	*dǎng shēn*	12 g	*Radix Codonopsis*
白术	*bái zhú*	9 g	*Rhizoma Atractylodis Macrocephalae*
茯苓	*fú líng*	9 g	*Poria*
补骨脂	*bǔ gǔ zhī*	9 g	*Fructus Psoraleae*
杜仲	*dù zhòng*	9 g	*Cortex Eucommiae*
牛膝	*niú xī*	9 g	*Radix Achyranthis Bidentatae*
泽泻	*zé xiè*	15 g	*Rhizoma Alismatis*
豨莶草	*xī xiān cǎo*	15 g	*Herba Siegesbeckiae*

Modifications

- For severe edema in the lower limbs, combine with *zhū líng* (猪苓, *Polyporus*) 15 g and *chē qián zǐ* (车前子, *Semen Plantaginis*) 15 g (wrapped).
- For severe fatigue, combine with *huáng qí* (黄芪, *Radix Astragali*) 15 g and *shān yào* (山药, *Rhizoma Dioscoreae*) 9 g.
- For nausea and vomiting, combine with *bàn xià* (半夏, *Rhizoma Pinelliae*) 9 g and *chén pí* (陈皮, *Pericarpium Citri Reticulatae*) 9 g.
- For severe joint pain, combine with *zhì cǎo wū* (制草乌, *Radix Aconiti Kusnezoffii Praeparata*) 9 g (decoct first) and *zhì chuān wū* (制川乌, *Radix Aconiti Praeparata*) 9 g (decoct first).

QUESTIONS

1. Describe the main clinical symptoms of gout.
2. Describe the pattern identifications and treatment principle of gout in Chinese medicine.
3. *Case study*. Try to make a pattern identification and give a prescription for the following case:

Mr. Liang, 60, suffered from gout for years and experienced recent joint pain after contraction of cold. The pain could be relieved by warmth and was especially located at the big toe, causing restricted movement. Other symptoms included cold intolerance and cold limbs. The tongue was pale, with a thin white coating. The pulse was wiry and thready.

COMMON ENDOCRINE SYSTEM CONDITIONS

Hyperthyroidism

Overview

Hyperthyroidism is a condition in which an overactive thyroid gland is producing an excessive amount of thyroid hormones that circulate in the blood. It is characterized by an enlarged thyroid, an increased metabolic rate of the body and disturbance of the autonomic nervous system. Etiologically, hyperthyroidism can be categorized into four patterns: thyroid hyperthyroidism, pituitary hyperthyroidism, heterologŏus TSH syndrome and struma ovarii (goiter of the ovary). Clinically, toxic diffuse goiter (also known as diffuse goiter or exophthalmic goiter) is most common. Usually, more females than males are affected (at a ratio of approximately 4–6:1). The condition can develop at any age but is most common between the ages of 20 and 40.

In Chinese medicine, hyperthyroidism falls under the category of "ying (goiter) *qi*." The main contributing factors include emotional disturbance and congenital deficiency. Long-term emotional depression coupled with sudden psychological trauma may affect the function of the liver in maintaining the free flow of *qi*, resulting in liver *qi* stagnation and subsequent phlegm and blood stasis. Over time, phlegm *qi* stagnation may result in goiter. Congenital kidney yin deficiency may cause hyperactivity of liver fire, leading to phlegm. Failure of kidney yang to transform fluid may produce phlegm as well.

Clinical manifestations

Common symptoms of hyperthyroidism are an enlarged thyroid, exophthalmos and tremor. A diffuse soft symmetrical swelling may occur on both sides of the neck. The goiter may be soft, painless and movable on swallowing. Exophthalmos can involve one or both eyes. Tremor is often seen in the hands, tongue and eyelids, especially upon mental nervousness and physical exertion. Other symptoms may include heat intolerance, excessive sweating (worsened by exertion), restlessness, irritability, rapid hunger with an increased appetite and weight loss.

Pattern identification and treatment

Liver qi stagnation

Signs and symptoms

Mild enlargement of the thyroid, chest tightness, pain in the hypochondriac regions, mental depression, emotion-related restlessness and excessive sweating, nausea, vomiting and occasional diarrhea or loose stools.

Tongue: red, with a thin coating
Pulse: wiry and rapid

Treatment principle

Soothe the liver, clear heat, regulate *qi* and relieve depression.

Formula

Modified *Dān Zhī Xiāo Yáo Sǎn* (丹栀逍遥散, "Cortex Moutan and Gardenia Free Wanderer Powder").

牡丹皮	*mŭ dān pí*	9 g	Cortex Moutan
山栀	*shān zhī*	9 g	Fructus Gardeniae
柴胡	*chái hú*	9 g	Radix Bupleuri
当归	*dāng guī*	9 g	Radix Angelicae Sinensis
白术	*bái zhú*	9 g	Rhizoma Atractylodis Macrocephalae
白芍	*bái sháo*	9 g	Radix Paeoniae Alba
茯苓	*fú líng*	9 g	Poria
薄荷	*bò hé*	6 g	Herba Menthae (decoct later)
夏枯草	*xià kū căo*	9 g	Spica Prunellae

Modifications

- For frequent belching, combine with *xuán fù huā* (旋覆花, *Flos Inulae*) 9 g (wrapped) and *dài zhě shí* (代赭石, *Haematitum*) 15 g (decoct first).

- For severe nausea and vomiting, combine with *jiāng bàn xià* (姜半夏, *Rhizoma Pinelliae Praeparatum*) 9 g and *jiāng zhú rú* (姜竹茹, *Caulis Bambusae in Taenia Praeparatum*) 9 g.

- For a severe bitter taste in the mouth, combine with *huáng lián* (黄连, *Rhizoma Coptidis*) 3 g and *huáng qín* (黄芩, *Radix Scutellariae*) 9 g.

- For constipation, combine with *dà huáng* (大黄, *Radix et Rhizoma Rhei*) 9 g (decoct later) and *má rén* (麻仁, *Fructus Cannabis*) 9 g.

Hyperactivity of liver fire

Signs and symptoms

Mild or moderate enlargement of the thyroid, mood swings, a red face, feverish sensations of the palms, soles and chest, a dry mouth with a bitter taste, tremor of the hands and tongue, and poor sleep.

Tongue: red, with a thin yellow coating
Pulse: wiry and rapid

Treatment principle

Clear liver fire, promote regeneration of fluids and remove masses.

Formula

Modified *Lóng Dǎn Xiè Gān Tāng* (龙胆泻肝汤, "Gentian Liver-Draining Decoction")

龙胆草	*lóng dǎn cǎo*	9 g	*Radix et Rhizoma Gentianae*
黄芩	*huáng qín*	9 g	*Radix Scutellariae*
山栀	*shān zhī*	9 g	*Fructus Gardeniae*
泽泻	*zé xiè*	9 g	*Rhizoma Alismatis*
木通	*mù tōng*	6 g	*Caulis Akebiae*
车前子	*chē qián zǐ*	15 g	*Semen Plantaginis* (wrapped)
当归	*dāng guī*	9 g	*Radix Angelicae Sinensis*
柴胡	*chái hú*	9 g	*Radix Bupleuri*
生地	*shēng dì*	12 g	*Radix Rehmanniae*
玄参	*xuán shēn*	15 g	*Radix Scrophulariae*
甘草	*zhì gān cǎo*	6 g	*Radix et Rhizoma Glycyrrhizae*

Modifications

- For a severe red face and eyes, combine with *gōu téng* (钩藤, *Ramulus Uncariae Cum Uncis*) 12 g (decoct later) and *shí jué míng* (石决明, *Concha Haliotidis*) 15 g (decoct first).
- For mouth or tongue ulcerations, combine with *huáng lián* (黄连, *Rhizoma Coptidis*) 3 g and *huáng bǎi* (黄柏, *Cortex Phellodendri Chinensis*) 9 g.
- For a dry mouth and fast hunger with an increased appetite, combine with *shí gāo* (石膏, *Gypsum Fibrosum*) 30 g (grinded and decoct first), *zhī mǔ* (知母, *Rhizoma Anemarrhenae*) 12 g and *tiān huā fěn* (天花粉, *Radix Trichosanthis*) 9 g.
- For severe insomnia, combine with *suān zǎo rén* (酸枣仁, *Semen Ziziphi Spinosae*) 9 g and *bǎi zǐ rén* (柏子仁, *Semen Platycladi*) 9 g.

Hyperactivity of liver yang

Signs and symptoms

Mild enlargement of the thyroid, palpitations, restlessness, irritability, a dry mouth with a bitter taste, tremor of the hands and tongue, dizziness, blurred vision, fast hunger with an increased appetite and weight loss.

Tongue: red, with a thin yellow coating
Pulse: wiry and powerful

Treatment principle

Soothe the liver, expel wind, resolve stasis and remove masses.

Formula

Modified *Zhēn Zhū Mǔ Wán* (珍珠母丸, *"Concha Margaritiferae Usta* Pill").

当归	*dāng guī*	9 g	*Radix Angelicae Sinensis*
珍珠母	*zhēn zhū mǔ*	30 g	*Concha Margaritiferae Usta* (decoct first)
龙齿	*lóng chǐ*	30 g	*Dens Draconis* (decoct first)
龙骨	*lóng gǔ*	30 g	*Os Draconis* (decoct first)
牡蛎	*mǔ lì*	30 g	*Concha Ostreae* (decoct first)
熟地黄	*shú dì huáng*	15 g	*Radix Rehmanniae Praeparata*
酸枣仁	*suān zǎo rén*	9 g	*Semen Ziziphi Spinosae*
柏子仁	*bǎi zǐ rén*	9 g	*Semen Platycladi*
海浮石	*hǎi fú shí*	15 g	*Pumex*
茯神	*fú shén*	9 g	*Sclerotium Poriae Pararadicis*
夏枯草	*xià kū cǎo*	9 g	*Spica Prunellae*

Modifications

- For dizziness with severe tremors, combine with *shān yáng jiǎo* (山羊角, *Radix et Rhizoma Sophorae Tonkinensis*) 30 g (decoct first) and *shí jué míng* (石决明, *Concha Haliotidis*) 30 g (decoct first).
- For fast hunger with an increased appetite, combine with *zhī mǔ* (知母, *Rhizoma Anemarrhenae*) 9 g and *shí gāo* (石膏, *Gypsum Fibrosum*) 30 g (decoct first).
- For palpitations and restlessness, combine with a powder of *líng yáng jiǎo* (羚羊角, *Cornu Saigae Tataricae*) 0.6 g and *dài mào* (玳瑁, *Carapax Eretmochelydis*) 15 g (decoct first).
- For blurred vision, combine with *jué míng zǐ* (决明子, *Semen Cassiae*) 15 g and *gǔ jīng cǎo* (谷精草, *Flos Eriocauli*) 9 g.

Deficiency of qi and yin

Signs and symptoms

Mild enlargement of the thyroid, palpitations, shortness of breath, restlessness, poor sleep, spontaneous sweating, night sweats, a sallow complexion, weight loss, fatigue, and tremor of the hands and tongue.

Tongue: dry and red, with a scanty coating
Pulse: thready and rapid

Treatment principle

Supplement *qi*, nourish yin, promote regeneration of fluid and remove masses.

Formula

Modified *Shēng Mài Sǎn* (生脉散, "Pulse-Engendering Powder") and *Èr Dōng Tāng* (二冬汤, "Asparagi and Ophiopogonis Decoction").

太子参	*tài zǐ shēn*	15 g	*Radix Pseudostellariae*
麦冬	*mài dōng*	9 g	*Radix Ophiopogonis*
五味子	*wǔ wèi zǐ*	9 g	*Fructus Schisandrae Chinensis*
天冬	*tiān dōng*	9 g	*Radix Asparagi*
天花粉	*tiān huā fěn*	9 g	*Radix Trichosanthis*
北沙参	*běi shā shēn*	9 g	*Radix Glehniae*
酸枣仁	*suān zǎo rén*	9 g	*Semen Ziziphi Spinosae*
丹参	*dān shēn*	15 g	*Radix et Rhizoma Salviae Miltiorrhizae*
玄参	*xuán shēn*	15 g	*Radix Scrophulariae*
知母	*zhī mǔ*	9 g	*Rhizoma Anemarrhenae*

Modifications

- For tinnitus and lumbar soreness, combine with *gǒu qǐzǐ* (枸杞子, *Fructus Lycii*) 9 g and *guī bǎn* (龟板, *Plastrum Testudinis*) 15 g (decoct first).
- For loose stools, combine with *shān yào* (山药, *Rhizoma Dioscoreae*) 9 g and *bái biān dòu* (白扁豆, *Semen Lablab Album*) 9 g.

- For persistent sweating, combine with *má huáng gēn* (麻黄根, *Radix et Rhizoma Ephedrae*) 9 g and *fú xiǎo mài* (浮小麦, *Fructus Tritici Levis*) 15 g.
- For restlessness and irritability, combine with *zhēn zhū mǔ* (珍珠母, *Concha Margaritiferae Usta*) 30 g and *lóng dǎn cǎo* (龙胆草, *Radix et Rhizoma Gentianae*) 9 g.

Phlegm–dampness stagnation

Signs and symptoms

Moderate enlargement of the thyroid, exophthalmos, chest tightness, bloating, difficulty in swallowing, heat intolerance, excessive sweating, a reduced appetite and loose stools.

Tongue: pale, with a greasy coating
Pulse: soft and slippery

Treatment principle

Regulate *qi*, resolve phlegm and soften masses.

Formula

Modified *Sì Hǎi Shū Yù Wán* (四海疏郁丸, "Four Seas Stagnation-Relieving Pill").

青木香	qīng mù xiāng	9 g	Radix Aristolochiae
陈皮	chén pí	9 g	Pericarpium Citri Reticulatae
半夏	bàn xià	9 g	Rhizoma Pinelliae
昆布	kūn bù	9 g	Thallus Laminariae
海藻	hǎi zǎo	9 g	Sargassum
莪术	é zhú	15 g	Rhizoma Curcumae
黄药子	huáng yào zǐ	9 g	Rhizoma Dioscoreae Bulbiferae
郁金	yù jīn	9 g	Radix Curcumae
香附	xiāng fù	9 g	Rhizoma Cyperi

Modifications

- For chest tightness with a pain in the hypochondriac region, combine with *yán hú suǒ* (延胡索, *Rhizoma Corydalis*) 9 g and *chuān liàn zǐ* (川楝子, *Fructus Toosendan*) 9 g.
- For loose stools and fatigue, combine with *shān yào* (山药, *Rhizoma Dioscoreae*) 9 g and *bái biǎn dòu* (白扁豆, *Semen Lablab Album*) 9 g.
- For a severe greasy tongue coating, combine with *cāng zhú* (苍术, *Rhizoma Atractylodis*) 9 g and *dǎn nán xīng* (胆南星, *Arisaema cum Bile*) 9 g.
- For painful goiter, combine with *shān cí gū* (山慈菇, *Pseudobulbus Cremastrae seu Pleiones*) 9 g and *xià kū cǎo* (夏枯草, *Spica Prunellae*) 9 g.

QUESTIONS

1. Describe the main clinical symptoms of hyperthyroidism.
2. Describe the pattern identifications and treatment method of hyperthyroidism in Chinese medicine.
3. *Case study.* Try to make a pattern identification and give a prescription for the following case:

Ms. Lin, 30, suffered for five years from hyperthyroidism that did not respond well to integrative Chinese and Western medical therapies. Recently she experienced restlessness, irritability, poor sleep, excessive sweating after mild exertion, red face and eyes, a dry mouth with a bitter taste, and tremor of the hands and tongue that was worsened by emotions. She also had an earlier menstrual period and symmetrical enlargement of the thyroid manifesting as soft, smooth and painless. The tongue was red. The pulse was wiry and rapid.

COMMON INFECTIOUS CONDITIONS

Viral Hepatitis

Overview

Viral hepatitis is a systemic infectious condition with distinctive liver inflammation caused by multiple hepatotropic viruses. Etiologically, viral hepatitis can be categorized into seven patterns: hepatitis A, hepatitis B, hepatitis C, hepatitis D, hepatitis E, hepatitis F and non-A-G hepatitis. Clinically, viral hepatitis can be categorized into acute hepatitis (jaundice and nonjaundice), chronic hepatitis (persistent and active), severe hepatitis (acute severe and subacute severe) and cholestatic hepatitis.

In Chinese medicine, viral hepatitis falls under the category of "jaundice," "pain in the hypochondriac region," "chronic consumption" and "abdominal masses". The main contributing factors are contraction of damp–heat and epidemic toxins with deficiency of antipathogenic *qi*. Acute hepatitis often presents with damp-heat and blockage of *qi* activities, whereas chronic hepatitis often presents with lingering dampness, blockage of collaterals and deficiency of the liver and kidneys. Severe hepatitis presents with exuberance of epidemic toxins and collapse of antipathogenic *qi*. Cholestatic hepatitis presents with retention of damp–heat, blood stasis and spleen deficiency.

Clinical manifestations

Common symptoms of viral hepatitis are fatigue, a poor appetite, nausea, vomiting, pain in the hypochondriac regions, bloating, hepatomegaly, fever and jaundice.

Acute hepatitis causes mental fatigue, a poor appetite, nausea, vomiting, distending pain in the right hypochondriac region, fever and jaundice.

Chronic hepatitis causes fatigue, a poor appetite, dull pain in the hepatic area, bloating, a low-grade fever, liver palm and spider angioma.

Severe hepatitis causes fever, jaundice, nausea, vomiting, nasal bleeding, hematemesis, ascites and somnolence. Restlessness, delirium, coma and convulsions may also be present.

Cholestatic hepatitis causes persistent jaundice, fatigue, skin itching and hepatomegaly.

Pattern identification and treatment

Retention of damp–heat

Signs and symptoms

Yellow face, eyes and body skin, gastric or abdominal fullness and distension, dull pain in the right hypochondriac region, nausea, vomiting, fever, a bitter taste, dark-yellow urine and constipation or loose stools.

Tongue: red on the tip, with a yellow greasy coating
Pulse: wiry and slippery

Treatment principle

Clear heat, resolve dampness and remove yellowness.

Formula

Supplemented *Yīn Chén Hāo Tāng* (茵陈蒿汤, "Artemisiae Scopariae Decoction").

茵陈	*yīn chén*	30 g	*Herba Artemisiae Scopariae*
山栀	*shān zhī*	9 g	*Fructus Gardeniae*
大黄	*dà huáng*	9 g	*Radix et Rhizoma Rhei* (decoct later)
田基黄	*tián jī huáng*	30 g	*Herba Hyperici Japonici*
白术	*bái zhú*	9 g	*Rhizoma Atractylodis Macrocephalae*
茯苓	*fú líng*	9 g	*Poria*
车前子	*chē qián zǐ*	30 g	*Semen Plantaginis (wrapped)*
板蓝根	*bǎn lán gēn*	30 g	*Radix Isatidis*

Modifications

- For excessive heat, combine with *huáng lián* (黄连, *Rhizoma Coptidis*) 3 g and *huáng qín* (黄芩, *Radix Scutellariae*) 9 g.

- For severe dampness, combine with *cāng zhú* (苍术, *Rhizoma Atractylodis*) 9 g and *hòu pò* (厚朴, *Cortex Magnoliae Officinalis*) 9 g.
- For severe nausea and vomiting, combine with *bàn xià* (半夏, *Rhizoma Pinelliae*) 9 g, *chén pí* (陈皮, *Pericarpium Citri Reticulatae*) 9 g and *zhú rú* (竹茹, *Caulis Bambusae in Taenia*) 9 g.

Liver qi stagnation

Signs and symptoms

Distending pain in the hypochondriac regions, gastric or abdominal distension, nausea, belching, a poor appetite, fatigue, fever and constipation.

Tongue: light-red, with a thin yellow coating
Pulse: wiry

Treatment principle

Soothe the liver, regulate *qi* and clear heat.

Formula

Modified *Chái Hú Shū Gān Sǎn* (柴胡疏肝散, "Bupleurum Liver-Soothing Powder").

柴胡	*chái hú*	9 g	*Radix Bupleuri*
枳壳	*zhǐ qiào*	9 g	*Fructus Aurantii*
白芍	*bái sháo*	9 g	*Radix Paeoniae Alba*
郁金	*yù jīn*	9 g	*Radix Curcumae*
香附	*xiāng fù*	9 g	*Rhizoma Cyperi*
田基黄	*tián jī huáng*	30 g	*Herba Hyperici Japonici*
大黄	*dà huáng*	9 g	*Radix et Rhizoma Rhei*
甘草	*gān cǎo*	6 g	*Radix et Rhizoma Glycyrrhizae*

Modifications

- For intense pain, combine with *yán hú suǒ* (延胡索, *Rhizoma Corydalis*) 9 g and *chuān liàn zǐ* (川楝子, *Fructus Toosendan*) 9 g.
- For a bitter taste due to heat, combine with *huáng lián* (黄连, *Rhizoma Coptidis*) 3 g and *huáng qín* (黄芩, *Radix Scutellariae*) 9 g.

- For nausea and belching, combine with *jiāng bàn xià* (姜半夏, *Rhizoma Pinelliae Praeparatum*) 9 g, *xuán fù huā* (旋覆花, *Flos Inulae*) 9 g (wrapped) and *jiāng zhú rú* (姜竹茹, *Caulis Bambusae in Taenia Praeparatum*) 9 g.

Spleen deficiency with internal dampness

Signs and symptoms

Dull pain in the right hypochondriac region, gastric or abdominal fullness and distension, a general heaviness sensation, pallor, nausea, a poor appetite and loose stools.

Tongue: pale, with a white greasy coating
Pulse: soft and thready

Treatment principle

Strengthen the spleen, harmonize the stomach and resolve dampness.

Formula

Modified *Xiāng Shā Liù Jūn Zǐ Tāng* (香砂六君子汤, "Costusroot and Amomum Six Gentlemen Decoction").

党参	*dǎng shēn*	12 g	*Radix Codonopsis*
苍术	*cāng zhú*	9 g	*Rhizoma Atractylodis*
白术	*bái zhú*	9 g	*Rhizoma Atractylodis Macrocephalae*
茯苓	*fú líng*	9 g	*Poria*
半夏	*bàn xià*	9 g	*Rhizoma Pinelliae*
陈皮	*chén pí*	9 g	*Pericarpium Citri Reticulatae*
木香	*mù xiāng*	6 g	*Radix Aucklandiae*
砂仁	*shā rén*	6 g	*Fructus Amomi* (decoct later)
山药	*shān yào*	15 g	*Rhizoma Dioscoreae*
鸡内金	*jī nèi jīn*	9 g	*Endothelium Corneum Gigeriae Galli*
甘草	*gān cǎo*	6 g	*Radix et Rhizoma Glycyrrhizae*

Modifications

- For a greasy tongue coating due to dampness, combine with *huò xiāng* (藿香, *Herba Agastachis*) 9 g and *pèi lán* (佩兰, *Herba Eupatorii*) 9 g.

- For severe pain in the right hypochondriac region, combine with *yán hú suǒ* (延胡索, *Rhizoma Corydalis*) 9 g and *chuān liàn zǐ* (川楝子, *Fructus Toosendan*) 9 g.
- For lassitude and loose stools, combine with *bái biǎn dòu* (白扁豆, *Semen Lablab Album*) 9 g and *yì yǐ rén* (薏苡仁, *Semen Coicis*) 9 g.

Yin deficiency of the liver and kidneys

Signs and symptoms

Dull pain in the hypochondriac regions, dizziness, tinnitus, blurred vision, restlessness, insomnia, feverish sensations on the palms and soles, dry lips and mouth, and soreness and weakness of the low back and knee joints.

Tongue: red, with a scanty or no coating
Pulse: wiry, thready and rapid

Treatment principle

Nourish yin, emolliate the liver and relieve pain.

Formula

Modified *Yī Guàn Jiān* (一贯煎, "Effective Integration Decoction").

生地	*shēng dì*	12 g	*Radix Rehmanniae*
熟地黄	*shú dì huáng*	9 g	*Radix Rehmanniae Praeparata*
枸杞子	*gǒu qǐ zǐ*	9 g	*Fructus Lycii*
北沙参	*běi shā shēn*	9 g	*Radix Glehniae*
麦冬	*mài dōng*	9 g	*Radix Ophiopogonis*
山茱萸	*shān zhū yú*	9 g	*Fructus Corni*
石斛	*shí hú*	9 g	*Caulis Dendrobii*
川楝子	*chuān liàn zǐ*	9 g	*Fructus Toosendan*
白芍	*bái sháo*	9 g	*Radix Paeoniae Alba*
牡丹皮	*mǔ dān pí*	9 g	*Cortex Moutan*

Modifications

- For severe pain in the hypochondriac regions, combine with *yán hú suǒ* (延胡索, *Rhizoma Corydalis*) 9 g and *bā yuè zhā* (八月札, *Fructus Akebiae*) 15 g.

- For severe restlessness and insomnia, combine with *huáng lián* (黄连, *Rhizoma Coptidis*) 6 g, *suān zǎo rén* (酸枣仁, *Semen Ziziphi Spinosae*) 9 g and *wǔ wèi zǐ* (五味子, *Fructus Schisandrae Chinensis*) 9 g.
- For dizziness and severe lumbar soreness, combine with *lǜ dòu yī* (绿豆衣, *Testa Glycinis*) 12 g, *nǚ zhēn zǐ* (女贞子, *Fructus Ligustri Lucidi*) 9 g and *guī bǎn* (龟板, *Plastrum Testudinis*) 15 g (decoct first).

Exuberance of toxic heat

Signs and symptoms

A high-grade fever, restlessness, aggravated jaundice, pain in the hypochondriac regions, bloating, dark-yellow urine and constipation; coma, delirium, convulsions or bloody stools may also be present.

Tongue: dark-red, with a dry yellow coating
Pulse: wiry, slippery and rapid

Treatment principle

Clear heat, remove toxins and cool the *ying*.

Formula

Modified *Xī Jiǎo Sǎn* (犀角散, "Rhinoceros Horn Powder").

水牛角	*shuǐ niú jiǎo*	30 g	*Cornu Bubali* (decoct first)
黄连	*huáng lián*	3 g	*Rhizoma Coptidis*
山栀	*shān zhī*	9 g	*Fructus Gardeniae*
牡丹皮	*mǔ dān pí*	9 g	*Cortex Moutan*
白茅根	*bái máo gēn*	30 g	*Rhizoma Imperatae*
赤芍	*chì sháo*	9 g	*Radix Paeoniae Rubra*
石斛	*shí hú*	9 g	*Caulis Dendrobii*
板蓝根	*bǎn lán gēn*	30 g	*Radix Isatidis*

Modifications

- For coma and delirium, combine with one pill of *Ān Gōng Niú Huáng Wán* (安宫牛黄丸, "Peaceful Palace Bovine Bezoar Pill").

- For severe convulsions, combine with a powder of *líng yáng jiǎo* (羚羊角, *Cornu Saigae Tataricae*) 0.6 g.
- For constipation with bloating, combine with *dà huáng* (大黄, *Radix et Rhizoma Rhei*) 9 g (decoct later) and *máng xiāo* (芒硝, *Natrii Sulfas*) 9 g.
- For dysuria or with ascites, combine with *chē qián zǐ* (车前子, *Semen Plantaginis*) 15 g (wrapped) and *hú lú* (葫芦, *Fructus Lagenariae*) 30 g.

QUESTIONS

1. Describe the main clinical symptoms of viral hepatitis.
2. Describe the signs and symptoms of viral hepatitis due to liver *qi* stagnation, as well as the treatment method.
3. *Case study*. Try to make a pattern identification and give a prescription for the following case:

Mr. Chen, 40, suffered from yellow skin and sclera for a week. Other symptoms included intolerable skin itching, distending pain in the right hypochondriac region, a poor appetite, intolerance of fatty food, dark-yellow urine and constipation. Findings of liver function tests: bilirubin was 4.8 mg the icteric index was 60 and GPT was 1300.

Bacillary Dysentery

Overview

Bacillary dysentery, commonly referred to as dysentery, is an acute inflammatory disorder of the intestine caused by *Shigella dysenteriae*. It especially involves the colon and results in systemic poisoning, abdominal pain and diarrhea. This condition can occur all year around, but is more common in summer and autumn. It can develop at any age, particularly in children and young adults. Toxic dysentery is often seen in children. Bacillary dysentery can be acute or chronic (longer than two months). By severity, acute dysentery can be subdivided into four patterns: mild dysentery, common dysentery, severe dysentery and toxic dysentery.

In Chinese medicine, dysentery falls under the category of "irregular bowel movements" or "intestinal disorder." The main contributing factors include contraction of damp–heat and epidemic toxins with an improper diet.

Ingestion of unclean food or overintake of cold fatty food may damage the spleen and stomach, leading to internal retention of damp–heat and subsequent irregular bowel movements. Damp–heat coupled with epidemic toxins may block the circulation of *qi* and blood within the intestine, leading to abdominal pain, tenesmus and stools containing mucus or blood.

Clinical manifestations

Alimentary tract symptoms of dysentery are abdominal pain, tenesmus and diarrhea containing mucus and/or blood in the feces. Some patients may also present with nausea and vomiting. Patients with a mild condition may have 4–5 times of bowel movements a day, whereas those with a severe condition may have more than 10 times. The diarrhea begins with yellow loose watery stools and later contains mucus and/or blood. Patients may also experience tenderness in the left lower abdomen and hyperactive bowel sounds. Toxic dysentery may not cause diarrhea or diarrhea mixed with mucus and/or blood. Consequently, the amount of mucus and/or blood in the feces cannot indicate the severity of damage to the colon.

Other than alimentary tract symptoms, systemic poisoning signs may be present. These include a low- or moderate-grade fever, dizziness, fatigue and a poor appetite. In severe cases, a high-grade fever, sluggishness and restlessness may be present. In extremely rare cases, fatal signs such as pallor, cold limbs, a drop in blood pressure, coma, convulsions or cyanosis may be present.

Pattern identification and treatment

Accumulation of damp–heat

Signs and symptoms

Abdominal pain, diarrhea containing mucus and/or blood, tenesmus, a burning sensation around the anus, chest tightness, gastric fullness, a poor appetite and scanty dark-yellow urine; fever or chills may also be present.

Tongue: a (slightly) yellow and greasy coating
Pulse: slippery and rapid

Treatment principle

Clear heat, resolve dampness, circulate *qi* and invigorate blood.

Formula

Modified *Sháo Yào Tāng* (芍药汤, "Peony Decoction").

赤芍	*chì sháo*	9 g	*Radix Paeoniae Rubra*
当归	*dāng guī*	9 g	*Radix Angelicae Sinensis*
黄连	*huáng lián*	3 g	*Rhizoma Coptidis*
黄芩	*huáng qín*	9 g	*Radix Scutellariae*
木香	*mù xiāng*	9 g	*Radix Aucklandiae*
槟榔	*bīng láng*	9 g	*Semen Arecae*
金银花	*jīn yín huā*	9 g	*Flos Lonicerae Japonicae*
甘草	*gān cǎo*	6 g	*Radix et Rhizoma Glycyrrhizae*

Modifications

- For severe toxic heat, combine with *bái tóu wēng* (白头翁, *Radix Pulsatillae*) 15 g and *huáng bǎi* (黄柏, *Cortex Phellodendri Chinensis*) 9 g.
- For severe turbid dampness, combine with *cāng zhú* (苍术, *Rhizoma Atractylodis*) 9 g and *chē qián zǐ* (车前子, *Semen Plantaginis*) 15 g (wrapped).
- For severe abdominal pain, combine with *yán hú suǒ* (延胡索, *Rhizoma Corydalis*) 9 g and *chuān liàn zǐ* (川楝子, *Fructus Toosendan*) 9 g.
- For chills and fever, combine with *gé gēn* (葛根, *Radix Puerariae Lobatae*) 9 g and *huò xiāng* (藿香, *Herba Agastachis*) 9 g.

Epidemic toxins entering the interior

Signs and symptoms

A sudden onset of intense abdominal pain, feces containing mucus and purple-red blood, tenesmus, a high-grade fever with a red face, headache and restlessness; pallor, cold limbs, coma and convulsions may also be present.

Tongue: dark-red, with a yellow coating
Pulse: slippery and rapid

Treatment principle

Clear the *ying*, cool blood, dry dampness and remove toxins.

Formula

Modified *Qīng Yíng Tāng* (清营汤, "*Ying* Level Clearing Decoction") and *Bái Tóu Wēng Tāng* (白头翁汤, "Pulsatilla Decoction").

水牛角	*shuǐ niú jiǎo*	30 g	*Cornu Bubali* (decoct first)
金银花	*jīn yín huā*	9 g	*Flos Lonicerae Japonicae*
黄芩	*huáng qín*	9 g	*Radix Scutellariae*
黄柏	*huáng bǎi*	9 g	*Cortex Phellodendri Chinensis*
黄连	*huáng lián*	3 g	*Rhizoma Coptidis*
牡丹皮	*mǔ dān pí*	9 g	*Cortex Moutan*
秦皮	*qín pí*	9 g	*Cortex Fraxini*

Modifications

- For a severe high-grade fever, combine with *Zǐ Xuě Dān* (紫雪丹, "*Purple Snow Elixir*") 6 g.
- For convulsions, combine with a powder of *líng yáng jiǎo* (羚羊角, *Cornu Saigae Tataricae*) 0.6 g and *shí jué míng* (石决明, *Concha Haliotidis*) 15 g (decoct first).
- For severe persistent abdominal pain, combine with *bīng láng* (槟榔, *Semen Arecae*) 9 g and *dà fù pí* (大腹皮, *Pericarpium Arecae*) 9 g.

- For life-threatening cold limbs, use *Shēn Fù Tāng* (参附汤, "Ginseng and Aconite Decoction") for an emergency and then combine with *Bái Tóu Wēng Tāng* (白头翁汤, "Pulsatilla Decoction").

Cold–dampness in the large intestine

Signs and symptoms

Diarrhea mixed with more white than red mucus (or white mucus alone), abdominal pain, tenesmus, a poor appetite, gastric or abdominal distension and a general heaviness sensation.

Tongue: pale, with a white greasy coating
Pulse: deep and moderate

Treatment principle

Warm the middle *jiao*, dissipate cold, circulate *qi* and resolve dampness.

Formula

Modified *Wèi Líng Tāng* (胃苓汤, "Stomach-Calming Poria Decoction").

苍术	*cāng zhú*	9 g	*Rhizoma Atractylodis*
白术	*bái zhú*	9 g	*Rhizoma Atractylodis Macrocephalae*
木香	*mù xiāng*	9 g	*Radix Aucklandiae*
肉桂	*ròu guì,*	4.5 g	*Cortex Cinnamomi* (decoct later)
厚朴	*hòu pò*	9 g	*Cortex Magnoliae Officinalis*
猪苓	*zhū líng*	9 g	*Polyporus*
茯苓	*fú lín*	9 g	*Poria*
焦山楂	*jiāo shān zhā*	9 g	*Fructus Crataegi Praeparata*
车前草	*chē qián cǎo*	15 g	*Herba Plantaginis*
陈皮	*chén pí*	9 g	*Pericarpium Citri Reticulatae*

Modifications

- For severe abdominal pain, combine with *dāng guī* (当归, *Radix Angelicae Sinensis*) 12 g and *bái sháo* (白芍, *Radix Paeoniae Alba*) 9 g.

- For severe tenesmus, combine with *bīng láng* (槟榔, *Semen Arecae*) 9 g and *zhǐ shí* (枳实, *Fructus Aurantii Immaturus*) 9 g.
- For cold intolerance, combine with *gān jiāng* (干姜, *Rhizoma Zingiberis*) 4.5 g and *wú zhū yú* (吴茱萸, *Fructus Evodiae*) 6 g.
- For cold limbs, combine with *páo fù zǐ* (炮附子, *Radix Aconiti Lateralis Praeparata*) 6 g (decoct first) and *páo jiāng* (炮姜, *Rhizoma Zingiberis Praeparata*) 6 g.

Sinking of clean yang

Signs and symptoms

Persistent diarrhea containing turbid or thin clear mucus, fecal incontinence, lassitude, lack of energy, reluctance to talk, a sallow complexion and a poor appetite.

Tongue: pale, with a white coating
Pulse: soft and thready

Treatment principle

Supplement *qi*, strengthen the spleen and lift up spleen *qi*.

Formula

Modified *Bǔ Zhōng Yì Qì Tāng* (补中益气汤, "Center-Supplementing and *Qi*-Boosting Decoction").

黄芪	huáng qí	15 g	Radix Astragali
党参	dǎng shēn	9 g	Radix Codonopsis
白术	bái zhú	9 g	Rhizoma Atractylodis Macrocephalae
葛根	gé gēn	9 g	Radix Puerariae Lobatae
升麻	shēng má	9 g	Rhizoma Cimicifugae
柴胡	chái hú	9 g	Radix Bupleuri
枳实	zhǐ shí	9 g	Fructus Aurantii Immaturus
当归	dāng guī	9 g	Radix Angelicae Sinensis
陈皮	chén pí	9 g	Pericarpium Citri Reticulatae
甘草	gān cǎo	6 g	Radix et Rhizoma Glycyrrhizae

Modifications

- For severe turbid diarrhea, combine with *huáng lián* (黄连, *Rhizoma Coptidis*) 3 g and *huáng bǎi* (黄柏, *Cortex Phellodendri Chinensis*) 9 g.
- For gastric or abdominal pain with a cold sensation, combine with *gān jiāng* (干姜, *Rhizoma Zingiberis*) 4.5 g and *ròu guì* (肉桂, *Cortex Cinnamomi*) 4.5 g (decoct later).
- For severe fatigue, combine with *shān yào* (山药, *Rhizoma Dioscoreae*) 9 g and *bái biǎn dòu* (白扁豆, *Semen Lablab Album*) 9 g.
- For a severe poor appetite, combine with *mài yá* (麦芽, *Fructus Hordei Germinatus*) 30 g and *tán xiāng* (檀香, *Lignum Santali Albi*) 3 g (decoct later).

Deficiency and cold in the spleen and kidneys

Signs and symptoms

Persistent intermittent diarrhea of thin clear stools, fecal incontinence, abdominal pain with a preference for warmth and pressure, tenesmus, a lusterless complexion, cold limbs, mental fatigue and a poor appetite.

Tongue: pale, with a thin white coating
Pulse: deep and thready

Treatment principle

Warm and tonify the spleen and kidneys, astringe the intestine and stop diarrhea.

Formula

Modified *Zhēn Rén Yǎng Zàng Tāng* (真人养脏汤, "Enlightened Master Viscera-Nourishing Decoction") and *Sì Shén Wán* (四神丸, "Four Spirits Pill").

党参	*dǎng shēn*	15 g	*Radix Codonopsis*
白术	*bái zhú*	9 g	*Rhizoma Atractylodis Macrocephalae*
肉桂	*ròu guì,*	4.5 g	*Cortex Cinnamomi* (decoct later)
当归	*dāng guī*	9 g	*Radix Angelicae Sinensis*

木香	*mù xiāng*	6 g	*Radix Aucklandiae*
肉豆蔻	*ròu dòu kòu*	6 g	*Semen Myristicae*
诃子	*hē zǐ*	9 g	*Fructus Chebulae*
白芍	*bái sháo*	9 g	*Radix Paeoniae Alba*
五味子	*wǔ wèi zǐ*	6 g	*Fructus Schisandrae Chinensis*
补骨脂	*bǔ gǔ zhī*	9 g	*Fructus Psoraleae*
吴茱萸	*wú zhū yú*	6 g	*Fructus Evodiae*
甘草	*gān cǎo*	6 g	*Radix et Rhizoma Glycyrrhizae*

Modifications

- For cold limbs, combine with *páo fù zǐ* (炮附子, *Radix Aconiti Lateralis Praeparata*) 6 g (decoct first) and *páo jiāng* (炮姜, *Rhizoma Zingiberis Praeparata*) 6 g.
- For severe abdominal pain, combine with *yán hú suǒ* (延胡索, *Rhizoma Corydalis*) 9 g and *chuān liàn zǐ* (川楝子, *Fructus Toosendan*) 9 g.
- For diarrhea mixed with turbid feces, combine with *bái tóu wēng* (白头翁, *Radix Pulsatillae*) 15 g and *huáng bǎi* (黄柏, *Cortex Phellodendri Chinensis*) 9 g.

QUESTIONS

1. Describe the main clinical symptoms of dysentery.
2. Describe the treatment principle for dysentery due to deficiency and cold in the spleen and kidneys.
3. *Case study.* Try to make a pattern identification and give a prescription for the following case:

Mr. Liang, 20, experienced sudden intense abdominal pain, nausea, vomiting and over 10 times of diarrhea containing mucus and blood after eating at a food stall the night before. He was treated with fluid infusion and a symptom-oriented method. Other symptoms included dull abdominal pain, five times of bowel movements containing mucus and blood, chest tightness, a poor appetite and dark-yellow urine. The tongue coating was yellow and greasy. The pulse was slippery and rapid.

Pulmonary Tuberculosis

Overview

Pulmonary tuberculosis is an infectious lung disease caused by the bacterium *Mycobacterium tuberculosis* (*M. tuberculosis*). It most commonly affects infants, adolescents and young adults. Women and the elderly are also prone it. This condition often follows diabetes mellitus, silicosis, gastrectomy, measles and whooping cough. If is also often seen in immunosuppressed persons, including immunosuppression conditions or administration of immunosuppressive agents. It is mainly spread through the air, when people who have on active MTB infection cough, sneeze or spit. Clinically, pulmonary tuberculosis can be categorized into four patterns: primary tuberculosis, hematogenous extensive tuberculosis and secondary tuberculosis.

In Chinese medicine, pulmonary tuberculosis is mainly due to infection by *M. tuberculosis* (*láo chóng* in Chinese medicine) and deficiency of *qi* and blood.

M. tuberculosis may damage the essence blood, consume *qi* and impair the lung collaterals. Congenital weakness, excessive consumption of alcohol, mental overexertion, a chronic condition or poor nutrition may all impair the healthy *qi*, making people more susceptible to pulmonary tuberculosis. The disease usually involves the lungs, but may spread to the spleen, kidneys, heart and liver, especially the spleen and kidneys.

Clinical manifestations

Common symptoms of pulmonary tuberculosis are cough, hemoptysis, tidal fever, night sweats and weight loss. This condition is often slow in onset. However, some patients may experience a sudden onset with rapid progression. The cough often starts off mild, unproductive or with production of scanty sticky sputum, and becomes aggravated after that, particularly in the afternoon or at night, coupled with yellow or white sputum. Hemoptysis usually begins as blood-tinged sputum. Some patients may cough up blood. The tidal fever presents with low-grade feverish sensations on the soles and palms, usually in the afternoon or at night; the fever, subsides in the morning. The night sweats are also progressive. So is the weight loss. In severe cases, emaciation may also be present.

Pattern identification and treatment

Lung yin deficiency

Signs and symptoms

Unproductive cough or cough with scanty or blood-tinged sputum, dull chest pain, a low-grade fever in the afternoon, rosy cheeks, feverish sensations of the palms and soles, a dry mouth and throat, and occasional night sweats.

Tongue: red on the tip, with a thin coating
Pulse: thready or thready–rapid

Treatment principle

Nourish yin, moisten the lungs, resolve phlegm and stop the coughing.

Formula

Modified *Yuè Huá Wán* (月华丸, "Lung Yin Nourishing Pill").

生地	*shēng dì*	15 g	*Radix Rehmanniae*
熟地黄	*shú dì huáng*	15 g	*Radix Rehmanniae Praeparata*
北沙参	*běi shā shēn*	12 g	*Radix Glehniae*
天冬	*tiān dōng*	9 g	*Radix Asparagi*
麦冬	*mài dōng*	9 g	*Radix Ophiopogonis*
百部	*bǎi bù*	9 g	*Radix Stemonae*
獭肝	*tǎ gān*	15 g	*Jecur Lutrae*
川贝母	*chuān bèi mǔ*	9 g	*Bulbus Fritillariae Cirrhosae*
白及	*bái jí*	3 g	*Rhizoma Bletillae* (swallow)
茯苓	*fú líng*	9 g	*Poria*
三七	*sān qī*	2 g	*Radix et Rhizoma Notoginseng*
山药	*shān yào*	15 g	*Rhizoma Dioscoreae*

Modifications

- For severe coughing, combine with *xìng rén* (杏仁, *Semen Armeniacae Amarum*) 9 g and *guā lóu* (瓜蒌, *Fructus Trichosanthis*) 15 g.
- For severe chest pain, combine with *yù jīn* (郁金, *Radix Curcumae*) 9 g and *yán hú suǒ* (延胡索, *Rhizoma Corydalis*) 9 g.
- For hemoptysis, combine with *bái máo gēn* (白茅根, *Rhizoma Imperatae*) 15 g and *xiān hè cǎo* (仙鹤草, *Herba Agrimoniae*) 15 g.
- For bone-steaming tidal fever, combine with *yín chái hú* (银柴胡, *Radix Stellariae*) 9 g and *gōng láo yè* (功劳叶, *Folium Ilicis*) 15 g.

Hyperactivity of fire due to yin deficiency

Signs and symptoms

Coughing, shortness of breath, production of scanty yellow sticky sputum, occasional hemoptysis (in a bright red color), feverish sensations on the palms and soles, bone-steaming tidal fever, night sweats, nocturnal emissions, irregular menstruation and gradual weight loss.

Tongue: dry and dark-red, with a thin, yellow or peeled coating
Pulse: thready, wiry and rapid

Treatment principle

Nourish yin, reduce fire, moisten the lungs and arrest bleeding.

Formula

Bǎi Hé Gù Jīn Tāng (百合固金汤, "Lily Bulb Metal-Securing Decoction") and *Qín Jiāo Biē Jiǎ Sǎn* (秦艽鳖甲散, "*Gentianae Macrophyllae* Turtle Shell Powder").

百合	*bǎi hé*	12 g	*Bulbus Lilii*
麦冬	*mài dōng*	9 g	*Radix Ophiopogonis*
玄参	*xuán shēn*	9 g	*Radix Scrophulariae*
生地	*shēng dì*	15 g	*Radix Rehmanniae*
熟地黄	*shú dì huáng*	9 g	*Radix Rehmanniae Praeparata*
鳖甲	*biē jiǎ*	15 g	*Carapax Trionycis* (decoct first)

知母	zhī mǔ	9 g	Rhizoma Anemarrhenae
秦艽	qín jiāo	9 g	Radix Gentianae Macrophyllae
地骨皮	dì gǔ pí	9 g	Cortex Lycii
川贝母	chuān bèi mǔ	9 g	Bulbus Fritillariae Cirrhosae
鱼腥草	yú xīng cǎo	15 g	Herba Houttuyniae
白及	bái jí	3 g	Rhizoma Bletillae (swallow)
白茅根	bái máo gēn	30 g	Rhizoma Imperatae

Modifications

- For cough with profuse yellow sputum, combine with *guā lóu* (瓜蒌, *Fructus Trichosanthis*) 15 g and *huáng qín* (黄芩, *Radix Scutellariae*) 9 g.
- For constipation with bloating, combine with *dà huáng* (大黄, *Radix et Rhizoma Rhei*) 9 g (decoct later) and *má rén* (麻仁, *Fructus Cannabis*) 9 g.
- For severe night sweats, combine with *wū méi* (乌梅, *Fructus Mume*) 9 g and *bì táo gàn* (碧桃干, *Fructus Persicae Immaturus*) 9 g.
- For severe hemoptysis, combine with *xiān hè cǎo* (仙鹤草, *Herba Agrimoniae*) 15 g and *zǐ zhū cǎo* (紫珠草, *Herba Callicarpae Pedunculatae*) 12 g.

Deficiency of qi and yin

Signs and symptoms

Coughing, shortness of breath, (light-red) blood-tinged sputum, tidal fever in the afternoon, a low weak voice, a dry mouth and throat, a bright pale complexion and rosy cheeks.

Tongue: light-red, with a thin coating
Pulse: soft and thready

Treatment principle

Supplement *qi*, nourish yin, moisten the lungs and stop the coughing.

Formulas

Modified *Bǎo Zhēn Tāng* (保真汤, "Genuine *Qi*-Preserving Decoction").

太子参	*tài zǐ shēn*	12 g	*Radix Pseudostellariae*
黄芪	*huáng qí*	30 g	*Radix Astragali*
白术	*bái zhú*	9 g	*Rhizoma Atractylodis Macrocephalae*
炙甘草	*zhì gān cǎo*	9 g	*Radix et Rhizoma Glycyrrhizae Praeparata cum Melle*
天冬	*tiān dōng*	9 g	*Radix Asparagi*
麦冬	*mài dōng*	9 g	*Radix Ophiopogonis*
生地	*shēng dì*	12 g	*Radix Rehmanniae*
熟地黄	*shú dì huáng*	12 g	*Radix Rehmanniae Praeparata*
白芍	*bái sháo*	9 g	*Radix Paeoniae Alba*
当归	*dāng guī*	9 g	*Radix Angelicae Sinensis*
地骨皮	*dì gǔ pí*	9 g	*Cortex Lycii*
黄柏	*huáng bǎi*	9 g	*Cortex Phellodendri Chinensis*
知母	*zhī mǔ*	9 g	*Rhizoma Anemarrhenae*
百部	*bǎi bù*	9 g	*Radix Stemonae*
白及	*bái jí*	3 g	*Rhizoma Bletillae* (swallow)

Modifications

- For a dry throat and a red tongue, combine with *guī bǎn* (龟板, *Plastrum Testudinis*) 15 g (decoct first) and *biē jiǎ* (鳖甲, *Carapax Trionycis*) 15 g (decoct first).
- For severe cough, combine with *zǐ wǎn* (紫菀, *Radix et Rhizoma Asteris*) 9 g and *kuǎn dōng huā* (款冬花, *Flos Farfarae*) 9 g.
- For severe mental fatigue, combine with *shān yào* (山药, *Rhizoma Dioscoreae*) 9 g and *bái biǎn dòu* (白扁豆, *Semen Lablab Album*) 9 g.
- For night sweats and spontaneous sweating, combine with *fú xiǎo mài* (浮小麦, *Fructus Tritici Levis*) 15 g and *duàn mǔ lì* (煅牡蛎, *Concha Ostreae Praeparatum*) 30 g (decoct first).

Deficiency of yin and yang

Signs and symptoms

Choking cough, hemoptysis, a dark-gray complexion, tidal fever, night sweats, spontaneous sweating, cold intolerance, weight loss, hoarseness, a poor appetite, loose stools, palpations and purple lips.

Tongue: Dry and red
Pulse: thready

Treatment principle

Nourish yin and tonify yang.

Formula

Modified *Bǔ Tiān Dà Zào Wán* (补天大造丸, "Earth-Tonifying Regenerating Pill").

太子参	*tài zǐ shēn*	12 g	*Radix Pseudostellariae*
黄芪	*huáng qí*	30 g	*Radix Astragali*
山药	*shān yào*	15 g	*Rhizoma Dioscoreae*
枸杞子	*gǒu qǐ zǐ*	9 g	*Fructus Lycii*
龟板	*guī bǎn*	15 g	*Plastrum Testudinis*
鹿角胶	*lù jiǎo jiāo*	12 g	*Colla Cornus Cervi*
紫河车	*zǐ hé chē*	3 g	*Placenta Hominis*
熟地黄	*shú dì huáng*	15 g	*Radix Rehmanniae Praeparata*
麦冬	*mài dōng*	9 g	*Radix Ophiopogonis*
阿胶	*ē jiāo*	9 g	*Colla Corii Asini* (melted)
当归	*dāng guī*	9 g	*Radix Angelicae Sinensis*
五味子	*wǔ wèi zǐ*	6 g	*Fructus Schisandrae Chinensis*

Modifications

- For severe shortness of breath, combine with *dōng chóng xià cǎo* (冬虫夏草, Cordyceps) 3 g and *ròu guì* (肉桂, *Cortex Cinnamomi*) 4.5 g (decoct later).
- For severe palpations, combine with *zǐ shí yīng* (紫石英, *Fluoritum*) 15 g and *dān shēn* (丹参, *Radix et Rhizoma Salviae Miltiorrhizae*) 15 g.
- For edema in the lower limbs, combine with *zhū líng* (猪苓, *Polyporus*) 15 g and *chē qián zǐ* (车前子, *Semen Plantaginis*) 15 g (wrapped).
- For diarrhea before dawn, combine with *ròu dòu kòu* (肉豆蔻, *Semen Myristicae*) and *bǔ gǔ zhī* (补骨脂, *Fructus Psoraleae*) 9 g.

Stagnant blood obstructing the collaterals

Signs and symptoms

Coughing, persistent hemoptysis with dark blood clots, a stabbing chest pain in a fixed position, fever in the afternoon or at night, rough scaly skin, a dark complexion and weight loss.

Tongue: dark, with ecchymosis
Pulse: thready and hesitant

Treatment principle

Invigorate blood, resolve stasis, moisten the lungs and stop the coughing.

Formula

Modified *Dà Huáng Zhè Chóng Wán* (大黄蟅虫丸, "Rhubarb and Eupolyphaga Pill").

大黄	*dà huáng*	9 g	*Radix et Rhizoma Rhei*
蟅虫	*zhé chóng*	6 g	*Eupolyphaga seu Steleophaga*
桃仁	*táo rén*	9 g	*Semen Persicae*
红花	*hóng huā*	9 g	*Flos Carthami*
丹参	*dān shēn*	15 g	*Radix et Rhizoma Salviae Miltiorrhizae*
生地	*shēng dì*	12 g	*Radix Rehmanniae*
杏仁	*xìng rén*	9 g	*Semen Armeniacae Amarum*
川贝母	*chuān bèi mǔ*	9 g	*Bulbus Fritillariae Cirrhosae*
百部	*bǎi bù*	9 g	*Radix Stemonae*
黄芩	*huáng qín*	9 g	*Radix Scutellariae*
当归	*dāng guī*	9 g	*Radix Angelicae Sinensis*
甘草	*gān cǎo*	6 g	*Radix et Rhizoma Glycyrrhizae*

Modifications

- For persistent hemoptysis, combine with a powder of *sān qī* (三七, *Radix et Rhizoma Notoginseng*) 2 g (swallow) and *huā ruǐ shí* (花蕊石, *Ophicalcitum*) 30 g.

- For fever in the afternoon, combine with *dì gǔ pí* (地骨皮, *Cortex Lycii*) 9 g and *yín chái hú* (银柴胡, *Radix Stellariae*) 9 g.
- For a dry mouth and throat, combine with *běi shâ shēn* (北沙参, *Radix Glehniae*) 9 g and *mài dōng* (麦冬, *Radix Ophiopogonis*) 9 g.
- For severe chest pain, combine with *yù jīn* (郁金, *Radix Curcumae*) 9 g and *yán hú suǒ* (延胡索, *Rhizoma Corydalis*) 9 g.

QUESTIONS

1. How does pulmonary tuberculosis spread?
2. Describe the pattern identifications of pulmonary tuberculosis as well as the treatment principles.
3. *Case study*. Try to make a pattern identification and give a prescription for the following case:

Ms. Zhong, 65, suffered from pulmonary tuberculosis for over 40 years and discontinued medications after clinical recovery. However, she started to experience coughing with shortness of breath recently, along with production of yellow, sticky, (bright red) blood-tinged sputum. Other symptoms included restlessness, irritability, feverish sensations on the palms and soles, tidal fever in the afternoon, rosy cheeks, night sweats and dry stools. The tongue was dark-red, with a peeled coating. The pulse was wiry, thready and rapid.

MALIGNANT CANCERS

Primary Bronchial Cancer

Overview

Primary bronchial cancer, often referred to as lung cancer, is the most common malignant lung cancer. According to cell differentiation and morphological features, lung cancer can be categorized into six patterns: squamous cell lung carcinoma, adenocarcinoma, small-cell undifferentiated carcinoma, large-cell undifferentiated carcinoma, bronchioloalveolar carcinoma and a mixed type of lung cancer. Squamous epithelial cell cancer accounts for 40%–50% of lung cancers. Small-cell undifferentiated carcinoma accounts for 20% (secondary to squamous epithelial cell cancer and adenocarcinoma in terms of incidence) of lung cancers and has the highest malignancy risk. The incidence of lung cancer tends to increase with age, starting from the age of 40 and significantly higher from the age of 50 to 60. Usually, more males than females are affected (at a ratio of approximately 2:1). Cigarette smoking is by far the biggest contributor to lung cancer. Smoking is estimated to account for 80%–85% of squamous cell lung carcinoma. Small-cell undifferentiated lung cancer is also strongly associated with smoking. Surgical resection is the first option once a diagnosis is confirmed.

In Chinese medicine, lung cancer falls under the category of "lung masses," "chest pain," "cough," "hemoptysis" and "dyspnea." The main contributing factors include toxins attacking the lungs, internal buildup of phlegm dampness and lung yin deficiency.

The lungs are known as the tender organs and are therefore prone to be attacked by pathogenic toxins. As a result, the dispersing and descending of lung *qi* can be impaired, followed by blood stasis and subsequent masses. An improper diet or emotional disturbance may impair the transportation and transformation of the spleen and stomach, leading to internal phlegm dampness affecting the lungs, which results in stagnation of *qi* and blood. Those with congenital or acquired lung yin deficiency are susceptible to contraction of internal or external pathogens.

Clinical manifestations

The main clinical symptoms of lung cancer are choking cough, hemoptysis, chest pain, shortness of breath and fever. The choking cough is often paroxysmal, irritant and unproductive. Production of scanty or a large amount of sputum may also be present. Bloody sputum can be intermittent. The chest pain is often intermittent at early stages and has no fixed positions. The pain can be oppressive or dull. However, intense persistent pain can occur at the later stages. The dyspnea (shortness of breath) is progressive, starting off with chest tightness and rapid breathing and gradually presenting with panting and cyanosis of the lips. The fever (normally 38°C) may or may not respond to drugs.

Pattern identification and treatment

Spleen deficiency with retention of phlegm dampness

Signs and symptoms

Coughing with white sticky sputum, chest tightness, shortness of breath, mental fatigue, a poor appetite, a bright pale complexion and loose stools.

Tongue: pale and swollen, with a white greasy coating
Pulse: soft and moderate

Treatment principle

Supplement *qi*, strengthen the spleen, regulate *qi* and resolve phlegm.

Formula

Modified *Liù Jūn Zǐ Tāng* (六君子汤, "Six Gentlemen Decoction").

党参	dǎng shēn	15 g	Radix Codonopsis
白术	bái zhú	9 g	Rhizoma Atractylodis Macrocephalae
茯苓	fú líng	9 g	Poria
甘草	gān cǎo	9 g	Radix et Rhizoma Glycyrrhizae
半夏	bàn xià	12 g	Rhizoma Pinelliae
陈皮	chén pí	9 g	Pericarpium Citri Reticulatae
胆南星	dǎn nán xīng	9 g	Arisaema cum Bile
枳壳	zhǐ qiào	9 g	Fructus Aurantii
紫菀	zǐ wǎn	9 g	Radix et Rhizoma Asteris
款冬花	kuǎn dōng huā	9 g	Flos Farfarae

Modifications

- For profuse phlegm turbidity, combine with *cāng zhú* (苍术, *Rhizoma Atractylodis*) 9 g and *hòu pò* (厚朴, *Cortex Magnoliae Officinalis*) 9 g.
- For yellow sticky sputum, combine with *huáng qín* (黄芩, *Radix Scutellariae*) 9 g and *yú xīng cǎo* (鱼腥草, *Herba Houttuyniae*) 15 g.

- For profuse blood in the sputum, combine with *bái jí* (白及, *Rhizoma Bletillae*) 9 g and *xiān hè cǎo* (仙鹤草, *Herba Agrimoniae*) 15 g.
- For chest pain, combine with *rm xiāng* (乳香, *Olibanum*) 6 g and *mò yào* (没药, *Myrrha*) 6 g.

Qi stagnation and blood stasis

Signs and symptoms

Coughing with bloody sputum, rapid breathing, distending or stabbing pain in the chest or hypochondriac regions with a fixed position, constipation and dark-purple lips and nails.

Tongue: dark with ecchymosis and a thin coating
Pulse: wiry and hesitant

Treatment principle

Circulate *qi*, invigorate blood, resolve phlegm and remove masses.

Formula

Modified *Fù Yuán Huó Xuè Tāng* (复元活血汤, "Original *Qi*-Restoring and Blood-Moving Decoction").

桃仁	*táo rén*	9 g	*Semen Persicae*
红花	*hóng huā*	9 g	*Flos Carthami*
当归	*dāng guī*	9 g	*Radix Angelicae Sinensis*
穿山甲	*chuān shān jiǎ*	9 g	*Squama Manitis* (decoct first)
大黄	*dà huáng*	9 g	*Radix et Rhizoma Rhei* (decoct later)
瓜蒌	*guā lóu*	9 g	*Fructus Trichosanthis*
蒲黄	*pú huáng*	9 g	*Pollen Typhae* (wrapped)
半夏	*bàn xià*	9 g	*Rhizoma Pinelliae*
陈皮	*chén pí*	9 g	*Pericarpium Citri Reticulatae*

Modifications

- For profuse blood in the sputum, combine with *sān qī* (三七, *Radix et Rhizoma Notoginseng*) 9 g and *ǒu jié tàn* (藕节炭, *Nodus Nelumbinis Rhizomatis Carbonisatus*) 9 g.

- For intense chest pain, combine with *yù jīn* (郁金, *Radix Curcumae*) 9 g and *yán hú suǒ* (延胡索, *Rhizoma Corydalis*) 9 g.
- For a low-grade fever, combine with *qīng hāo* (青蒿, *Herba Artemisiae Annuae*) 9 g and *dì gǔ pí* (地骨皮, *Cortex Lycii*) 9 g.
- For excessive sputum, combine with *dǎn nán xīng* (胆南星, *Arisaema cum Bile*) 9 g and *zhú rú* (竹茹, *Caulis Bambusae in Taenia*) 9 g.

Exuberance of toxic heat

Signs and symptoms

A high-grade fever, rapid breathing, coughing with yellow sputum containing fresh blood, chest pain, a dry mouth with a bitter taste, dark-yellow urine and constipation.

Tongue: red, with a thin coating
Pulse: surging and rapid

Treatment principle

Remove toxins, clear heat in the lungs and resolve phlegm.

Formula

Modified *Wǔ Wèi Xiāo Dú Yǐn* (五味消毒饮, "Five Ingredient Toxin-Removing Beverage") and *Qīng Fèi Huà Tán Tāng* (清肺化痰汤, "*Qi*-Clearing and Phlegm-Transforming Decoction").

金银花	*jīn yín huā*	9 g	*Flos Lonicerae Japonicae*
野菊花	*yě jú huā*	9 g	*Flos Chrysanthemi Indici*
蒲公英	*pú gōng yīng*	15 g	*Herba Taraxaci*
紫花地丁	*zǐ huā dì dīng*	15 g	*Herba Violae*
龙葵	*lóng kuí*	30 g	*Herba Solani Nigri*
黄芩	*huáng qín*	9 g	*Radix Scutellariae*
桑白皮	*sāng bái pí*	9 g	*Cortex Mori*
山栀	*shān zhī*	9 g	*Fructus Gardeniae*
贝母	*bèi mǔ*	9 g	*Bulbus Fritillaria*
瓜蒌	*guā lóu*	9 g	*Fructus Trichosanthis*
知母	*zhī mǔ*	9 g	*Rhizoma Anemarrhenae*
甘草	*gān cǎo*	6 g	*Radix et Rhizoma Glycyrrhizae*

Modifications

- For constipation with severe bloating, combine with *dà huáng* (大黄, *Radix et Rhizoma Rhei*) 9 g (decoct later) and *máng xiāo* (芒硝, *Natrii Sulfas*) 9 g.
- For severe coughing, combine with *xìng rén* (杏仁, *Semen Armeniacae Amarum*) 9 g and *mǎ dôu líng* (马兜铃, *Fructus Aristolochiae*) 9 g.
- For yellow sticky sputum, combine with *tiān zhú huáng* (天竺黄, *Concretio Silicea Bambusae*) 9 g and *yú xīng cǎo* (鱼腥草, *Herba Houttuyniae*) 15 g.
- For a high-grade fever, combine with *shí gāo* (石膏, *Gypsum Fibrosum*) 30 g (decoct first) and *Zǐ Xu ě Dān* (紫雪丹, "Purple Snow Elixir") 6 g.

Internal heat due to yin deficiency

Signs and symptoms

Unproductive coughs or coughing with scanty, sticky or bloody sputum, restlessness, insomnia, a dry mouth and throat, tidal fever, night sweats and dry stools.

Tongue: red, with a scanty or peeled coating
Pulse: thready and rapid

Treatment principle

Nourish yin, promote regeneration of fluids, moisten the lungs and resolve phlegm.

Formula

Shā Shēn Mài Dōng Tāng (沙参麦冬汤, "*Adenophorae seu Glehniae* and *Ophiopogon Decoction*") and *Qīng Gǔ Sǎn* (清骨散, "Bone-Clearing Powder").

北沙参	*běi shā shēn*	9 g	*Radix Glehniae*
麦冬	*mài dōng*	9 g	*Radix Ophiopogonis*
天花粉	*tiān huā fěn*	9 g	*Radix Trichosanthis*

玉竹	yù zhú	12 g	Rhizoma Polygonati Odorati
银柴胡	yín chái hú	9 g	Radix Stellariae
胡黄连	hú huáng lián	6 g	Rhizoma Picrorhizae
鳖甲	biē jiǎ	15 g	Carapax Trionycis (decoct first)
知母	zhī mǔ	9 g	Rhizoma Anemarrhenae
甘草	gān cǎo	6 g	Radix et Rhizoma Glycyrrhizae
阿胶	ē jiāo	9 g	Colla Corii Asini (melted)

Modifications

- For restlessness with insomnia, combine with *wǔ wèi zǐ* (五味子, *Fructus Schisandrae Chinensis*) 9 g and *yè jiāo téng* (夜交藤, *Caulis Polygoni Multiflori*) 15 g.

- For severe night sweats, combine with *fú xiǎo mài* (浮小麦, *Fructus Tritici Levis*) 15 g and *bì táo gàn* (碧桃干, *Fructus Persicae Immaturus*) 9 g.

- For constipation, combine with *dà huáng* (大黄, *Radix et Rhizoma Rhei*) 9 g (decoct later) and *má rén* (麻仁, *Fructus Cannabis*) 9 g.

- For severe coughing, combine with *chuān bèi mǔ* (川贝母, *Bulbus Fritillariae Cirrhosae*) 9 g and *zǐ wǎn* (紫菀, *Radix et Rhizoma Asteris*) 9 g.

Deficiency of qi and yin

Signs and symptoms

Coughing with rapid breathing, low and weak coughs with blood-stripped sputum, mental fatigue, a bright pale complexion, weight loss, intolerance of wind, spontaneous sweating, night sweats and a dry mouth with a desire to drink water.

Tongue: red, with a scanty coating
Pulse: thready and weak

Treatment principle

Supplement *qi*, nourish yin, clear heat and resolve phlegm.

Formula

Supplemented *Shēng Mài Sǎn* (生脉散, "Pulse-Engendering Powder").

太子参	tài zǐ shēn	9 g	Radix Pseudostellariae
麦冬	mài dōng	15 g	Radix Ophiopogonis
五味子	wǔ wèi zǐ	9 g	Fructus Schisandrae Chinensis
黄芪	huáng qí	30 g	Radix Astragali
生地	shēng dì	15 g	Radix Rehmanniae
百部	bǎi bù	9 g	Radix Stemonae
川贝母	chuān bèi mǔ	9 g	Bulbus Fritillariae Cirrhosae
黄芩	huáng qín	9 g	Radix Scutellariae
杏仁	xìng rén	9 g	Semen Armeniacae Amarum
黄精	huáng jīng	12 g	Rhizoma Polygonati
甘草	gān cǎo	6 g	Radix et Rhizoma Glycyrrhizae

Modifications

- For severe coughing, combine with *zǐ wǎn* (紫菀, *Radix et Rhizoma Asteris*) 9 g and *kuān dōng huā* (款冬花, *Flos Farfarae*) 9 g.
- For severe hemoptysis, combine with *bái máo gēn* (白茅根, *Rhizoma Imperatae*) 30 g and *sān qī* (三七, *Radix et Rhizoma Notoginseng*) 9 g.
- For severe mental fatigue, combine with *shān yào* (山药, *Rhizoma Dioscoreae*) 9 g and *bái biǎn dòu* (白扁豆, *Semen Lablab Album*) 9 g.
- For profuse sweating, combine with *nuò dào gēn* (糯稻根, *Radix Oryzae Glutinosae*) 30 g and *duàn mǔ lì* (煅牡蛎, *Concha Ostreae Praeparatum*) 30 g (decoct first).

QUESTIONS

1. Describe the main clinical manifestations of lung cancer.
2. Describe the pattern identifications of lung cancer and highlight the pattern with the highest incidence and malignancy.
3. *Case study.* Try to make a pattern identification and give a prescription for the following case:

Mr. Wang, 68, suffered from chronic bronchitis for 20 years. Two months prior to treatment, he suddenly presented with blood in the sputum and was diagnosed with central bronchogenic carcinoma. The symptoms included frequent coughing with fresh blood and mucus in the sputum, chest tightness, shortness of breath, fatigue, a poor appetite and loose stools. The tongue was pale, with a white greasy coating. The pulse was soft and thready.

Gastric Cancer

Overview

Gastric cancer, often referred to as stomach cancer, is one of the most common malignant cancers in China and ranks No. 1 among all the alimentary tract cancers. Stomach cancer causes half of the deaths. Usually, more males than females are affected (at a ratio of approximately 2.3–3.6:1). It can develop at any age but is most common between the ages of 50 and 60. It rarely affects adults under 30. Stomach cancer can develop in any part of the stomach. The most common parts are the gastric antrum, the lesser curvature of the stomach, the anterior–posterior walls and the cardiac region. It rarely occurs in the gastric corpus. According to the tissue structures, stomach cancer can be categorized into four patterns: adenocarcinoma, undifferentiated carcinoma, mucocellular carcinoma and special carcinoma. Surgical resection is the first option once a diagnosis is confirmed.

In Chinese medicine, stomach cancer falls under the category of "stomachache," "dysphagia," "acid reflux" or "abdominal masses." The main contributing factors include an improper diet, emotional disturbances and constitutional deficiency.

Excessive consumption of alcohol and overingestion of hot spicy dry food may cause heat retention in the stomach to consume yin, leading to insufficiency of yin fluids and blood. Worry or anxiety may impair the spleen, leading to phlegm. Anger may damage the liver, causing liver *qi* stagnation. Consequently, stagnation of *qi* and blood may result in stasis and subsequent masses. Constitutional deficiency of the spleen may cause internal phlegm *qi* stagnation.

Clinical manifestations

The main clinical manifestations of stomach cancer are epigastric fullness, distension, discomfort or pain, a poor appetite, unexplained weight loss and black stools. The epigastric fullness, distension and discomfort often begin with an intermittent onset and do not seem to be associated with food intake. The stomach pain appears progressive, persistent and irregular. A poor appetite, especially intolerance of meats, is a distinctive early sign of stomach cancer. Weight loss is also progressive. Black stools can be intermittent or persistent. Hemoptysis may also be present. Other symptoms include nausea, acid regurgitation, belching, a burning sensation (heartburn) and fatigue.

Pattern identification and treatment

Disharmony between the liver and the stomach

Signs and symptoms

Gastric distension, fullness, discomfort or pain, frequent belching, hiccups, nausea, vomiting and a poor appetite.

Tongue: light-red, with a thin white or thin yellow coating
Pulse: wiry

Treatment principle

Soothe the liver, harmonize the stomach, downregulate stomach *qi* and relieve pain.

Formula

Modified *Chái Hú Shū Gān Sǎn* (柴胡疏肝散, "Bupleurum Liver-Soothing Powder") and *Xuán Fù Dài Zhě Tāng* (旋覆代赭汤, "Inula and Hematite Decoction").

柴胡	*chái hú*	9 g	*Radix Bupleuri*
枳壳	*zhǐ qiào*	9 g	*Fructus Aurantii*
白芍	*bái sháo*	9 g	*Radix Paeoniae Alba*
木香	*mù xiāng*	6 g	*Radix Aucklandiae*
郁金	*yù jīn*	9 g	*Radix Curcumae*
厚朴	*hòu pò*	9 g	*Cortex Magnoliae Officinalis*
沉香	*chén xiāng*	3 g	*Lignum Aquilariae Resinatum* (decoct later)
半夏	*bàn xià*	12 g	*Rhizoma Pinelliae*
旋覆花	*xuán fù huā*	9 g	*Flos Inulae* (wrapped)
代赭石	*dài zhě shí*	30 g	*Haematitum* (decoct first)
甘草	*gān cǎo*	6 g	*Radix et Rhizoma Glycyrrhizae*

Modifications

- For severe stomach pain, combine with *yán hú suŏ* (延胡索, *Rhizoma Corydalis*) 9 g and *chuān liàn zĭ* (川楝子, *Fructus Toosendan*) 9 g.
- For heartburn, combine with *zhī mŭ* (知母, *Rhizoma Anemarrhenae*) 9 g and *huáng lián* (黄连, *Rhizoma Coptidis*) 6 g.
- For a dry mouth with a desire to drink water, combine with *shēng dì* (生地, *Radix Rehmanniae*) 15 g and *mài dōng* (麦冬, *Radix Ophiopogonis*) 9 g.
- For dry stools, combine with *má rén* (麻仁, *Fructus Cannabis*) 9 g and *yù lĭ rén* (郁李仁, *Semen Pruni*) 9 g.

Phlegm qi stagnation

Signs and symptoms

Chest or gastric fullness, distension or pain, loss of appetite (especially for meat), dysphagia and vomiting of saliva.

Tongue: light-red, with a white greasy coating
Pulse: wiry and slippery

Treatment principle

Regulate *qi*, resolve phlegm, promote digestion and remove masses.

Formula

Modified *Hăi Zăo Yù Hú Tāng* (海藻玉壶汤, "Sargassum Jade Kettle Decoction").

海藻	*hăi zăo*	9 g	*Sargassum*
昆布	*kūn bù*	9 g	*Thallus Laminariae*
半夏	*bàn xià*	9 g	*Rhizoma Pinelliae*
陈皮	*chén pí*	9 g	*Pericarpium Citri Reticulatae*
牡蛎	*mŭ lì*	30 g	*Concha Ostreae*
枳实	*zhĭ shí*	9 g	*Fructus Aurantii Immaturus*
山楂	*shān zhā*	9 g	*Fructus Crataegi*

神曲	shén qū	9 g	Massa Medicata Fermentata
茯苓	fú líng	9 g	Poria
制天南星	zhì tiān nán xīng	9 g	Rhizoma Arisaematis praeparatum
贝母	bèi mǔ	9 g	Bulbus Fritillaria

Modifications

- For severe gastric distension and pain, combine with *xiāng yuán* (香橼, *Fructus Citri*) 9 g and *bā yuè zhā* (八月札, *Fructus Akebiae*) 15 g.
- For a severe poor appetite, combine with *jī nèi jīn* (鸡内金, *Endothelium Corneum Gigeriae Galli*) 9 g and *mài yá* (麦芽, *Fructus Hordei Germinatus*) 15 g.
- For severe nausea, combine with *xuán fù huā* (旋覆花, *Flos Inulae*) 9 g (wrapped) and *dài zh shí* (代赭石, *Haematitum*)15 g (decoct first).
- For stomach pain with a burning sensation, combine with *bái huā shé shé cǎo* (白花蛇舌草, *Herba Hedyotis Diffusae*) 30 g and *pú gōng yīng* (蒲公英, *Herba Taraxaci*) 30 g.

Toxic heat with phlegm stasis

Signs and symptoms

Gastric pain with a burning sensation, fever, a dry mouth with a desire to drink water, nausea, vomiting of saliva or undigested food that resembles red beans, black stools, dark-yellow urine and dry rough skin.

Tongue: dark-purple or with ecchymosis and a yellow greasy coating
Pulse: slippery and rapid

Treatment principle

Clear heat, remove toxins and resolve phlegm stasis.

Formula

Modified *Sì Miào Yǒng Ān Tāng* (四妙勇安汤, "Four Wonderfully Effective Heroes Decoction").

金银花	*jīn yín huā*	9 g	*Flos Lonicerae Japonicae*
玄参	*xuán shēn*	12 g	*Radix Scrophulariae*
当归	*dāng guī*	9 g	*Radix Angelicae Sinensis*
莪术	*é zhú*	9 g	*Rhizoma Curcumae*
蛇莓	*shé méi*	30 g	*Herba Duchesneae Indicae*
夏枯草	*xià kū cǎo*	9 g	*Spica Prunellae*
三七	*sān qī*	9 g	*Radix et Rhizoma Notoginseng*
甘草	*gān cǎo*	6 g	*Radix et Rhizoma Glycyrrhizae*
半夏	*bàn xià*	9 g	*Rhizoma Pinelliae*
陈皮	*chén pí*	9 g	*Pericarpium Citri Reticulatae*

Modifications

- For a yellow thick greasy coating, combine with *yì yǐ rén* (薏苡仁, *Semen Coicis*) 15 g and *bái huā shé shé cǎo* (白花蛇舌草, *Herba Hedyotis Diffusae*) 30 g.
- For severe black stools, remove *é zhú* (*Rhizoma Curcumae*) and *dāng guī* (*Radix Angelicae Sinensis*) and combine with *bái jí* (白及, *Rhizoma Bletillae*) 9 g and *xiān hè cǎo* (仙鹤草, *Herba Agrimoniae*) 15 g.
- For severe stomach pain, combine with *lù lù tōng* (路路通, *Fructus Liquidambaris*) 9 g and *jim xiāng chóng* (九香虫, *Aspongopus*) 6 g.
- For a dark-purple tongue due to severe blood stasis, combine with *sān léng* (三棱, *Rhizoma Sparganii*) and *shuǐ zhì* (水蛭, *Hirudo*) 6 g.

Stomach yin deficiency

Signs and symptoms

Gastric pain, weight loss, dry skin, palpable abdominal masses, a dry mouth and throat, tidal fever, night sweats and dry stools.

Tongue: red, with no or a scanty coating
Pulse: thready and rapid

Treatment principle

Nourish yin, benefit the stomach, unblock collaterals and remove masses.

Formula

Yī Guàn Jiān (一贯煎, "Effective Integration Decoction") and *Shī Xiào Sǎn* (失笑散, "Sudden Smile Powder").

北沙参	*běi shā shēn*	12 g	Radix Glehniae
麦冬	*mài dōng*	9 g	Radix Ophiopogonis
生地	*shēng dì*	9 g	Radix Rehmanniae
枸杞子	*gǒu qǐ zǐ*	9 g	Fructus Lycii
当归	*dāng guī*	9 g	Radix Angelicae Sinensis
川楝子	*chuān liàn zǐ*	9 g	Fructus Toosendan
五灵脂	*wǔ líng zhī*	9 g	Faeces Trogopterori (wrapped)
蒲黄	*pú huáng*	9 g	Pollen Typhae (wrapped)
夏枯草	*xià kū cǎo*	9 g	Spica Prunellae
八月札	*bā yuè zhā*	9 g	Fructus Akebiae

Modifications

- For stomach pain with a burning sensation, combine with *pú gōng yīng* (蒲公英, *Herba Taraxaci*) 15 g and *zhī mǔ* (知母, *Rhizoma Anemarrhenae*) 9 g.
- For solid painful abdominal masses, combine with *sān léng* (三棱, *Rhizoma Sparganii*) and *é zhú* (莪术, *Rhizoma Curcumae*) 9 g.
- For constipation, combine with *má rén* (麻仁, *Fructus Cannabis*) 9 g and *yù lǐ rén* (郁李仁, *Semen Pruni*) 9 g.
- For a dry mouth with a desire to drink water, combine with *tiān huā fěn* (天花粉, *Radix Trichosanthis*) 9 g and *xuán shēn* (玄参, *Radix Scrophulariae*) 9 g.

Deficiency and cold in the spleen and stomach

Signs and symptoms

Dull gastric pain, a bright pale complexion, debilitation, eating food in the morning but vomiting up in the evening, loss of appetite, abdominal masses, cold limbs and edema in the lower limbs.

Tongue: pale, with a white coating
Pulse: deep and thready

Treatment principle

Warm the middle *jiao*, dissipate cold, strengthen the spleen and relieve pain.

Formula

Modified *Zhěng Yáng Lǐ Láo Tāng* (拯阳理劳汤, "Yang-Saving and Fatigue-Improving Decoction").

党参	*dǎng shēn*	15 g	*Radix Codonopsis*
黄芪	*huáng qí*	30 g	*Radix Astragali*
白术	*bái zhú*	9 g	*Rhizoma Atractylodis Macrocephalae*
陈皮	*chén pí*	9 g	*Pericarpium Citri Reticulatae*
肉桂	*ròu guì,*	4.5 g	*Cortex Cinnamomi* (decoct later)
炮附子	*páo fù zǐ*	9 g	*Radix Aconiti Lateralis Praeparata* (decoct first)
当归	*dāng guī*	9 g	*Radix Angelicae Sinensis*
丁香	*dīng xiāng*	4.5 g	*Flos Caryophylli*
延胡索	*yán hú suǒ*	9 g	*Rhizoma Corydalis*
炙甘草	*zhì gān cǎo*	9 g	*Radix et Rhizoma Glycyrrhizae Praeparata cum Melle*

Modifications

- For severe cold intolerance and cold limbs, combine with *xiān máo* (仙茅, *Rhizoma Curculiginis*) 9 g and *xiān líng pí* (仙灵脾, *Herba Epimedii*) 9 g.
- For severe edema in the lower limbs, combine with *zhū líng* (猪苓, *Polyporus*) 15 g and *chē qián zǐ* (车前子, *Semen Plantaginis*) 15 g (wrapped).
- For severe vomiting, combine with *bàn xià* (半夏, *Rhizoma Pinelliae*) 9 g and *dài zh shí* (代赭石, *Haematitum*) 15 g (decoct first).
- For loose stools, combine with *páo jiāng* (炮姜, *Rhizoma Zingiberis Praeparatum*) 6 g and *shān yào* (山药, *Rhizoma Dioscoreae*) 9 g.

QUESTIONS

1. Describe the main clinical manifestations of stomach cancer.
2. Describe the treatment principle for stomach cancer due to toxic heat with phlegm stasis.
3. *Case study.* Try to make a pattern identification and give a prescription for the following case:

Mr. Zhang, 55, suffered from chronic gastritis for years and recently experienced progressive gastric distension and discomfort that did not respond to drugs. Other symptoms included nausea, loss of appetite and dry stools. The tongue was light-red, with a thin white coating. The pulse was wiry. The patient was later diagnosed with stomach cancer by gastroscope.

Primary Carcinoma of the Liver

Overview

Primary carcinoma of the liver is one of the most common malignancies in China. It causes high mortality. Its incidence is secondary only to those of gastric cancer and esophageal cancer. Usually, more males than females are affected (at a ratio of approximately 2–5:1). This condition can develop at any age but is most common between the ages of 40 and 49. Approximately four out of five primary carcinoma of the liver are hepatocellular carcinomas (also known as malignant hepatomas). The rest, one out of five, are intrahepatic cholangiocellular carcinomas. A combination of the two is extremely rare. Life-threatening complications may occur at the later stages. They include hepatic coma, alimentary tract hemorrhage, hemorrhage following carcinoma nodules, bloody ascites and secondary infections. Surgical resection is the first option once a diagnosis is confirmed.

In Chinese medicine, primary carcinoma of the liver falls under the category of "abdominal masses," "jaundice," "abdominal tympanites" or pain in the hypochondriac regionst." The main contributing factors include an improper diet, emotional disturbance and the subsequent blood stasis, damp–heat and toxic fire.

Excessive consumption of alcohol or an improper diet may damage the spleen and stomach, causing turbid dampness and toxic heat to impair the transportation and transformation, which results in bloating, a poor appetite, nausea, vomiting and fatigue. The damp–heat may further affect the liver and gallbladder, leading to jaundice and pain in the hypochondriac regions. Emotional disturbance such as anger may damage the liver, causing liver *qi* stagnation, blood stasis and subsequent masses. Liver *qi* stagnation may either compromise the spleen or transform into fire to further cause intense pain. Over time, the enlarged masses may block the *qi* activities and result in ascites. Failure of the spleen to transport and transform coupled with kidney deficiency may cause fluid retention, leading to abdominal tympanites. Buildup of stagnant blood may cause fever and jaundice. The fire transformed from liver *qi* stagnation or damp–heat may in turn consume fluids, resulting in hyperactivity of deficient fire and subsequent hemorrhage. Eventually, consumption of the fluid and blood may cause toxic fire to ascend and disturb the mind, leading to coma.

Clinical manifestations

Primary carcinoma of the liver is clinically characterized by hepatalgia, hepatomegaly, jaundice, ascites and unintentional weight loss. Hepatalgia is the most common symptom. Patients may experience intermittent or persistent dull pain that can radiate to the right shoulder and low back. Hepatomegaly is often progressive and tender, appearing solid with an irregular surface and border, as well as nodules in varying sizes. Jaundice is present in approximately 50% of the patients. Ascites occurs at the later stages, coupled with rapid progression of yellowish or bloody masses. The weight loss is also progressive. In rare cases, alimentary tract hemorrhage or cachexia may also be present. Other symptoms include upper abdominal distension, a poor appetite, nausea, vomiting and mental fatigue.

Pattern identification and treatment

Liver qi stagnation

Signs and symptoms

Distending pain in the right hypochondriac region, belching, chest tightness, abdominal bloating, a poor appetite, a sallow complexion, lassitude and loose stools.

Tongue: red, with a thin coating
Pulse: wiry

Treatment principle

Soothe the liver, regulate *qi*, invigorate blood and relieve pain.

Formula

Modified *Xiāo Yáo Sǎn* (逍遥散, "Free Wanderer Powder").

柴胡	*chái hú*	9 g	*Radix Bupleuri*
当归	*dāng guī*	9 g	*Radix Angelicae Sinensis*
赤芍	*chì sháo*	9 g	*Radix Paeoniae Rubra*
白芍	*bái sháo*	9 g	*Radix Paeoniae Alba*
枳壳	*zhǐ qiào*	9 g	*Fructus Aurantii*
白术	*bái zhú*	9 g	*Rhizoma Atractylodis Macrocephalae*
茯苓	*fú líng*	9 g	*Poria*
陈皮	*chén pí*	6 g	*Pericarpium Citri Reticulatae*
桃仁	*táo rén*	9 g	*Semen Persicae*
郁金	*yù jīn*	9 g	*Radix Curcumae*
甘草	*gān cǎo*	6 g	*Radix et Rhizoma Glycyrrhizae*

Modifications

- For severe pain in the hypochondriac regions, combine with *chuān liàn zǐ* (川楝子, *Fructus Toosendan*) 9 g and *yán hú suǒ* (延胡索, *Rhizoma Corydalis*) 9 g.

- For a poor appetite, combine with *mài yá* (麦芽, *Fructus Hordei Germinatus*) 12 g and *jī nèi jīn* (鸡内金, *Endothelium Corneum Gigeriae Galli*) 9 g.
- For a bitter taste and a thin yellow tongue coating, combine with *bái huā shé shé cǎo* (白花蛇舌草, *Herba Hedyotis Diffusae*) 30 g and *lóng kuí* (龙葵, *Herba Solani Nigri*) 30 g.
- For palpable masses in the hypochondrium, combine with *hǎi zǎo* (海藻, *Sargassum*) 15 g and *é zhú* (莪术, *Rhizoma Curcumae*) 9 g.

Damp–heat with toxic stasis

Signs and symptoms

Solid masses in the hypochondrium with a stabbing pain, gastric or abdominal fullness and distension, drumlike abdominal tympanites, jaundice, a dark-gray complexion, rough scaly skin, a high-grade fever, thirst dark-yellow urine and dry black stools.

Tongue: red, with ecchymosis and a yellow greasy coating
Pulse: wiry, slippery and rapid

Treatment principle

Clear heat, resolve dampness, remove toxins and resolve stasis.

Formula

Modified *Yīn Chén Hāo Tāng* (茵陈蒿汤, "Artemisiae Scopariae Decoction") and *Táo Hóng Sì Wù Tāng* (桃红四物汤, "Peach Kernel and Carthamus Four Substances Decoction").

茵陈	*yīn chén*	30 g	*Herba Artemisiae Scopariae*
山栀	*shān zhī*	9 g	*Fructus Gardeniae*
大黄	*dà huáng*	9 g	*Radix et Rhizoma Rhei* (decoct later)
桃仁	*táo rén*	9 g	*Semen Persicae*
红花	*hóng huā*	9 g	*Flos Carthami*
当归	*dāng guī*	9 g	*Radix Angelicae Sinensis*
赤芍	*chì sháo*	9 g	*Radix Paeoniae Rubra*
川芎	*chuān xiōng*	9 g	*Rhizoma Chuanxiong*
石见穿	*shí jiàn chuān*	30 g	*Herba Salviae Chinensis*
白花蛇舌草	*bái huā shé shé cǎo*	30 g	*Herba Hedyotis Diffusae*

Modifications

- For severe ascites, combine with *hú lú* (葫芦, *Fructus Lagenariae*) 30 g and *bīng láng* (槟榔, *Semen Arecae*) 12 g.
- For severe pain in the hypochondriac regions, combine with *yán hú suǒ* (延胡索, *Rhizoma Corydalis*) 9 g and *rǒ xiāng* (乳香, *Olibanum*) 9 g.
- For nausea, combine with *bàn xià* (半夏, *Rhizoma Pinelliae*) 9 g and *zhú rú* (竹茹, *Caulis Bambusae in Taenia*) 9 g.
- For a poor appetite, combine with *shén qū* (神曲, *Massa Medicata Fermentata*) 9 g and *shān zhā* (山楂, *Fructus Crataegi*) 9 g.

Toxic blood stasis

Signs and symptoms

Huge masses in the hypochondrium with aggravated distension and fixed pain that can radiate to the low back, worsened gastric or abdominal distension and jaundice.

Tongue: dark-purple, with ecchymosis or petechiae
Pulse: wiry and hesitant

Treatment principle

Invigorate blood, resolve stasis, remove masses and remove toxins.

Formula

Modified *Gé Xià Zhú Yū Tāng* (膈下逐瘀汤, "Expelling Stasis Below the Diaphragm Decoction").

桃仁	táo rén	9 g	Semen Persicae
红花	hóng huā	9 g	Flos Carthami
赤芍	chì sháo	9 g	Radix Paeoniae Rubra
五灵脂	wǔ líng zhī	9 g	Faeces Trogopterori
蒲黄	pú huáng	9 g	Pollen Typhae (wrapped)
土鳖虫	tǔ biē chóng	6 g	Eupolyphaga seu Steleophaga
穿山甲	chuān shān jiǎ	9 g	Squama Manitis
白花蛇舌草	bái huā shé shé cǎo	30 g	Herba Hedyotis Diffusae
石见穿	shí jiàn chuān	30 g	Herba Salviae Chinensis

Modifications

- For severe pain in the hypochondriac regions, combine with *yán hú suǒ* (延胡索, *Rhizoma Corydalis*) 9 g and *é zhú* (莪术, *Rhizoma Curcumae*) 9 g; Alternatively, apply *chán sū* (蟾酥, *Venenum Bufonis*) ointment to the painful area.
- For severe bloating, combine with *bīng láng* (槟榔, *Semen Arecae*) 9 g and *dà fù pí* (大腹皮, *Pericarpium Arecae*) 9 g.
- For severe jaundice, combine with *yīn chén* (茵陈, *Herba Artemisiae Scopariae*) 15 g and *shān zhī* (山栀, *Fructus Gardeniae*) 9 g.
- For severe ascites, combine with *chē qián zǐ* (车前子, *Semen Plantaginis*) 15 g (wrapped) and *hú lú* (葫芦, *Fructus Lagenariae*) 30 g.

Toxic heat damaging yin

Signs and symptoms

Solid masses, drum like abdominal tympanites, significant weight loss, pain in the hypochondriac regions, dizziness, tinnitus, tidal fever and night sweats. Alternatively, a high-grade fever, thirst, nasal or gum bleeding, yellow eyes and face, dry stools and scanty dark-yellow urine may be present.

Tongue: dry and red, with a peeled coating
Pulse: thready, wiry and rapid

Treatment principle

Nourish yin, clear heat, remove toxins and resolve stasis.

Formula

Modified *Xī Jiǎo Dì Huáng Tāng* (犀角地黄汤, "Rhinoceros Horn and Rehmannia Decoction").

水牛角	*shuǐ niú jiǎo*	30 g	*Cornu Bubali* (decoct first)
生地	*shēng dì*	15 g	*Radix Rehmanniae*
赤芍	*chì sháo*	9 g	*Radix Paeoniae Rubra*

牡丹皮	*mǔ dān pí*	9 g	*Cortex Moutan*
鳖甲	*biē jiǎ*	15 g	*Carapax Trionycis* (decoct first)
金银花	*jīn yín huā*	12 g	*Flos Lonicerae Japonicae*
徐长卿	*xú cháng qīng*	9 g	*Radix et Rhizoma Cynanchi Paniculati*
白花蛇舌草	*bái huā shé shé cǎo*	30 g	*Herba Hedyotis Diffusae*
女贞子	*nǔ zhēn zǐ*	9 g	*Fructus Ligustri Lucidi*

Modifications

- For hematemesis and black stools, combine with *sān qī* (三七, *Radix et Rhizoma Notoginseng*) 9 g and *huái huā* (槐花, *Flos Sophorae*) 15 g.

- For severe jaundice, combine with *hǔ zhàng* (虎杖, *Rhizoma Polygoni Cuspidati*) 9 g and *yīn chén* (茵陈, *Herba Artemisiae Scopariae*) 15 g.

- For severe ascites, combine with *chē qián zǐ* (车前子, *Semen Plantaginis*) 15 g (wrapped) and *hú lú* (葫芦, *Fructus Lagenariae*) 30 g.

- For a severe dry mouth, combine with *mài dōng* (麦冬, *Radix Ophiopogonis*) 9 g and *shí hú* (石斛, *Caulis Dendrobii*) 9 g.

- For constipation, combine with *má rén* (麻仁, *Fructus Cannabis*) 9 g and *yù lǐ rén* (郁李仁, *Semen Pruni*) 9 g.

Spleen deficiency with retention of dampness

Signs and symptoms

Pain in the hypochondriac regions, palpable masses below the ribs, mental fatigue, indigestion, gastric or abdominal distension, loose stools and a bright pale complexion.

Tongue: pale, with a white greasy coating
Pulse: soft and thready

Treatment principle

Strengthen the spleen, supplement *qi* and dry dampness.

Formula

Modified *Xiāng Shā Liù Jūn Zǐ Tāng* (香砂六君子汤, "Costus Root and Amomum Six Gentlemen Decoction") and *Píng Wèi Sǎn* (平胃散, "Stomach-Calming Powder").

党参	*dǎng shēn*	9 g	*Radix Codonopsis*
苍术	*cāng zhú*	9 g	*Rhizoma Atractylodis*
白术	*bái zhú*	9 g	*Rhizoma Atractylodis Macrocephalae*
茯苓	*fú líng*	9 g	*Poria*
陈皮	*chén pí*	9 g	*Pericarpium Citri Reticulatae*
厚朴	*hòu pò*	9 g	*Cortex Magnoliae Officinalis*
砂仁	*shā rén*	6 g	*Fructus Amomi* (decoct later)
木香	*mù xiāng*	6 g	*Radix Aucklandiae*
莪术	*é zhú*	9 g	*Rhizoma Curcumae*
炙甘草	*zhì gān cǎo*	9 g	*Radix et Rhizoma Glycyrrhizae Praeparata cum Melle*

Modifications

- For severe pain in the hypochondriac regions, combine with *yán hú suǒ* (延胡索, *Rhizoma Corydalis*) 9 g and *sān qī* (三七, *Radix et Rhizoma Notoginseng*) 9 g.
- For significant bloating, combine with *dà fù pí* (大腹皮, *Pericarpium Arecae*) 9 g and *zhǐ shí* (枳实, *Fructus Aurantii Immaturus*) 9 g.
- For severe loose stools, combine with *shān yào* (山药, *Rhizoma Dioscoreae*) 9 g and *bái biǎn dòu* (白扁豆, *Semen Lablab Album*) 9 g.
- For a yellow greasy tongue coating, combine with *huáng lián* (黄连, *Rhizoma Coptidis*) 3 g and *huáng bǎi* (黄柏, *Cortex Phellodendri Chinensis*) 9 g.

QUESTIONS

1. Describe the common complications of primary carcinoma of the liver.
2. Describe the main clinical manifestations of primary carcinoma of the liver.
3. *Case study*. Try to make a pattern identification and give a prescription for the following case:

Mr. Huang, 45, suffered from hepatitis B for 10 years and recently experienced distension, pain and discomfort in the right hypochondriac region with a suspected mass. He was diagnosed with primary carcinoma of the liver. Other symptoms included pain, distension and discomfort in the right hypochondriac region, mental fatigue, a poor appetite, loose stools and poor sleep. The tongue was pale and swollen, with tooth marks and a thin white coating. The pulse was soft and thready.

Index to the Formulas

Bā Zhèng Sǎn (八正散, "Eight Corrections Powder"), from *Beneficial Formulas from the Taiping Imperial Pharmacy (Tài Píng Huì Mín Hé Jì Jú Fāng,* 太平惠民和剂局方)

Ingredients: *Qú mài* (瞿麦, *Herba Dianthi*), *biǎn xù* (萹蓄, *Herba Polygoni Avicularis*), *huá shí* (滑石, *Talcum*), *shān zhī* (山栀, *Fructus Gardeniae*), *mù tōng* (木通, *Caulis Akebiae*), *chē qián zǐ* (车前子, *Semen Plantaginis*), *dà huáng* (大黄, *Radix et Rhizoma Rhei*), *zhì gān cǎo* (炙甘草, *Radix et Rhizoma Glycyrrhizae Praeparata cum Melle*) and *dēng xīn cǎo* (灯心草, *Medulla Junci*).

Bǎi Hé Gù Jīn Tāng (百合固金汤, "Lily Bulb Metal-Securing Decoction"), from *Medical Formulas Collected and Analyzed (Yī Fāng Jí Jiě,* 医方集解)

Ingredients: *Shēng dì* (生地, *Radix Rehmanniae*), *shú dì huáng* (熟地黄, *Radix Rehmanniae Praeparata*), *mài dōng* (麦冬, *Radix Ophiopogonis*), *bèi mǔ* (贝母, *Bulbus Fritillaria*), *bǎi hé* (百合, *Bulbus Lilii*), *dāng guī* (当归, *Radix Angelicae Sinensis*), *sháo yào* (芍药, *Radix Paeoniae*), *xuán shēn* (玄参, *Radix Scrophulariae*) and *jié gěng* (桔梗, *Radix Platycodonis*)

Bái Tóu Wēng Tāng (白头翁汤, "Pulsatilla Decoction"), from *Treatise on Cold Damage (Shāng Hán Lùn,* 伤寒论)

Ingredients: *Bái tóu wēng* (白头翁, *Radix Pulsatillae*), *qín pí* (秦皮, *Cortex Fraxini*), *huáng lián* (黄连, *Rhizoma Coptidis*) and *huáng bǎi* (黄柏, *Cortex Phellodendri Chinensis*)

Bàn Xià Bái Zhú Tiān Má Tāng (半夏白术天麻汤, "Pinellia, Atractylodes Macrocephala and Gastrodia Decoction"), from *Medical Revelations (Yī Xué Xīn Wù,* 医学心悟)

Ingredients: *Bàn xià* (半夏, *Rhizoma Pinelliae*), *bái zhú* (白术, *Rhizoma Atractylodis Macrocephalae*), *tiān má* (天麻, *Rhizoma Gastrodiae*), *chén pí* (陈皮, *Pericarpium Citri Reticulatae*), *fú líng* (茯苓, *Poria*), *gān cǎo*

(甘草, *Radix et Rhizoma Glycyrrhizae*), *shēng jiāng* (生姜, *Rhizoma Zingiberis Recens*) and *dà zǎo* (大枣, *Fructus Jujubae*)

Bǎo Zhēn Tāng (保真汤, "Genuine-*Qi*-Preserving Decoction"), from *Beneficial Formulas from the Taiping Imperial Pharmacy* (*Tài Píng Huì Mín Hé Jì Jú Fāng*, 太平惠民和剂局方)

Ingredients: *Gǎo běn* (藁本, *Rhizoma Ligustici*), *chuān xiōng* (川芎, *Rhizoma Chuanxiong*), *gān cǎo* (甘草, *Radix et Rhizoma Glycyrrhizae*) and *cāng zhú* (苍术, *Rhizoma Atractylodis*)

Bǔ Tiān Dà Zào Wán (补天大造丸, "Earth-Tonifying Regenerating Pill"), from *The Origin of Miscellaneous Diseases* (*Zá Bìng Yuán*, 杂病源)

Ingredients: *Shú dì huáng* (熟地黄, *Radix Rehmanniae Praeparata*), *huí xiāng* (茴香, *Foeniculum Valgare*), *huáng bǎi* (黄柏, *Cortex Phellodendri Chinensis*), *bái zhú* (白术, *Rhizoma Atractylodis Macrocephalae*), *shēng dì* (生地, *Radix Rehmanniae*), *niú xī* (牛膝, *Radix Achyranthis Bidentatae*), *mài dōng* (麦冬, *Radix Ophiopogonis*), *dù zhòng* (杜仲, *Cortex Eucommiae*), *wǔ wèi zǐ* (五味子, *Fructus Schisandrae Chinensis*), *gǒu qǐ zǐ* (枸杞子, *Fructus Lycii*), *chén pí* (陈皮, *Pericarpium Citri Reticulatae*), *gān jiāng* (干姜, *Rhizoma Zingiberis*), *cè bǎi yè* (侧柏叶, *Cacumen Platycladi*) and *zǐ hé chē* (紫河车, *Placenta Hominis*)

Bǔ Yáng Huán Wǔ Tāng (补阳还五汤, "Yang-Supplementing and Five-Returning Decoction"), from *Correction of Errors in Medical Works* (*Yī Lín Gǎi Cuò*, 医林改错)

Ingredients: *Dāng guī* (当归, *Radix Angelicae Sinensis*), *chuān xiōng* (川芎, *Rhizoma Chuanxiong*), *huáng qí* (黄芪, *Radix Astragali*), *táo rén* (桃仁, *Semen Persicae*), *dì lóng* (地龙, *Pheretima*), *chì sháo* (赤芍, *Radix Paeoniae Rubra*) and *hóng huā* (红花, *Flos Carthami*)

Bǔ Zhōng Yì Qì Tāng (补中益气汤, "Center-Supplementing and *Qi*-Boosting Decoction"), from *Treatise on the Spleen and Stomach* (*Pí Wèi Lùn*, 脾胃论)

Ingredients: *Rén shēn* (人参, *Radix et Rhizoma Ginseng*), *huáng qí* (黄芪, *Radix Astragali*), *bái zhú* (白术, *Rhizoma Atractylodis Macrocephalae*), *gān cǎo* (甘草, *Radix et Rhizoma Glycyrrhizae*), *dāng guī* (当归, *Radix Angelicae Sinensis*), *chén pí* (陈皮, *Pericarpium Citri Reticulatae*), *shēng má* (升麻, *Rhizoma Cimicifugae*) and *chái hú* (柴胡, *Radix Bupleuri*)

Chái Hú Shū Gān Sǎn (柴胡疏肝散, "Bupleurum Liver-Soothing Powder"), from *The Complete Works of [Zhang] Jing-yue* (*Jǐng Yuè Quán Shū*, 景岳全书)

Ingredients: *Chái hú* (柴胡, *Radix Bupleuri*), *zhǐ qiào* (枳壳, *Fructus Aurantii*), *sháo yào* (芍药, *Radix Paeoniae*), *gān cǎo* (甘草, *Radix et Rhizoma Glycyrrhizae*), *xiāng fù* (香附, *Rhizoma Cyperi*) and *chuān xiōng* (川芎, *Rhizoma Chuanxiong*)

Dà Bǔ Yīn Wán (大补阴丸, "Major Yin-Supplementing Pill"), from *Teachings of [Zhu] Dan-xi* (*Dān Xī Xīn Fǎ*, 丹溪心法)

Ingredients: *Zhī mǔ* (知母, *Rhizoma Anemarrhenae*), *huáng bǎi* (黄柏, *Cortex Phellodendri Chinensis*), *shú dì huáng* (熟地黄, *Radix Rehmanniae Praeparata*) and *guī bǎn* (龟板, *Plastrum Testudinis*)

Dà Bǔ Yuán Jiān (大补元煎, "Major *Yuan*-Supplementing Decoction"), from *Complete Works of [Zhang] Jing-yue* (*Jǐng Yuè Quán Shū*, 景岳全书)

Ingredients: *Rén shēn* (人参, *Radix et Rhizoma Ginseng*), *shān yào* (山药, *Rhizoma Dioscoreae*), *shú dì huáng* (熟地黄, *Radix Rehmanniae Praeparata*), *dù zhòng* (杜仲, *Cortex Eucommiae*), *gǒu qǐ zǐ* (枸杞子, *Fructus Lycii*), *dāng guī* (当归, *Radix Angelicae Sinensis*), *shān zhū yú* (山茱萸, *Fructus Corni*) and *gān cǎo* (甘草, *Radix et Rhizoma Glycyrrhizae*)

Dà Chái Hú Tāng (大柴胡汤, "Major Bupleurum Decoction") from *Treatise on Cold Damage* (*Shāng Hán Lùn*, 伤寒论)

Ingredients: *Chái hú* (柴胡, *Radix Bupleuri*), *huáng qín* (黄芩, *Radix Scutellariae*), *bàn xià* (半夏, *Rhizoma Pinelliae*), *zhǐ shí* (枳实, *Fructus Aurantii Immaturus*), *bái sháo* (白芍, *Radix Paeoniae Alba*), *dà huáng* (大黄, *Radix et Rhizoma Rhei*), *shēng jiāng* (生姜, *Rhizoma Zingiberis Recens*) and *dà zǎo* (大枣, *Fructus Jujubae*)

Dà Chéng Qì Tāng (大承气汤, "Major Purgative Decoction"), from *Treatise on Cold Damage* (*Shāng Hán Lùn*, 伤寒论)

Ingredients: *Dà huáng* (大黄, *Radix et Rhizoma Rhei*), *hòu pò* (厚朴, *Cortex Magnoliae Officinalis*), *zhǐ shí* (枳实, *Fructus Aurantii Immaturus*) and *máng xiāo* (芒硝, *Natrii Sulfas*)

Dà Huáng Zhè Chóng Wán (大黄蟅虫丸, "Rhubarb and Eupolyphaga Pill"), from *Essentials from the Golden Cabinet* (*Jīn Guì Yào Lüè*, 金匮要略)

Ingredients: *Dà huáng* (大黄, *Radix et Rhizoma Rhei*), *zhé chóng* (蛰虫, *Eupolyphaga seu Steleophaga*), *gān qī* (干漆, *Resina Toxicodendri*), *shēng dì* (生地, *Radix Rehmanniae*), *gān cǎo* (甘草, *Radix et Rhizoma Glycyrrhizae*), *shuǐ zhì* (水蛭, *Hirudo*), *sháo yào* (芍药, *Radix Paeoniae*), *huáng qín* (黄芩, *Radix Scutellariae*), *táo rén* (桃仁, *Semen Persicae*), *xìng rén* (杏仁, *Semen Armeniacae Amarum*), *méng chóng* (虻虫, *Tabanus*) and *qí cáo* (蛴螬, *Larva Holotrichiae*)

Dà Wū Tóu Jiān (大乌头煎, "Aconiti Decoction"), from *Essentials from the Golden Cabinet* (*Jīn Guì Yào Lüè*, 金匮要略)

Ingredients: *Chuān wū* (川乌, *Radix Aconiti*)

Dài Gé Sǎn (黛蛤散, "*Indigo Naturalis* and *Concha Meretricis seu Cyclinae Powder*") (experienced formula)

Ingredients: *Qīng dài* (青黛, *Indigo Naturalis*) and *hǎi gé qiào* (海蛤壳, *Concha Meretricis seu Cyclinae*)

Dān Shēn Yǐn (丹参饮, "Salvia Beverage"), from *Golden Mirror of the Medical Tradition* (*Yī Zōng Jīn Jiàn*, 医宗金鉴)

Ingredients: *Dān shēn* (丹参, *Radix et Rhizoma Salviae Miltiorrhizae*), *tán xiāng* (檀香, *Lignum Santali Albi*) and *shā rén* (砂仁, *Fructus Amomi*)

Dān Zhī Xiāo Yáo Sǎn (丹栀逍遥散, "*Cortex Moutan* and Gardenia Free Wanderer Powder"), from *Xue's Case Records* (*Xuē Shì Yī Àn*, 薛氏医案)

Ingredients: *Dāng guī* (当归, *Radix Angelicae Sinensis*), *bái sháo* (白芍, *Radix Paeoniae Alba*), *bái zhú* (白术, *Rhizoma Atractylodis Macrocephalae*), *chái hú* (柴胡, *Radix Bupleuri*), *fú líng* (茯苓, *Poria*), *zhì gān cǎo* (炙甘草, *Radix et Rhizoma Glycyrrhizae Praeparata cum Melle*), *shēng jiāng* (生姜, *Rhizoma Zingiberis Recens*), *bò hé* (薄荷, *Herba Menthae*), *mǔ dān pí* (牡丹皮, *Cortex Moutan*) and *zhī zǐ* (栀子, *Fructus Gardeniae*)

Dāng Guī Sì Nì Tāng (当归四逆汤, "Angelicae and Frigid Extremities Decoction"), from *Treatise on Cold Damage* (*Shāng Hán Lùn*, 伤寒论)

Ingredients: *Dāng guī* (当归, *Radix Angelicae Sinensis*), *guì zhī* (桂枝, *Ramulus Cinnamomi*), *sháo yào* (芍药, *Radix Paeoniae*), *xì xīn* (细辛, *Radix et Rhizoma Asari*), *gān cǎo* (甘草, *Radix et Rhizoma Glycyrrhizae*), *tōng cǎo* (通草, *Medulla Tetrapanacis*) and *dà zǎo* (大枣, *Fructus Jujubae*)

Dǎo Chì Chéng Qì Tāng (导赤承气汤, "*Paeoniae Rubra* Purgative Decoction"), from *Systematic Differentiation of Warm Diseases* (*Wēn Bìng Tiáo Biàn*, 温病条辨)

Ingredients: *Chì sháo* (赤芍, *Radix Paeoniae Rubra*), *shēng dì* (生地, *Radix Rehmanniae*), *dà huáng* (大黄, *Radix et Rhizoma Rhei*), *huáng lián* (黄连, *Rhizoma Coptidis*), *huáng bǎi* (黄柏, *Cortex Phellodendri Chinensis*) and *máng xiāo* (芒硝, *Natrii Sulfas*)

Dǎo Tán Tāng (导痰汤, "Phlegm-Expelling Decoction"), from *Formulas to Aid the Living* (*Jì Shēng Fāng*, 济生方)

Ingredients: *Bàn xià* (半夏, *Rhizoma Pinelliae*), *chén pí* (陈皮, *Pericarpium Citri Reticulatae*), *zhǐ shí* (枳实, *Fructus Aurantii Immaturus*), *fú líng* (茯苓, *Poria*), *gān cǎo* (甘草, *Radix et Rhizoma Glycyrrhizae*) and *zhì tiān nán xīng* (制天南星, *Rhizoma Arisaematis praeparatum*)

Dì Huáng Yǐn Zǐ (地黄饮子, "Rehmannia Drink"), from *An Elucidation of Formulas* (*Xuān Míng Lùn Fāng*, 宣明论方)

Ingredients: *Shēng dì* (生地, *Radix Rehmanniae*), *bā jǐ tiān* (巴戟天, *Radix Morindae Officinalis*), *shān zhū yú* (山茱萸, *Fructus Corni*), *shí hú* (石斛, *Caulis Dendrobii*), *ròu cōng róng* (肉苁蓉, *Herba Cistanches*), *wǔ wèi zǐ* (五味子, *Fructus Schisandrae Chinensis*), *ròu guì* (肉桂, *Cortex Cinnamomi*), *fú líng* (茯苓, *Poria*), *mài dōng* (麦冬, *Radix Ophiopogonis*), *páo fù zǐ* (炮附子, *Radix Aconiti Lateralis Praeparata*), *shí chāng pú* (石菖蒲, *Rhizoma Acori Tatarinowii*) and *yuǎn zhì* (远志, *Radix Polygalae*)

Dí Tán Tāng (涤痰汤, "Phlegm-Flushing Decoction"), from *Formulas to Aid the Living* (*Jì Shēng Fāng*, 济生方)

Ingredients: *Zhì bàn xià* (制半夏, *Rhizoma Pinelliae Praeparata*), *zhì tiān nán xīng* (制天南星, *Rhizoma Arisaematis praeparatum*), *chén pí* (陈皮, *Pericarpium Citri Reticulatae*), *zhǐ shí* (枳实, *Fructus Aurantii Immaturus*), *fú líng* (茯苓, *Poria*), *rén shēn* (人参, *Radix et Rhizoma Ginseng*), *shí chāng pú* (石菖蒲, *Rhizoma Acori Tatarinowii*), *zhú rú* (竹茹, *Caulis Bambusae in Taenia*), *gān cǎo* (甘草, *Radix et Rhizoma Glycyrrhizae*) and *shēng jiāng* (生姜, *Rhizoma Zingiberis Recens*)

Dìng Chuǎn Tāng (定喘汤, "Arrest Wheezing Decoction"), from *Standards for Diagnosis and Treatment* (*Zhèng Zhì Zhǔn Shéng*, 证治准绳)

Ingredients: *Bái guǒ* (白果, *Semen Ginkgo*), *má huáng* (麻黄, *Herba Ephedrae*), *sāng bái pí* (桑白皮, *Cortex Mori*), (款冬花, *Flos Farfarae*), *bàn xià* (半夏, *Rhizoma Pinelliae*), *xìng rén* (杏仁, *Semen Armeniacae Amarum*), *zǐ sū zǐ* (紫苏子, *Fructus Perillae*), *huáng qín* (黄芩, *Radix Scutellariae*) and *gān cǎo* (甘草, *Radix et Rhizoma Glycyrrhizae*)

Èr Chén Tāng (二陈汤, "Two Matured Substances Decoction"), from *Beneficial Formulas from the Taiping Imperial Pharmacy* (*Tài Píng Huì Mín Hé Jì Jú Fāng*, 太平惠民和剂局方)

Ingredients: *Bàn xià* (半夏, *Rhizoma Pinelliae*), *jú hóng* (橘红, *Exocarpium Citri Rubrum*), *fú líng* (茯苓, *Poria*) and *gān cǎo* (甘草, *Radix et Rhizoma Glycyrrhizae*)

Èr Dōng Tāng (二冬汤, "Asparagi and Ophiopogonis Decoction"), from *Medical Revelations* (*Yī Xué Xīn Wù*, 医学心悟)

Ingredients: *Tiān dōng* (天冬, *Radix Asparagi*), *mài dōng* (麦冬, *Radix Ophiopogonis*), *tiān huā fěn* (天花粉, *Radix Trichosanthis*), *huáng qín*

(黄芩, *Radix Scutellariae*), *zhī mǔ* (知母, *Rhizoma Anemarrhenae*), *hé yè* (荷叶, *Folium Nelumbinis*), *rén shēn* (人参, *Radix et Rhizoma Ginseng*) and *gān cǎo* (甘草, *Radix et Rhizoma Glycyrrhizae*),

Èr Shén Sàn (二神散, "*Spora Lygodii* and *Talcum Powder*"), from *Extracts of Internal Medicine* (*Nèi Kē Zhāi Yào*, 内科摘要*)

Ingredients: *Bǔ gǔ zhī* (补骨脂, *Fructus Psoraleae*) and *ròu dòu kòu* (肉豆蔻, *Semen Myristicae*)

Èr Xiān Tāng (二仙汤, "*Chong* and *Ren–Regulating Decoction*"), from *Clinical Manuals of TCM Formulas* (*Zhōng Yī Fāng Jì Lín Chuáng Shǒu Cè*, 中医方剂临床手册)

Ingredients: *Xiān máo* (仙茅, *Rhizoma Curculiginis*), *xiān líng pí* (仙灵脾, *Herba Epimedii*), *dāng guī* (当归, *Radix Angelicae Sinensis*), *bā jǐ tiān* (巴戟天, *Radix Morindae Officinalis*), *huáng bǎi* (黄柏, *Cortex Phellodendri Chinensis*) and *zhī mǔ* (知母, *Rhizoma Anemarrhenae*)

Fù Yuán Huó Xuè Tāng (复元活血汤, "Original *Qi*-Restoring and Blood-Moving Decoction"), from *Inventions of Medicine* (*Yī Xué Fā Míng*, 医学发明)

Ingredients: *Bái zhú* (白术, *Rhizoma Atractylodis Macrocephalae*), *Guā lóu gēn* (瓜蒌根, *Radix Trichosanthis*), *dāng guī* (当归, *Radix Angelicae Sinensis*), *hóng huā* (红花, *Flos Carthami*), *gān cǎo* (甘草, *Radix et Rhizoma Glycyrrhizae*), *chuān shān jiǎ* (穿山甲, *Squama Manitis*), *dà huáng* (大黄, *Radix et Rhizoma Rhei*) and *táo rén* (桃仁, *Semen Persicae*)

Fù Zǐ Lǐ Zhōng Wán (附子理中丸, "Aconite Center-Regulating Pill"), from *Beneficial Formulas from the Taiping Imperial Pharmacy* (*Tài Píng Huì Mín Hé Jì Jú Fāng*, 太平惠民和剂局方)

Ingredients: *Pào fù zǐ* (炮附子, *Radix Aconiti Lateralis Praeparata*), *rén shēn* (人参, *Radix et Rhizoma Ginseng*), *bái zhú* (白术, *Rhizoma Atractylodis Macrocephalae*), *páo jiāng* (炮姜, *Rhizoma Zingiberis Praeparatum*) and *zhì gān cǎo* (炙甘草, *Radix et Rhizoma Glycyrrhizae Praeparata cum Melle*)

Fù Zǐ Tāng (附子汤, "Aconite Decoction"), from *Treatise on Cold Damage* (*Shāng Hán Lùn*, 伤寒论)

Ingredients: *Fù zǐ* (附子, *Radix Aconiti Lateralis*), *fú líng* (茯苓, *Poria*), *rén shēn* (人参, *Radix et Rhizoma Ginseng*), *bái zhú* (白术, *Rhizoma Atractylodis Macrocephalae*) and *sháo yào* (芍药, *Radix Paeoniae*)

Gé Xià Zhú Yū Tāng (膈下逐瘀汤, "Expelling Stasis Below the Diaphragm Decoction"), from *Correction of Errors in Medical Works* (*Yī Lín Gǎi Cuò*, 医林改错)

Ingredients: *Wŭ líng zhī* (五灵脂, *Faeces Trogopterori*), *dāng guī* (当归, *Radix Angelicae Sinensis*), *chuān xiōng* (川芎, *Rhizoma Chuanxiong*), *táo rén* (桃仁, *Semen Persicae*), *mŭ dān pí* (牡丹皮, *Cortex Moutan*), *chì sháo* (赤芍, *Radix Paeoniae Rubra*), *wū yào* (乌药, *Radix Linderae*), *yán hú suŏ* (延胡索, *Rhizoma Corydalis*), *gān căo* (甘草, *Radix et Rhizoma Glycyrrhizae*), *xiāng fù* (香附, *Rhizoma Cyperi*), *hóng huā* (红花, *Flos Carthami*) and *zhĭ qiào* (枳壳, *Fructus Aurantii*)

Guā Lóu Xiè Bái Bái Jiŭ Tāng (瓜蒌薤白白酒汤, "Trichosanthes, Chinese Chives and White Wine Decoction"), from the *Treatise on Cold Damage* (*Shāng Hán Lùn*, 伤寒论)

Ingredients: *Guā lóu* (瓜蒌, *Fructus Trichosanthis*), *xiè bái* (薤白, *Bulbus Allii Macrostemi*) and *bái jiŭ* (白酒, *White Wine*)

Guī Pí Tāng (归脾汤, "Spleen-Restoring Decoction"), from *Formulas to Aid the Living* (*Jì Shēng Fāng*, 济生方)

Ingredients: *Dăng shēn* (党参, *Radix Codonopsis*), *huáng qí* (黄芪, *Radix Astragali*), *bái zhú* (白术, *Rhizoma Atractylodis Macrocephalae*), *fú shén* (茯神, *Sclerotium Poriae Pararadicis*), *suān zăo rén* (酸枣仁, *Semen Ziziphi Spinosae*), *lóng yăn ròu* (龙眼肉, *Arillus Longan*), *mù xiāng* (木香, *Radix Aucklandiae*), *zhì gān căo* (炙甘草, *Radix et Rhizoma Glycyrrhizae Praeparata cum Melle*), *yuăn zhì* (远志, *Radix Polygalae*), *dāng guī* (当归, *Radix Angelicae Sinensis*), *shēng jiāng* (生姜, *Rhizoma Zingiberis Recens*) and *dà zăo* (大枣, *Fructus Jujubae*)

Guì Zhī Tāng (桂枝汤, "Cinnamon Twig Decoction Plus Peony"), from *Treatise on Cold Damage* (*Shāng Hán Lùn*, 伤寒论)

Ingredients: *Guì zhī* (桂枝, *Ramulus Cinnamomi*), *sháo yào* (芍药, *Radix Paeoniae*), *shēng jiāng* (生姜, *Rhizoma Zingiberis Recens*), *zhì gān căo* (炙甘草, *Radix et Rhizoma Glycyrrhizae Praeparata cum Melle*) and *dà zăo* (大枣, *Fructus Jujubae*)

Hăi Zăo Yù Hú Tāng (海藻玉壶汤, "Sargassum Jade Kettle Decoction"), from *The Golden Mirror of the Medical Tradition* (*Yī Zōng Jīn Jiàn*, 医宗金鉴)

Ingredients: *Hăi zăo* (海藻, *Sargassum*), *kūn bù* (昆布, *Thallus Laminariae*), *hăi dài căo* (海带草, *Herba Zosterae Marinae*), *bàn xià* (半夏, *Rhizoma Pinelliae*), *chén pí* (陈皮, *Pericarpium Citri Reticulatae*), *qīng pí* (青皮, *Pericarpium Citri Reticulatae Viride*), *lián qiào* (连翘, *Fructus Forsythiae*), *bèi mŭ* (贝母, *Bulbus Fritillaria*), *chuān xiōng* (川芎, *Rhizoma Chuanxiong*), *dú huó* (独活, *Radix Angelicae Pubescentis*) and *gān căo* (甘草, *Radix et Rhizoma Glycyrrhizae*)

Hé Táo Chéng Qì Tāng (核桃承气汤, "Semen Juglandis Purgative Decoction"), from the *Treatise on Cold Damage* (*Shāng Hán Lùn*, 伤寒论)

Ingredients: *Hé táo rén* (核桃仁, Semen Juglandis), *dà huáng* (大黄, *Radix et Rhizoma Rhei*), *guì zhī* (桂枝, *Ramulus Cinnamomi*), *gān cǎo* (甘草, *Radix et Rhizoma Glycyrrhizae*) and *máng xiāo* (芒硝, *Natrii Sulfas*)

Huà Bān Tāng (化斑汤, "Stasis-Resolving Decoction"), from *Systematic Differentiation of Warm Diseases* (*Wēn Bìng Tiáo Biàn*, 温病条辨)

Ingredients: *Shí gāo* (石膏, *Gypsum Fibrosum*), *zhī mǔ* (知母, *Rhizoma Anemarrhenae*), *gān cǎo* (甘草, *Radix et Rhizoma Glycyrrhizae*), *xuán shēn* (玄参, *Radix Scrophulariae*), *jīng mǐ* (粳米, *Oryza Sativa L.*) and *xī jiǎo* (犀角, *Cornu Rhinocerotis*)

Huà Gān Jiān (化肝煎, "Liver-Benefiting Decoction"), from the *Complete Works of [Zhang] Jing-yue* (*Jǐng Yuè Quán Shū*, 景岳全书)

Ingredients: *Qīng pí* (青皮, *Pericarpium Citri Reticulatae Viride*), *chén pí* (陈皮, *Pericarpium Citri Reticulatae*), *sháo yào* (芍药, *Radix Paeoniae*), *mǔ dān pí* (牡丹皮, *Cortex Moutan*), *zé xiè* (泽泻, *Rhizoma Alismatis*) and *bèi mǔ* (贝母, *Bulbus Fritillaria*)

Huà Yū Tāng (化瘀汤, "Stasis-Resolving Decoction") (experienced formula)

Ingredients: *Dāng guī* (当归, *Radix Angelicae Sinensis*), *chì sháo* (赤芍, *Radix Paeoniae Rubra*), *mǔ dān pí* (牡丹皮, *Cortex Moutan*), *táo rén* (桃仁, *Semen Persicae*), *hóng huā* (红花, *Flos Carthami*), *dān shēn* (丹参, *Radix et Rhizoma Salviae Miltiorrhizae*), *chuān shān jiǎ* (穿山甲, *Squama Manitis*), *bái zhú* (白术, *Rhizoma Atractylodis Macrocephalae*), *zé xiè* (泽泻, *Rhizoma Alismatis*), *qīng pí* (青皮, *Pericarpium Citri Reticulatae Viride*) and *mǔ lì* (牡蛎, *Concha Ostreae*)

Huáng Lián Jiě Dú Tāng (黄连解毒汤, "Coptis Toxin-Resolving Decoction"), from *Arcane Essentials from the Imperial Library* (*Wài Tái Mì Yào*, 外台秘要)

Ingredients: *Huáng lián* (黄连, *Rhizoma Coptidis*), *huáng qín* (黄芩, *Radix Scutellariae*), *huáng bǎi* (黄柏, *Cortex Phellodendri Chinensis*) and *shān zhī* (山栀, *Fructus Gardeniae*)

Huáng Qí Bǔ Zhōng Tāng (黄芪补中汤, "Astragalus Center-Tonifying Decoction"), from *Ten Selected Texts by Li Dong-Yuan* (*Dōng Yuán Shí Shū*, 东垣十书)

Ingredients: *Huáng qí* (黄芪, *Radix Astragali*), *rén shēn* (人参, *Radix et Rhizoma Ginseng*), *gān cǎo* (甘草, *Radix et Rhizoma Glycyrrhizae*), *bái zhú* (白术, *Rhizoma Atractylodis Macrocephalae*), *cāng zhú* (苍术, *Rhizoma Atractylodis*), *zé xiè* (泽泻, *Rhizoma Alismatis*), *zhū líng* (猪苓, *Polyporus*) and *fú líng* (茯苓, *Poria*)

Huáng Qí Jiàn Zhōng Tāng (黄芪建中汤, "Astragalus Center-Fortifying Decoction"), from *Essentials from the Golden Cabinet* (*Jīn Guì Yào Lüè*, 金匮要略)

Ingredients: *Huáng qí* (黄芪, *Radix Astragali*), *bái sháo* (白芍, *Radix Paeoniae Alba*), *guì zhī* (桂枝, *Ramulus Cinnamomi*), *zhì gān cǎo* (炙甘草, *Radix et Rhizoma Glycyrrhizae Praeparata cum Melle*), *shēng jiāng* (生姜, *Rhizoma Zingiberis Recens*), *dà zǎo* (大枣, *Fructus Jujubae*) and *yí tang* (饴糖, *Saccharum Granorum*)

Huó Luò Xiào Líng Wán (活络效灵丸, "Effective Channel-Activating Pill"), from the *Records of Chinese Medicine with Reference to Western Medicine* (*Yī Xué Zhōng Zhōng Cān Xī Lù*, 医学衷中参西录)

Ingredients: *Dāng guī* (当归, *Radix Angelicae Sinensis*), *dān shēn* (丹参, *Radix et Rhizoma Salviae Miltiorrhizae*), *rǔ xiāng* (乳香, *Olibanum*) and *mò yào* (没药, *Myrrha*)

Jīn Guì Shèn Qì Wán (金匮肾气丸, "Golden Cabinet's Kidney *Qi* Pill"), from *Essentials from the Golden Cabinet* (*Jīn Guì Yào Lüè*, 金匮要略)

Ingredients: *Shú dì huáng* (熟地黄, *Radix Rehmanniae Praeparata*), *shān yào* (山药, *Rhizoma Dioscoreae*), *shān zhū yú* (山茱萸, *Fructus Corni*), *mǔ dān pí* (牡丹皮, *Cortex Moutan*), *fú líng* (茯苓, *Poria*), *zé xiè* (泽泻, *Rhizoma Alismatis*), *fù zǐ* (附子, *Radix Aconiti Lateralis Praeparata*) and *ròu guì* (肉桂, *Cortex Cinnamomi*)

Jīng Fáng Bài Dú Sǎn (荆防败毒散, "Schizonepeta and Saposhnikovia Toxin-Resolving Powder"), from *Numerous Miraculous Prescriptions for Health Cultivation* (*Shè Shēng Zhòng Miào Fāng*, 摄生众妙方)

Ingredients: *Jīng jiè* (荆芥, *Herba Schizonepetae*), *fáng fēng* (防风, *Radix Saposhnikoviae*), *qiāng huó* (羌活, *Rhizoma et Radix Notopterygii*), *dú huó* (独活, *Radix Angelicae Pubescentis*), *chái hú* (柴胡, *Radix Bupleuri*), *qián hú* (前胡, *Radix Peucedani*), *chuān xiōng* (川芎, *Rhizoma Chuanxiong*), *zhǐ qiào* (枳壳, *Fructus Aurantii*), *fú líng* (茯苓, *Poria*), *jié gěng* (桔梗, *Radix Platycodonis*) and *gān cǎo* (甘草, *Radix et Rhizoma Glycyrrhizae*)

Lǐ Zhōng Wán (理中丸, "Center-Regulating Pill"), from *Treatise on Cold Damage* (*Shāng Hán Lùn*, 伤寒论)

Ingredients: *Dǎng shēn* (党参, *Radix Codonopsis*), *bái zhú* (白术, *Rhizoma Atractylodis Macrocephalae*), *gān jiāng* (干姜, *Rhizoma Zingiberis*) and *gān cǎo* (甘草, *Radix et Rhizoma Glycyrrhizae*)

Líng Guì Zhú Gān Tāng (苓桂术甘汤, "Poria, Cinnamon Twig, Atractylodes Macrocephala and Licorice Decoction"), from *Essentials from the Golden Cabinet* (*Jīn Guì Yào Lüè*, 金匮要略)

Ingredients: *Fú líng* (茯苓, *Poria*), *guì zhī* (桂枝, *Ramulus Cinnamomi*), *zhū líng* (猪苓, *Polyporus*), *zé xiè* (泽泻, *Rhizoma Alismatis*), *bái zhú* (白术, *Rhizoma Atractylodis Macrocephalae*) and *gān cǎo* (甘草, *Radix et Rhizoma Glycyrrhizae*)

Líng Jiǎo Gōu Téng Tāng (羚角钩藤汤, "Antelope Horn and Uncaria Decoction"), from the *Popular Guide to the "Treatise on Cold Damage"* (*Tōng Sú Shāng Hán Lùn*, 通俗伤寒论)

Ingredients: *Líng yáng jiǎo* (羚羊角, *Cornu Saigae Tataricae*), *sāng yè* (桑叶, *Folium Mori*), *chuān bèi mǔ* (川贝母, *Bulbus Fritillariae Cirrhosae*), *shēng dì* (生地, *Radix Rehmanniae*), *gōu téng* (钩藤, *Ramulus Uncariae Cum Uncis*), *jú huā* (菊花, *Flos Chrysanthemi*), *bái sháo* (白芍, *Radix Paeoniae Alba*), *gān cǎo* (甘草, *Radix et Rhizoma Glycyrrhizae*), *zhú rú* (竹茹, *Caulis Bambusae in Taenia*) and *fú shén* (茯神, *Sclerotium Poriae Pararadicis*)

Líng Zǐ Sǎn (金铃子散, "Toosendan Powder"), from *Formulas from Benevolent Sages* (*Shèng Huì Fāng*, 圣惠方)

Ingredients: *Chuān liàn zǐ* (川楝子, *Fructus Toosendan*) and *yán hú suǒ* (延胡索, *Rhizoma Corydalis*)

Liù Jūn Zǐ Tāng (六君子汤, "Six Gentlemen Decoction"), from *Fine Formulas for Women* (*Fù Rén Liáng Fāng*, 妇人良方)

Ingredients: *Rén shēn* (人参, *Radix et Rhizoma Ginseng*), *bái zhú* (白术, *Rhizoma Atractylodis Macrocephalae*), *fú líng* (茯苓, *Poria*), *gān cǎo* (甘草, *Radix et Rhizoma Glycyrrhizae*), *chén pí* (陈皮, *Pericarpium Citri Reticulatae*) and *bàn xià* (半夏, *Rhizoma Pinelliae*)

Liù Wèi Dì Huáng Wán (六味地黄丸, "Six-Ingredient Rehmannia Pill"), from *The Key to Diagnosis and Treatment of Children's Diseases* (*Xiǎo Ér Yào Zhèng Zhí Jué*, 小儿药证直诀)

Ingredients: *Shú dì huáng* (熟地黄, *Radix Rehmanniae Praeparata*), *gān shān yào* (干山药, *Rhizoma Dioscoreae Recens*), *shān zhū yú* (山茱萸, *Fructus Corni*), *fú líng* (茯苓, *Poria*), *mǔ dān pí* (牡丹皮, *Cortex Moutan*) and *zé xiè* (泽泻, *Rhizoma Alismatis*)

Lóng Dǎn Xiè Gān Tāng (龙胆泻肝汤, "Gentian Liver-Draining Decoction"), from *Secrets from the Orchid Chamber* (*Lán Shì Mì Cáng*, 兰室秘藏)

Ingredients: *Lóng dǎn cǎo* (龙胆草, *Radix et Rhizoma Gentianae*), *zé xiè* (泽泻, *Rhizoma Alismatis*), *mù tōng* (木通, *Caulis Akebiae*), *chē qián zǐ* (车前子, *Semen Plantaginis*), *dāng guī* (当归, *Radix Angelicae Sinensis*), *chái hú* (柴胡, *Radix Bupleuri*) and *shēng dì* (生地, *Radix Rehmanniae*) [plus *zhī zǐ* (栀子, *Fructus Gardeniae*) and *huáng qín* (黄芩, *Radix Scutellariae*)]

Má Huáng Fù Zǐ Xì Xīn Tāng (麻黄附子细辛汤, "Ephedra, Aconite and Asarum Decoction"), from the *Treatise on Cold Damage* (*Shāng Hán Lùn*, 伤寒论)

Ingredients: *Má huáng* (麻黄, *Herba Ephedrae*), *fù zǐ* (附子, *Radix Aconiti Lateralis Praeparata*) and *xì xīn* (细辛, *Radix et Rhizoma Asari*)

Má Xìng Shí Gān Tāng (麻杏石甘汤, "Ephedra, Apricot Kernel, Gypsum and Licorice Decoction"), from the *Treatise on Cold Damage* (*Shāng Hán Lùn*, 伤寒论)

Ingredients: *Má huáng* (麻黄, *Herba Ephedrae*), *xìng rén* (杏仁, *Semen Armeniacae Amarum*), *shí gāo* (石膏, *Gypsum Fibrosum*) and *zhì gān cǎo* (炙甘草, *Radix et Rhizoma Glycyrrhizae Praeparata cum Melle*)

Mù Xiāng Bīng Láng Wán (木香槟榔丸, "*Costus Root and Areca Pill*"), from the *Teachings of [Zhu] Dan-xi* (*Dān Xī Xīn Fǎ*, 丹溪心法)

Ingredients: *Mù xiāng* (木香, *Radix Aucklandiae*), *bīng láng* (槟榔, *Semen Arecae*), *qīng pí* (青皮, *Pericarpium Citri Reticulatae Viride*), *chén pí* (陈皮, *Pericarpium Citri Reticulatae*), *é zhú* (莪术, *Rhizoma Curcumae*), *zhǐ qiào* (枳壳, *Fructus Aurantii*), *huáng lián* (黄连, *Rhizoma Coptidis*), *huáng bǎi* (黄柏, *Cortex Phellodendri Chinensis*), *dà huáng* (大黄, *Radix et Rhizoma Rhei*), *xiāng fù* (香附, *Rhizoma Cyperi*) and *qiān niú zǐ* (牵牛子, *Semen Pharbitidis*)

Píng Wèi Sǎn (平胃散, "Stomach-Calming Powder"), from *Beneficial Formulas from the Taiping Imperial Pharmacy* (*Tài Píng Huì Mín Hé Jì Jú Fāng*, 太平惠民和剂局方)

Ingredients: *Cāng zhú* (苍术, *Rhizoma Atractylodis*), *hòu pò* (厚朴, *Cortex Magnoliae Officinalis*), *jú pí* (橘皮, *Pericarpium Citri Reticulatae*), *gān cǎo* (甘草, *Radix et Rhizoma Glycyrrhizae*), *shēng jiāng* (生姜, *Rhizoma Zingiberis Recens*) and *dà zǎo* (大枣, *Fructus Jujubae*)

Qī Bǎo Měi Rán Dān (七宝美髯丹, "Seven Treasures Beard-Blackening Elixir"), from *Medical Formulas Collected and Analyzed* (*Yī Fāng Jí Jiě*, 医方集解)

Ingredients: *Hé shŏu wū* (何首乌, *Radix Polygoni Multiflori*), *fú líng* (茯苓, *Poria*), *niú xī* (牛膝, *Radix Achyranthis Bidentatae*), *dāng guī* (当归, *Radix Angelicae Sinensis*), *gŏu qĭ zĭ* (枸杞子, *Fructus Lycii*), *tù sī zĭ* (菟丝子, *Semen Cuscutae*) and *bŭ gŭ zhī* (补骨脂, *Fructus Psoraleae*)

Qĭ Jú Dì Huáng Wán (杞菊地黄丸, "Lycium Berry, Chrysanthemum and Rehmannia Pill"), from *The Key to Diagnosis and Treatment of Children's Diseases* (*Xiăo Ér Yào Zhèng Zhí Jué*, 小儿药证直诀)

Ingredients: *Gŏu qĭ zĭ* (枸杞子, *Fructus Lycii*), *jú huā* (菊花, *Flos Chrysanthemi*), *shú dì huáng* (熟地黄, *Radix Rehmanniae Praeparata*), *shān zhū yú* (山茱萸, *Fructus Corni*), *shān yào* (山药, *Rhizoma Dioscoreae*), *zé xiè* (泽泻, *Rhizoma Alismatis*), *mŭ dān pí* (牡丹皮, *Cortex Moutan*) and *fú líng* (茯苓, *Poria*)

Qī Wèi Bái Zhú Sàn (七味白术散, "Seven-Ingredient *Atractylodis Macrocephalae Powder*"), from *The Key to Diagnosis and Treatment of Children's Diseases* (*Xiăo Ér Yào Zhèng Zhí Jué*, 小儿药证直诀)

Ingredients: *Rén shēn* (人参, *Radix et Rhizoma Ginseng*), *fú líng* (茯苓, *Poria*), *bái zhú* (白术, *Rhizoma Atractylodis Macrocephalae*), *gān căo* (甘草, *Radix et Rhizoma Glycyrrhizae*), *huò xiāng yè* (藿香叶, *Folium Agastachis*), *mù xiāng* (木香, *Radix Aucklandiae*) and *gé gēn* (葛根, *Radix Puerariae Lobatae*)

Qī Wèi Dū Qì Wán (七味都气丸, "Seven-Ingredient *Qi*-Restraining Pill"), from *Modified Readings from the Medical Ancestors* (*Yī Zōng Jĭ Rèn Piān*, 医宗己任篇)

Ingredients: *Dì huáng* (地黄, *Radix Rehmanniae*), *shān zhū yú* (山茱萸, *Fructus Corni*), *shān yào* (山药, *Rhizoma Dioscoreae*), *fú líng* (茯苓, *Poria*), *mŭ dān pí* (牡丹皮, *Cortex Moutan*), *zé xiè* (泽泻, *Rhizoma Alismatis*) and *wŭ wèi zĭ* (五味子, *Fructus Schisandrae Chinensis*)

Qiàn Gēn Sàn (茜根散, "Rubiae Powder"), from the *Complete Works of [Zhang] Jing-yue* (*Jĭng Yuè Quán Shū*, 景岳全书)

Ingredients: *Qiàn căo gēn* (茜草根, *Radix et Rhizoma Rubiae*), *huáng qín* (黄芩, *Radix Scutellariae*), *ē jiāo* (阿胶, *Colla Corii Asini*), *cè băi yè* (侧柏叶, *Cacumen Platycladi*), *shēng dì* (生地, *Radix Rehmanniae*) and *gān căo* (甘草, *Radix et Rhizoma Glycyrrhizae*)

Qiān Jīn Wĕi Jìng Tāng (千金苇茎汤, "Valuable Phragmites Stem Decoction"), from *Important Formulas Worth a Thousand Gold Pieces for Emergency* (*Bèi Jí Qiān Jīn Yào Fāng*, 备急千金要方)

Ingredients: *Lú gēn* (芦根, *Rhizoma Phragmitis*), *yì yǐ rén* (薏苡仁, *Semen Coicis*), *dōng guā zǐ* (冬瓜子, *Semen Benincasae*) and *táo rén* (桃仁, *Semen Persicae*)

Qín Jiāo Biē Jiǎ Sǎn (秦艽鳖甲散, "*Gentianae Macrophyllae* Turtle Shell Powder"), from *The Precious Mirror of Health* (*Wèi Shēng Bǎo Jiàn*, 卫生宝鉴)

Ingredients: *Dì gǔ pí* (地骨皮, *Cortex Lycii*), *chái hú* (柴胡, *Radix Bupleuri*), *qín jiāo* (秦艽, *Radix Gentianae Macrophyllae*), *zhī mǔ* (知母, *Rhizoma Anemarrhenae*), *dāng guī* (当归, *Radix Angelicae Sinensis*), *biē jiǎ* (鳖甲, *Carapax Trionycis*), *qīng hāo* (青蒿, *Herba Artemisiae Annuae*) and *wū méi* (乌梅, *Fructus Mume*)

Qīng Fèi Huà Tán Tāng (清肺化痰汤, "Lung-Clearing and Phlegm-Resolving Decoction"), from *General Formulas* (*Tǒng Zhǐ Fāng*, 统旨方)

Ingredients: *Huáng qín* (黄芩, *Radix Scutellariae*), *shān zhī* (山栀, *Fructus Gardeniae*), *jié gěng* (桔梗, *Radix Platycodonis*), *mài dōng* (麦冬, *Radix Ophiopogonis*), *sāng yè* (桑叶, *Folium Mori*), *bèi mǔ* (贝母, *Bulbus Fritillaria*), *zhī mǔ* (知母, *Rhizoma Anemarrhenae*), *guā lóu rén* (瓜蒌仁, *Semen Trichosanthis*), *jú hóng* (橘红, *Exocarpium Citri Rubrum*), *fú líng* (茯苓, *Poria*) and *gān cǎo* (甘草, *Radix et Rhizoma Glycyrrhizae*)

Qīng Gōng Tāng (清宫汤, "Heart-Clearing Decoction"), from *Systematic Differentiation of Warm Diseases* (*Wēn Bìng Tiáo Biàn*, 温病条辨)

Ingredients: *Xuán shēn* (玄参, *Radix Scrophulariae*), *lián zǐ xīn* (莲子心, *Plumula Nelumbinis*), *zhú yè xīn* (竹叶心, *Folium Pleioblasti*), *lián qiào* (连翘, *Fructus Forsythiae*), *xī jiǎo* (犀角, *Cornu Rhinocerotis*) and *mài dōng* (麦冬, *Radix Ophiopogonis*)

Qīng Gǔ Sǎn (清骨散, "Bone-Clearing Powder"), from *Standards for Diagnosis and Treatment* (*Zhèng Zhì Zhǔn Shéng*, 证治准绳)

Ingredients: *Yín chái hú* (银柴胡, *Radix Stellariae*), *hú huáng lián* (胡黄连, *Rhizoma Picrorhizae*), *qín jiāo* (秦艽, *Radix Gentianae Macrophyllae*), *biē jiǎ* (鳖甲, *Carapax Trionycis*), *dì gǔ pí* (地骨皮, *Cortex Lycii*), *qīng hāo* (青蒿, *Herba Artemisiae Annuae*), *zhī mǔ* (知母, *Rhizoma Anemarrhenae*) and *gān cǎo* (甘草, *Radix et Rhizoma Glycyrrhizae*)

Qīng Zhōng Tāng (清中汤, "Center-Clearing Decoction"), from *Categorized Patterns with Clear-Cut Treatments* (*Lèi Zhèng Zhì Cái*, 类证治裁)

Ingredients: *Huáng lián* (黄连, *Rhizoma Coptidis*), *shān zhī* (山栀, *Fructus Gardeniae*), *chén pí* (陈皮, *Pericarpium Citri Reticulatae*), *fú líng* (茯苓, *Poria*), *bàn xià* (半夏, *Rhizoma Pinelliae*), *gān cǎo* (甘草, *Radix et Rhizoma*

Glycyrrhizae), *cǎo dòu kòu* (草豆蔻, *Semen Alpiniae Katsumadai*) and *shēng jiāng* (生姜, *Rhizoma Zingiberis Recens*)

Sān Ào Tāng (三拗汤, "Rough and Ready Three Decoction"), from *Beneficial Formulas from the Taiping Imperial Pharmacy* (*Tài Píng Huì Mín Hé Jì Jú Fāng*, 太平惠民和剂局方)

Ingredients: *Má huáng* (麻黄, *Herba Ephedrae*), *xìng rén* (杏仁, *Semen Armeniacae Amarum*) and *gān cǎo* (甘草, *Radix et Rhizoma Glycyrrhizae*)

Sāng Jú Yǐn (桑菊饮, "Mulberry Leaf and Chrysanthemum Beverage"), from *Systematic Differentiation of Warm Diseases* (*Wēn Bìng Tiáo Biàn*, 温病条辨)

Ingredients: *Sāng yè* (桑叶, *Folium Mori*), *jú huā* (菊花, *Flos Chrysanthemi*), *lián qiào* (连翘, *Fructus Forsythiae*), *bò hé* (薄荷, *Herba Menthae*), *jié gěng* (桔梗, *Radix Platycodonis*), *xìng rén* (杏仁, *Semen Armeniacae Amarum*), *lú gēn* (芦根, *Rhizoma Phragmitis*) and *gān cǎo* (甘草, *Radix et Rhizoma Glycyrrhizae*)

Shā Shēn Mài Mén Dōng Tāng (沙参麦门冬汤, "*Adenophorae seu Glehniae* and *Ophiopogon* Decoction") from *Systematic Differentiation of Warm Diseases* (*Wēn Bìng Tiáo Biàn*, 温病条辨)

Ingredients: *Shā shēn* (沙参, *Radix Adenophorae seu Glehniae*), *mài dōng* (麦冬, *Radix Ophiopogonis*), *yù zhú* (玉竹, *Rhizoma Polygonati Odorati*), *sāng yè* (桑叶, *Folium Mori*), *gān cǎo* (甘草, *Radix et Rhizoma Glycyrrhizae*), *tiān huā fěn* (天花粉, *Radix Trichosanthis*) and *bái biǎn dòu* (白扁豆, *Semen Lablab Album*)

Shào Fǔ Zhú Yū Tāng (少腹逐瘀汤, "Lower Abdominal Stasis–Expelling Decoction"), from *Correction of Errors in Medical Works* (*Yī Lín Gǎi Cuò*, 医林改错)

Ingredients: *Xiǎo huí xiāng* (小茴香, *Fructus Foeniculi*), *gān jiāng* (干姜, *Rhizoma Zingiberis*), *yán hú suǒ* (延胡索, *Rhizoma Corydalis*), *mò yào* (没药, *Myrrha*), *dāng guī* (当归, *Radix Angelicae Sinensis*), *chuān xiōng* (川芎, *Rhizoma Chuanxiong*), *ròu guì* (肉桂, *Cortex Cinnamomi*), *chì sháo* (赤芍, *Radix Paeoniae Rubra*), *pú huáng* (蒲黄, *Pollen Typhae*) and *wǔ líng zhī* (五灵脂, *Faeces Trogopterori*)

Sháo Yào Tāng (芍药汤, "Peony Decoction"), from the *Collection of Writings on the Mechanism of Disease, Suitability of* Qi, *and the Safeguarding of Life as Discussed in the "Basic Questions"* (*Sù Wèn Bìng Jī Qì Yí Bǎo Mìng Jí*, 素问病机气宜保命集)

Ingredients: *Huáng qín* (黄芩, *Radix Scutellariae*), *sháo yào* (芍药, *Radix Paeoniae*), *zhì gān cǎo* (炙甘草, *Radix et Rhizoma Glycyrrhizae Praeparata cum Melle*), *huáng lián* (黄连, *Rhizoma Coptidis*), *dà huáng* (大黄, *Radix et Rhizoma Rhei*), *bīng láng* (槟榔, *Semen Arecae*), *dāng guī* (当归, *Radix Angelicae Sinensis*), *mù xiāng* (木香, *Radix Aucklandiae*) and *ròu guì* (肉桂, *Cortex Cinnamomi*)

Shè Gān Má Huáng Tāng (射干麻黄汤, "Belamcanda and Ephedra Decoction"), from *Essentials from the Golden Cabinet* (*Jīn Guì Yào Lüè*, 金匮要略)

Ingredients: *Shè gān* (射干, *Rhizoma Belamcandae*), *má huáng* (麻黄, *Herba Ephedrae*), *xì xīn* (细辛, *Radix et Rhizoma Asari*), *zǐ wǎn* (紫菀, *Radix et Rhizoma Asteris*), *kuǎn dōng huā* (款冬花, *Flos Farfarae*), *bàn xià* (半夏, *Rhizoma Pinelliae*), *wǔ wèi zǐ* (五味子, *Fructus Schisandrae Chinensis*), *shēng jiāng* (生姜, *Rhizoma Zingiberis Recens*) and *dà zǎo* (大枣, *Fructus Jujubae*)

Shēn Fù Lóng Mǔ Tāng (参附龙牡汤, "Ginseng, Aconite, *Os Draconis* and *Concha Ostreae* Decoction"), from *Effective Formulas from Generations of Physicians* (*Shì Yī Dé Xiào Fāng*, 世医得效方)

Ingredients: *Rén shēn* (人参, *Radix et Rhizoma Ginseng*), *fù zǐ* (附子, *Radix Aconiti Lateralis*), *lóng gǔ* (龙骨, *Os Draconis*) and *mǔ lì* (牡蛎, *Concha Ostreae*)

Shēn Fù Tāng (参附汤, "Ginseng and Aconite Decoction"), from *Effective Formulas from Generations of Physicians* (*Shì Yī Dé Xiào Fāng*, 世医得效方)

Ingredients: *Rén shēn* (人参, *Radix et Rhizoma Ginseng*) and *fù zǐ* (附子, *Radix Aconiti Lateralis*)

Shēn Líng Bái Zhú Sǎn (参苓白术散, "Ginseng, Poria and *Atractylodes Macrocephalae* Powder"), from *Beneficial Formulas from the Taiping Imperial Pharmacy* (*Tài Píng Huì Mín Hé Jì Jú Fāng*, 太平惠民和剂局方)

Ingredients: *Rén shēn* (人参, *Radix et Rhizoma Ginseng*), *fú líng* (茯苓, *Poria*), *bái zhú* (白术, *Rhizoma Atractylodis Macrocephalae*), *jié gěng* (桔梗, *Radix Platycodonis*), *shān yào* (山药, *Rhizoma Dioscoreae*), *gān cǎo* (甘草, *Radix et Rhizoma Glycyrrhizae*), *bái biǎn dòu* (白扁豆, *Semen Lablab Album*), *lián zǐ xīn* (莲子心, *Plumula Nelumbinis*), *shā rén* (砂仁, *Fructus Amomi*) and *yì yǐ rén* (薏苡仁, *Semen Coicis*)

Shēn Tòng Zhú Yū Tāng (身痛逐瘀汤, "Generalized Pain Stasis–Expelling Decoction"), from *Correction of Errors in Medical Works* (*Yī Lín Gǎi Cuò*, 医林改错)

Ingredients: *Qín jiāo* (秦艽, *Radix Gentianae Macrophyllae*), *chuān xiōng* (川芎, *Rhizoma Chuanxiong*), *táo rén* (桃仁, *Semen Persicae*), *hóng huā* (红花, *Flos Carthami*), *gān cǎo* (甘草, *Radix et Rhizoma Glycyrrhizae*), *qiāng huó* (羌活, *Rhizoma et Radix Notopterygii*), *mò yào* (没药, *Myrrha*), *xiāng fù* (香附, *Rhizoma Cyperi*), *wǔ líng zhī* (五灵脂, *Faeces Trogopterori*), *niú xī* (牛膝, *Radix Achyranthis Bidentatae*), *dì lóng* (地龙, *Pheretima*) and *dāng guī* (当归, *Radix Angelicae Sinensis*)

Shēng Mài Sǎn (生脉散, "Pulse-Engendering Powder"), from *Important Formulas Worth a Thousand Gold Pieces for Emergency* (*Bèi Jí Qiān Jīn Yào Fāng*, 备急千金要方)

Ingredients: *Rén shēn* (人参, *Radix et Rhizoma Ginseng*), *mài dōng* (麦冬, *Radix Ophiopogonis*) and *wǔ wèi zǐ* (五味子, *Fructus Schisandrae Chinensis*)

Shí Wěi Sàn (石苇散, "Pyrrosiae Powder"), from *Supplementary to Diagnosis and Treatment* (*Zhèng Zhì Huì Bǔ*, 证治汇补)

Ingredients: *Shí wéi* (石韦, *Folium Pyrrosiae*), *dōng kuí zǐ* (冬葵子, *Fructus Malvae*), *qú mài* (瞿麦, *Herba Dianthi*), *huá shí* (滑石, *Talcum*) and *chē qián zǐ* (车前子, *Semen Plantaginis*)

Shī Xiào Sǎn (失笑散, "Sudden Smile Powder"), from *Beneficial Formulas from the Taiping Imperial Pharmacy* (*Tài Píng Huì Mín Hé Jì Jú Fāng*, 太平惠民和剂局方)

Ingredients: *Wǔ líng zhī* (五灵脂, *Faeces Trogopterori*) and *pú huáng* (蒲黄, *Pollen Typhae*)

Shùn Qì Hé Zhōng Tāng (顺气和中汤, "Qi-Balancing and Middle Jiao–Harmonizing Decoction"), from *The Precious Mirror of Health* (*Wèi Shēng Bǎo Jiàn*, 卫生宝鉴)

Ingredients: *Huáng qí* (黄芪, *Radix Astragali*), *rén shēn* (人参, *Radix et Rhizoma Ginseng*), *gān cǎo* (甘草, *Radix et Rhizoma Glycyrrhizae*), *bái zhú* (白术, *Rhizoma Atractylodis Macrocephalae*), *chén pí* (陈皮, *Pericarpium Citri Reticulatae*), *dāng guī* (当归, *Radix Angelicae Sinensis*), *bái sháo* (白芍, *Radix Paeoniae Alba*), *shēng má* (升麻, *Rhizoma Cimicifugae*), *chái hú* (柴胡, *Radix Bupleuri*), *xì xīn* (细辛, *Radix et Rhizoma Asari*), *chuān xiōng* (川芎, *Rhizoma Chuanxiong*) and *màn jīng zǐ* (蔓荆子, *Fructus Viticis*)

Sì Hǎi Shū Yù Tāng (四海疏郁汤, "Four Seas Stagnation-Relieving Decoction"), from the *Great Collections of Sores* (*Yáng Yī Zhèng Zhì Dà Quán*, 疡医大全)

Ingredients: *Hǎi gé qiào* (海蛤壳, *Concha Meretricis seu Cyclinae*), *hǎi dài cǎo* (海带草, *Herba Zosterae Marinae*), *hǎi zǎo* (海藻, *Sargassum*), *hǎi piāo xiāo* (海螵蛸, *Endoconcha Sepiae*), *kūn bù* (昆布, *Thallus Laminariae*), *chén pí* (陈皮, *Pericarpium Citri Reticulatae*) and *qīng mù xiāng* (青木香, *Radix Aristolochiae*)

Sì Jūn Zǐ Tāng (四君子汤, "Four Gentlemen Decoction"), from *Beneficial Formulas from the Taiping Imperial Pharmacy* (*Tài Píng Huì Mín Hé Jì Jú Fāng*, 太平惠民和剂局方)

Ingredients: *Dǎng shēn* (党参, *Radix Codonopsis*), *bái zhú* (白术, *Rhizoma Atractylodis Macrocephalae*), *fú líng* (茯苓, *Poria*) and *gān cǎo* (甘草, *Radix et Rhizoma Glycyrrhizae*)

Sì Miào Wán (四妙丸, "Wonderfully Effective Four Pill"), from *Convenient Reader on Established Formulas* (*Chéng Fāng Biàn Dú*, 成方便读)

Ingredients: *Huáng bǎi* (黄柏, *Cortex Phellodendri Chinensis*), *cāng zhú* (苍术, *Rhizoma Atractylodis*), *yì yǐ rén* (薏苡仁, *Semen Coicis*) and *niú xī* (牛膝, *Radix Achyranthis Bidentatae*

Sì Nì Sǎn (四逆散, "Frigid Extremities Powder"), from *Treatise on Cold Damage* (*Shāng Hán Lùn*, 伤寒论)

Ingredients: *Chái hú* (柴胡, *Radix Bupleuri*), *gān cǎo* (甘草, *Radix et Rhizoma Glycyrrhizae*), *zhǐ shí* (枳实, *Fructus Aurantii Immaturus*) and *sháo yào* (芍药, *Radix Paeoniae*)

Sì Shén Wán (四神丸, "Four Spirits Pill"), from *Extracts of Internal Medicine* (*Nèi Kē Zhāi Yào*, 内科摘要)

Ingredients: *Bǔ gǔ zhī* (补骨脂, *Fructus Psoraleae*), *ròu dòu kòu* (肉豆蔻, *Semen Myristicae*), *wú zhū yú* (吴茱萸, *Fructus Evodiae*), *wǔ wèi zǐ* (五味子, *Fructus Schisandrae Chinensis*), *shēng jiāng* (生姜, *Rhizoma Zingiberis Recens*) and *dà zǎo* (大枣, *Fructus Jujubae*)

Sì Wù Tāng (四物汤, "Four-Substance Decoction"), from *Beneficial Formulas from the Taiping Imperial Pharmacy* (*Tài Píng Huì Mín Hé Jì Jú Fāng*, 太平惠民和剂局方)

Ingredients: *Dāng guī* (当归, *Radix Angelicae Sinensis*), *bái sháo* (白芍, *Radix Paeoniae Alba*), *chuān xiōng* (川芎, *Rhizoma Chuanxiong*) and *shú dì huáng* (熟地黄, *Radix Rehmanniae Praeparata*)

Táo Hóng Sì Wù Tāng (桃红四物汤, "Peach Kernel and Carthamus Four-Substance Decoction"), from *The Golden Mirror of the Medical Tradition* (*Yī Zōng Jīn Jiàn*, 医宗金鉴)

Ingredients: *Shú dì huáng* (熟地黄, *Radix Rehmanniae Praeparata*), *chuān xiōng* (川芎, *Rhizoma Chuanxiong*), *bái sháo* (白芍, *Radix Paeoniae Alba*), *dāng guī* (当归, *Radix Angelicae Sinensis*), *táo rén* (桃仁, *Semen Persicae*) and *hóng huā* (红花, *Flos Carthami*)

Tiān Má Gōu Téng Yǐn (天麻钩藤饮, "Gastrodia and Uncaria Beverage"), from *New Explanations for the Diagnosis and Treatment of Miscellaneous Diseases* (*Zá Bìng Zhèng Zhì Xīn Yì*, 杂病证治新义)

Ingredients: *Tiān má* (天麻, *Rhizoma Gastrodiae*), *gōu téng* (钩藤, *Ramulus Uncariae Cum Uncis*), *shí jué míng* (石决明, *Concha Haliotidis*), *niú xī* (牛膝, *Radix Achyranthis Bidentatae*), *sāng jì shēng* (桑寄生, *Herba Taxilli*), *dù zhòng* (杜仲, *Cortex Eucommiae*), *shān zhī* (山栀, *Fructus Gardeniae*), *huáng qín* (黄芩, *Radix Scutellariae*), *yì mǔ cǎo* (益母草, *Herba Leonuri*), *fú shén* (茯神, *Sclerotium Poriae Pararadicis*) and *yè jiāo téng* (夜交藤, *Caulis Polygoni Multiflori*)

Tōng Qiào Huó Xuè Tāng (通窍活血汤, "Orifice-Unblocking and Blood-Invigorating Decoction"), from *Correction of Errors in Medical Works* (*Yī Lín Gǎi Cuò*, 医林改错)

Ingredients: *Chì sháo* (赤芍, *Radix Paeoniae Rubra*), *chuān xiōng* (川芎, *Rhizoma Chuanxiong*), *táo rén* (桃仁, *Semen Persicae*), *hóng huā* (红花, *Flos Carthami*), *shè xiāng* (麝香, *Moschus*), *shēng jiāng* (生姜, *Rhizoma Zingiberis Recens*), *dà zǎo* (大枣, *Fructus Jujubae*) and *cōng bái* (葱白, *Bulbus Allii Fistulosi*)

Tòng Xiè Yào Fāng (痛泻药方, "Important Formula for Painful Diarrhea"), from *The Complete Works of [Zhang] Jing-yue* (*Jǐng Yuè Quán Shū*, 景岳全书)

Ingredients: *Bái zhú* (白术, *Rhizoma Atractylodis Macrocephalae*), *bái sháo* (白芍, *Radix Paeoniae Alba*), *fáng fēng* (防风, *Radix Saposhnikoviae*) and *chén pí* (陈皮, *Pericarpium Citri Reticulatae*)

Tòu Nóng Sǎn (透脓散, "Pus-Expelling Powder"), from *The Orthodox Lineage of External Medicine* (*Wài Kē Zhèng Zōng*, 外科正宗)

Ingredients: *Huáng qí* (黄芪, *Radix Astragali*), *dāng guī* (当归, *Radix Angelicae Sinensis*), *chuān shān jiǎ* (穿山甲, *Squama Manitis*), *zào jiǎo cì* (皂角刺, *Spina Gleditsiae*) and *chuān xiōng* (川芎, *Rhizoma Chuanxiong*)

Wèi Líng Tāng (胃苓汤, "Stomach-Calming Poria Decoction"), from *Teachings of [Zhu] Dan-xi* (*Dān Xī Xīn Fǎ*, 丹溪心法)

Ingredients: *Cāng zhú* (苍术, *Rhizoma Atractylodis*), *hòu pò* (厚朴, *Cortex Magnoliae Officinalis*), *chén pí* (陈皮, *Pericarpium Citri Reticulatae*), *gān cǎo* (甘草, *Radix et Rhizoma Glycyrrhizae*), *shēng jiāng* (生姜, *Rhizoma Zingiberis Recens*), *dà zǎo* (大枣, *Fructus Jujubae*), *guì zhī* (桂枝, *Ramulus*

Cinnamomi), *bái zhú* (白术, *Rhizoma Atractylodis Macrocephalae*), *zé xiè* (泽泻, *Rhizoma Alismatis*), *fú líng* (茯苓, *Poria*) and *zhū líng* (猪苓, *Polyporus*)

Wēn Dǎn Tāng (温胆汤, "Gallbladder-Warming Decoction"), from *Important Formulas Worth a Thousand Gold Pieces for Emergency* (*Bèi Jí Qiān Jīn Yào Fāng*, 备急千金要方)

Ingredients: *Bàn xià* (半夏, *Rhizoma Pinelliae*), *jú pí* (橘皮, *Pericarpium Citri Reticulatae*), *gān cǎo* (甘草, *Radix et Rhizoma Glycyrrhizae*), *zhǐ shí* (枳实, *Fructus Aurantii Immaturus*), *zhú rú* (竹茹, *Caulis Bambusae in Taenia*), *shēng jiāng* (生姜, *Rhizoma Zingiberis Recens*) and *fú líng* (茯苓, *Poria*)

Wēn Pí Tāng (温脾汤, "Spleen-Warming Decoction"), from *Important Formulas Worth a Thousand Gold Pieces for Emergency* (*Bèi Jí Qiān Jīn Yào Fāng*, 备急千金要方)

Ingredients: *Fù zǐ* (附子, *Radix Aconiti Lateralis Praeparata*), *rén shēn* (人参, *Radix et Rhizoma Ginseng*), *dà huáng* (大黄, *Radix et Rhizoma Rhei*), *gān jiāng* (干姜, *Rhizoma Zingiberis*) and *gān cǎo* (甘草, *Radix et Rhizoma Glycyrrhizae*)

Wú Bǐ Shān Yào Wán (无比山药丸, "Incomparable Dioscoreae Pill"), from *Important Formulas Worth a Thousand Gold Pieces for Emergency* (*Bèi Jí Qiān Jīn Yào Fāng*, 备急千金要方)

Ingredients: *Shan yào* (山药, *Rhizoma Dioscoreae*), *ròu cōng róng* (肉苁蓉, *Herba Cistanches*), *shú dì huáng* (熟地黄, *Radix Rehmanniae Praeparata*), *shān zhū yú* (山茱萸, *Fructus Corni*), *fú shén* (茯神, *Sclerotium Poriae Pararadicis*), *tù sī zǐ* (菟丝子, *Semen Cuscutae*), *wǔ wèi zǐ* (五味子, *Fructus Schisandrae Chinensis*), *chì shí zhī* (赤石脂, *Halloysitum Rubrum*), *bā jǐ tiān* (巴戟天, *Radix Morindae Officinalis*), *zé xiè* (泽泻, *Rhizoma Alismatis*), *dù zhòng* (杜仲, *Cortex Eucommiae*) and *niú xī* (牛膝, *Radix Achyranthis Bidentatae*)

Wǔ Líng Sǎn (五苓散, "Five-Substance Powder with Poria"), from the *Treatise on Cold Damage* (*Shāng Hán Lùn*, 伤寒论)

Ingredients: *Bái zhú* (白术, *Rhizoma Atractylodis Macrocephalae*), *fú líng* (茯苓, *Poria*), *zhū líng* (猪苓, *Polyporus*), *zé xiè* (泽泻, *Rhizoma Alismatis*) and *guì zhī* (桂枝, *Ramulus Cinnamomi*)

Wǔ Wèi Xiāo Dú Yǐn (五味消毒饮, "Five-Ingredient Toxin-Removing Beverage"), from *The Golden Mirror of the Medical Tradition* (*Yī Zōng Jīn Jiàn*, 医宗金鉴)

Ingredients: *Jīn yín huā* (金银花, *Flos Lonicerae Japonicae*), *yě jú huā* (野菊花, *Flos Chrysanthemi Indici*), *pú gōng yīng* (蒲公英, *Herba Taraxaci*), *zǐ huā dì dīng* (紫花地丁, *Herba Violae*) and *zǐ bèi tiān kuí* (紫背天葵, *Herba Semiaquilegiae*)

Xī Jiǎo Dì Huáng Tāng (犀角地黄汤, "Rhinoceros Horn and Rehmannia Decoction"), from *Important Formulas Worth a Thousand Gold Pieces for Emergency* (*Bèi Jí Qiān Jīn Yào Fāng*, 备急千金要方)

Ingredients: *Xī jiǎo* (犀角, *Cornu Rhinocerotis*), *shēng dì* (生地, *Radix Rehmanniae*), *mǔ dān pí* (牡丹皮, *Cortex Moutan*) and *chì sháo* (赤芍, *Radix Paeoniae Rubra*)

Xī Jiǎo Sǎn (犀角散, "Rhinoceros Horn Powder"), from *Important Formulas Worth a Thousand Gold Pieces for Emergency* (*Bèi Jí Qiān Jīn Yào Fāng*, 备急千金要方)

Ingredients: *Xī jiǎo* (犀角, *Cornu Rhinocerotis*), *huáng lián* (黄连, *Rhizoma Coptidis*), *shēng má* (升麻, *Rhizoma Cimicifugae*), *shān zhī* (山栀, *Fructus Gardeniae*) and *yīn chén* (茵陈, *Herba Artemisiae Scopariae*)

Xiāng Shā Liù Jūn Zǐ Tāng (香砂六君子汤, "Costus Root and Amomum Six Gentlemen Decoction"), from *Medical Formulas Collected and Analyzed* (*Yī Fāng Jí Jiě*, 医方集解)

Ingredients: *Rén shēn* (人参, *Radix et Rhizoma Ginseng*), *bái zhú* (白术, *Rhizoma Atractylodis Macrocephalae*), *fú líng* (茯苓, *Poria*), *gān cǎo* (甘草, *Radix et Rhizoma Glycyrrhizae*), *bàn xià* (半夏, *Rhizoma Pinelliae*), *chén pí* (陈皮, *Pericarpium Citri Reticulatae*), *mù xiāng* (木香, *Radix Aucklandiae*) and *shā rén* (砂仁, *Fructus Amomi*)

Xiāo Kě Fāng (消渴方, "Diabetes-Relieving Formula"), from the *Teachings of [Zhu] Dan-xi* (*Dān Xī Xīn Fǎ*, 丹溪心法)

Ingredients: *Huáng lián mò* (黄连末, "Powder of *Rhizoma Coptidis*"), *tiān huā fěn mò* (天花粉末, "Powder of *Radix Trichosanthis*"), *shēng dì zhī* (生地汁, *Succus Rehmanniae*), *ǒu zhī* (藕汁, *Succus Nelumbinis Rhizomatis*), *rǔ zhī* (乳汁, milk), *shēng jiāng zhī* (生姜汁, *Succus Rhizomatis Zingiberis*) and *fēng mì* (蜂蜜, *Mel*)

Xiǎo Qīng Lóng Tāng (小青龙汤, "Minor Green Dragon Decoction"), from the *Treatise on Cold Damage* (*Shāng Hán Lùn*, 伤寒论)

Ingredients: *Má huáng* (麻黄, *Herba Ephedrae*), *guì zhī* (桂枝, *Ramulus Cinnamomi*), *xì xīn* (细辛, *Radix et Rhizoma Asari*), *gān jiāng* (干姜, *Rhizoma Zingiberis*), *bàn xià* (半夏, *Rhizoma Pinelliae*), *wǔ wèi zǐ* (五味子,

Fructus Schisandrae Chinensis), *bái sháo* (白芍, *Radix Paeoniae Alba*) and *gān cǎo* (甘草, *Radix et Rhizoma Glycyrrhizae*)

Xiāo Yáo Sǎn (逍遥散, "Free Wanderer Powder"), from *Beneficial Formulas from the Taiping Imperial Pharmacy (Tài Píng Huì Mín Hé Jì Jú Fāng*, 太平惠民和剂局方)

Ingredients: *Chái hú* (柴胡, *Radix Bupleuri*), *bái zhú* (白术, *Rhizoma Atractylodis Macrocephalae*), *bái sháo* (白芍, *Radix Paeoniae Alba*), *dāng guī* (当归, *Radix Angelicae Sinensis*), *fú líng* (茯苓, *Poria*), *zhì gān cǎo* (炙甘草, *Radix et Rhizoma Glycyrrhizae Praeparata cum Melle*), *bò hé* (薄荷, *Herba Menthae*) and *wèi jiāng* (煨姜, *Rhizoma Zingiberis Rosc.*)

Xiè Bái Sàn (泻白散, "Mori Powder"), from *The Key to Diagnosis and Treatment of Children's Diseases (Xiǎo Ér Yào Zhèng Zhí Jué*, 小儿药证直诀)

Ingredients: *Sāng bái pí* (桑白皮, *Cortex Mori*), *dì gǔ pí* (地骨皮, *Cortex Lycii*), *gān cǎo* (甘草, *Radix et Rhizoma Glycyrrhizae*) and *jīng mǐ* (粳米, *Oryza Sativa L.*)

Xìng Sū Sǎn (杏苏散, "Apricot Kernel and Perilla Powder"), from *Systematic Differentiation of Warm Diseases (Wēn Bìng Tiáo Biàn*, 温病条辨)

Ingredients: *Xìng rén* (杏仁, *Semen Armeniacae Amarum*), *zǐ sū zǐ* (紫苏子, *Fructus Perillae*), *chén pí* (陈皮, *Pericarpium Citri Reticulatae*), *bàn xià* (半夏, *Rhizoma Pinelliae*), *shēng jiāng* (生姜, *Rhizoma Zingiberis Recens*), *jié gěng* (桔梗, *Radix Platycodonis*), *qián hú* (前胡, *Radix Peucedani*), *fú líng* (茯苓, *Poria*), *gān cǎo* (甘草, *Radix et Rhizoma Glycyrrhizae*) and *dà zǎo* (大枣, *Fructus Jujubae*)

Xuán Fù Dài Zhě Tāng (旋覆代赭汤, "Inula and Hematite Decoction"), from the *Treatise on Cold Damage (Shāng Hán Lùn*, 伤寒论)

Ingredients: *Xuán fù huā* (旋覆花, *Flos Inulae*), *dài zhě shí* (代赭石, *Haematitum*), *rén shēn* (人参, *Radix et Rhizoma Ginseng*), *bàn xià* (半夏, *Rhizoma Pinelliae*), *zhì gān cǎo* (炙甘草, *Radix et Rhizoma Glycyrrhizae Praeparata cum Melle*), *shēng jiāng* (生姜, *Rhizoma Zingiberis Recens*) and *dà zǎo* (大枣, *Fructus Jujubae*)

Xuè Fǔ Zhú Yū Tāng (血府逐瘀汤, "Blood Stasis–Expelling Decoction"), from *Correction of Errors in Medical Works (Yī Lín Gǎi Cuò*, 医林改错)

Ingredients: *Dāng guī* (当归, *Radix Angelicae Sinensis*), *shēng dì* (生地, *Radix Rehmanniae*), *táo rén* (桃仁, *Semen Persicae*), *hóng huā* (红花, *Flos Carthami*), *zhǐ qiào* (枳壳, *Fructus Aurantii*), *chì sháo* (赤芍, *Radix Paeoniae Rubra*), *chái hú* (柴胡, *Radix Bupleuri*), *gān cǎo* (甘草, *Radix et*

Rhizoma Glycyrrhizae), *jié gěng* (桔梗, *Radix Platycodonis*), *chuān xiōng* (川芎, *Rhizoma Chuanxiong*) and *niú xī* (牛膝, *Radix Achyranthis Bidentatae*)

Yī Guàn Jiān (一贯煎, "Effective Integration Decoction"), from *[Wei] Liu-zhou's Discourse on Medicine* (*Liǔ Zhōu Yī Huà*, 柳州医话)

Ingredients: *Běi shā shēn* (北沙参, *Radix Glehniae*), *mài dōng* (麦冬, *Radix Ophiopogonis*), *dāng guī* (当归, *Radix Angelicae Sinensis*), *shēng dì* (生地, *Radix Rehmanniae*), *gǒu qǐ zǐ* (枸杞子, *Fructus Lycii*) and *chuān liàn zǐ* (川楝子, *Fructus Toosendan*)

Yì Wèi Tāng (益胃汤, "Stomach-Benefiting Decoction"), from *Systematic Differentiation of Warm Diseases* (*Wēn Bìng Tiáo Biàn*, 温病条辨)

Ingredients: *Shā shēn* (沙参, *Radix Adenophorae seu Glehniae*), *mài dōng* (麦冬, *Radix Ophiopogonis*), *shēng dì* (生地, *Radix Rehmanniae*), *yù zhú* (玉竹, *Rhizoma Polygonati Odorati*) and *bīng táng* (冰糖, *Crystal Sugar*)

Yīn Chén Hāo Tāng (茵陈蒿汤, "Artemisiae Scopariae Decoction"), from *Treatise on Cold Damage* (*Shāng Hán Lùn*, 伤寒论)

Ingredients: *Yīn chén* (茵陈, *Herba Artemisiae Scopariae*), *zhī zǐ* (栀子, *Fructus Gardeniae*) and *dà huáng* (大黄, *Radix et Rhizoma Rhei*)

Yín Qiào Sǎn (银翘散, "Lonicera and Forsythia Powder"), from *Systematic Differentiation of Warm Diseases* (*Wēn Bìng Tiáo Biàn*, 温病条辨)

Ingredients: *Jīn yín huā* (金银花, *Flos Lonicerae Japonicae*), *lián qiào* (连翘, *Fructus Forsythiae*), *niú bàng zǐ* (牛蒡子, *Fructus Arctii*), *jié gěng* (桔梗, *Radix Platycodonis*), *bò hé* (薄荷, *Herba Menthae*), *zhú yè* (竹叶, *Folium Phyllostachydis Henonis*), *jīng jiè* (荆芥, *Herba Schizonepetae*), *dàn dòu chǐ* (淡豆豉, *Semen Sojae Praeparatum*), *gān cǎo* (甘草, *Radix et Rhizoma Glycyrrhizae*) and *lú gēn* (芦根, *Rhizoma Phragmitis*)

Yòu Guī Wán (右归丸, "Right-Restoring Pill"), from *Complete Works of [Zhang] Jing-yue* (*Jǐng Yuè Quán Shū*, 景岳全书)

Ingredients: *Shú dì huáng* (熟地黄, *Radix Rehmanniae Praeparata*), *shān yào* (山药, *Rhizoma Dioscoreae*), *shān zhū yú* (山茱萸, *Fructus Corni*), *gǒu qǐ zǐ* (枸杞子, *Fructus Lycii*), *dù zhòng* (杜仲, *Cortex Eucommiae*), *tù sī zǐ* (菟丝子, *Semen Cuscutae*), *zhì fù zǐ* (制附子, *Radix Aconiti Lateralis Praeparata*), *ròu guì* (肉桂, *Cortex Cinnamomi*), *dāng guī* (当归, *Radix Angelicae Sinensis*) and *lù jiǎo jiāo* (鹿角胶, *Colla Cornus Cervi*)

Yù Píng Fēng Sǎn (玉屏风散, "Jade Wind-Barrier Powder"), from *Effective Formulas from Generations of Physicians* (*Shì Yī Dé Xiào Fāng*, 世医得效方)

Ingredients: *Huáng qí* (黄芪, *Radix Astragali*), *bái zhú* (白术, *Rhizoma Atractylodis Macrocephalae*) and *fáng fēng* (防风, *Radix Saposhnikoviae*)

Yuè Bì Jiā Zhú Tāng (越婢加术汤, "Maidservant from Yue Decoction Plus Atractylodis Macrocephalae"), from *Essentials from the Golden Cabinet* (*Jīn Guì Yào Lüè*, 金匮要略)

Ingredients: *Má huáng* (麻黄, *Herba Ephedrae*), *shí gāo* (石膏, *Gypsum Fibrosum*), *gān cǎo* (甘草, *Radix et Rhizoma Glycyrrhizae*), *dà zǎo* (大枣, *Fructus Jujubae*), *bái zhú* (白术, *Rhizoma Atractylodis Macrocephalae*) and *shēng jiāng* (生姜, *Rhizoma Zingiberis Recens*)

Yuè Huá Wán (月华丸, "Lung Yin Nourishing Pill"), from *Medical Revelations* (*Yī Xué Xīn Wù*, 医学心悟)

Ingredients: *Tiān dōng* (天冬, *Radix Asparagi*), *mài dōng* (麦冬, *Radix Ophiopogonis*), *shēng dì* (生地, *Radix Rehmanniae*), *shú dì huáng* (熟地黄, *Radix Rehmanniae Praeparata*), *shān yào* (山药, *Rhizoma Dioscoreae*), *bǎi bù* (百部, *Radix Stemonae*), *shā shēn* (沙参, *Radix Adenophorae seu Glehniae*), *chuān bèi mǔ* (川贝母, *Bulbus Fritillariae Cirrhosae*), *fú líng* (茯苓, *Poria*), *ē jiāo* (阿胶, *Colla Corii Asini*), *sān qī* (三七, *Radix et Rhizoma Notoginseng*), *tǎ gān* (獭肝, *Jecur Lutrae*), *jú huā* (菊花, *Flos Chrysanthemi*) and *sāng yè* (桑叶, *Folium Mori*)

Zēng Yè Chéng Qì Tāng (增液承气汤, "Humor-Increasing Purgative Decoction"), from *Systematic Differentiation of Warm Diseases* (*Wēn Bìng Tiáo Biàn*, 温病条辨)

Ingredients: *Dà huáng* (大黄, *Radix et Rhizoma Rhei*), *máng xiāo* (芒硝, *Natrii Sulfas*), *xuán shēn* (玄参, *Radix Scrophulariae*), *mài dōng* (麦冬, *Radix Ophiopogonis*) and *shēng dì* (生地, *Radix Rehmanniae*)

Zhèn Gān Xī Fēng Tāng (镇肝熄风汤, "Liver-Sedating and Wind-Extinguishing Decoction"), from the *Records of Chinese Medicine with Reference to Western Medicine* (*Yī Xué Zhōng Zhōng Cān Xī Lù*, 医学衷中参西录)

Ingredients: *Niú xī* (牛膝, *Radix Achyranthis Bidentatae*), *lóng gǔ* (龙骨, *Os Draconis*), *bái sháo* (白芍, *Radix Paeoniae Alba*), *tiān dōng* (天冬, *Radix Asparagi*), *mài yá* (麦芽, *Fructus Hordei Germinatus*), *dài zhě shí* (代赭石, *Haematitum*), *mǔ lì* (牡蛎, *Concha Ostreae*), *xuán shēn* (玄参, *Radix Scrophulariae*), *chuān liàn zǐ* (川楝子, *Fructus Toosendan*), *yīn chén* (茵陈, *Herba Artemisiae Scopariae*) and *gān cǎo* (甘草, *Radix et Rhizoma Glycyrrhizae*)

Zhēn Rén Yǎng Zàng Tāng (真人养脏汤, "Enlightened Master Viscera-Nourishing Decoction"), from *Standards for Diagnosis and Treatment* (*Zhèng Zhì Zhǔn Shéng*, 证治准绳)

Ingredients: *Hē zǐ* (诃子, *Fructus Chebulae*), *yīng sù qiào* (罂粟壳, *Pericarpium Papaveris*), *ròu dòu kòu* (肉豆蔻, *Semen Myristicae*), *bái zhú* (白术, *Rhizoma Atractylodis Macrocephalae*), *rén shēn* (人参, *Radix et Rhizoma Ginseng*), *mù xiāng* (木香, *Radix Aucklandiae*), *ròu guì* (肉桂, *Cortex Cinnamomi*), *zhì gān cǎo* (炙甘草, *Radix et Rhizoma Glycyrrhizae Praeparata cum Melle*), *shēng jiāng* (生姜, *Rhizoma Zingiberis Recens*) and *dà zǎo* (大枣, *Fructus Jujubae*)

Zhēn Wǔ Tāng (真武汤, "True Warrior Decoction"), from the *Treatise on Cold Damage* (*Shāng Hán Lùn*, 伤寒论)

Ingredients: *Páo fù zǐ* (炮附子, *Radix Aconiti Lateralis Praeparata*), *bái zhú* (白术, *Rhizoma Atractylodis Macrocephalae*), *fú líng* (茯苓, *Poria*), *sháo yào* (芍药, *Radix Paeoniae*) and *shēng jiāng* (生姜, *Rhizoma Zingiberis Recens*)

Zhēn Zhū Mǔ Wán (珍珠母丸, "Concha Margaritiferae Usta Pill"), from *Experiential Formulas for Universal Relief* (*Pǔ Jì Běn Shì Fāng*, 普济本事方)

Ingredients: *Zhēn zhū mǔ* (珍珠母, *Concha Margaritiferae Usta*), *dāng guī* (当归, *Radix Angelicae Sinensis*), *shú dì huáng* (熟地黄, *Radix Rehmanniae Praeparata*), *rén shēn* (人参, *Radix et Rhizoma Ginseng*), *suān zǎo rén* (酸枣仁, *Semen Ziziphi Spinosae*), *bǎi zǐ rén* (柏子仁, *Semen Platycladi*), *xī jiǎo* (犀角, *Cornu Rhinocerotis*), *fú shén* (茯神, *Sclerotium Poriae Pararadicis*), *chén xiāng* (沉香, *Lignum Aquilariae Resinatum*) and *lóng chǐ* (龙齿, *Dens Draconis*)

Zhěng Yáng Lǐ Láo Tāng (拯阳理劳汤, "Yang-Saving and Fatigue-Improving Decoction"), from *Required Readings from the Medical Ancestors* (*Yī Zōng Bì Dú*, 医宗必读)

Ingredients: *Rén shēn* (人参, *Radix et Rhizoma Ginseng*), *huáng qí* (黄芪, *Radix Astragali*), *ròu guì* (肉桂, *Cortex Cinnamomi*), *dāng guī* (当归, *Radix Angelicae Sinensis*), *bái zhú* (白术, *Rhizoma Atractylodis Macrocephalae*), *gān cǎo* (甘草, *Radix et Rhizoma Glycyrrhizae*), *chén pí* (陈皮, *Pericarpium Citri Reticulatae*), *wǔ wèi zǐ* (五味子, *Fructus Schisandrae Chinensis*), *shēng jiāng* (生姜, *Rhizoma Zingiberis Recens*) and *dà zǎo* (大枣, *Fructus Jujubae*)

Zhī Bǎi Dì Huáng Wán (知柏地黄丸, "Anemarrhena, Phellodendron and Rehmannia Pill"), from *The Golden Mirror of the Medical Tradition* (*Yī Zōng Jīn Jiàn*, 医宗金鉴)

Ingredients: *Zhī mǔ* (知母, *Rhizoma Anemarrhenae*), *huáng bǎi* (黄柏, *Cortex Phellodendri Chinensis*), *shú dì huáng* (熟地黄, *Radix Rehmanniae Praeparata*), *shān zhū yú* (山茱萸, *Fructus Corni*), *shān yào* (山药, *Rhizoma Dioscoreae*), *mǔ dān pí* (牡丹皮, *Cortex Moutan*), *zé xiè* (泽泻, *Rhizoma Alismatis*) and *fú líng* (茯苓, *Poria*)

Zhōng Mǎn Fēn Xiāo Wán (中满分消丸, "Abdominal Fullness–Relieving Pill"), from *Secrets from the Orchid Chamber* (*Lán Shì Mì Cáng*, 兰室秘藏)

Ingredients: *Hòu pò* (厚朴, *Cortex Magnoliae Officinalis*), *zhǐ shí* (枳实, *Fructus Aurantii Immaturus*), *huáng lián* (黄连, *Rhizoma Coptidis*), *huáng qín* (黄芩, *Radix Scutellariae*), *zhī mǔ* (知母, *Rhizoma Anemarrhenae*), *bàn xià* (半夏, *Rhizoma Pinelliae*), *chén pí* (陈皮, *Pericarpium Citri Reticulatae*), *zé xiè* (泽泻, *Rhizoma Alismatis*), *fú líng* (茯苓, *Poria*), *shā rén* (砂仁, *Fructus Amomi*), *gān jiāng* (干姜, *Rhizoma Zingiberis*), *jiāng huáng* (姜黄, *Rhizoma Curcumae Longae*), *rén shēn* (人参, *Radix et Rhizoma Ginseng*), *bái zhú* (白术, *Rhizoma Atractylodis Macrocephalae*), *gān cǎo* (甘草, *Radix et Rhizoma Glycyrrhizae*) and *zhū líng* (猪苓, *Polyporus*)

Zhū Líng Tāng (猪苓汤, "Polyporus Decoction"), from *Treatise on Cold Damage* (*Shāng Hán Lùn*, 伤寒论)

Ingredients: *Zhū líng* (猪苓, *Polyporus*), *fú líng* (茯苓, *Poria*), *zé xiè* (泽泻, *Rhizoma Alismatis*), *ē jiāo* (阿胶, *Colla Corii Asini*) and *huá shí* (滑石, *Talcum*)

Zhú Yè Shí Gāo Tāng (竹叶石膏汤, "Lophatherum and Gypsum Decoction"), from the *Treatise on Cold Damage* (*Shāng Hán Lùn*, 伤寒论)

Ingredients: *Zhú yè* (竹叶, *Folium Phyllostachydis Henonis*), *shí gāo* (石膏, *Gypsum Fibrosum*), *mài dōng* (麦冬, *Radix Ophiopogonis*), *rén shēn* (人参, *Radix et Rhizoma Ginseng*), *bàn xià* (半夏, *Rhizoma Pinelliae*), *jīng mǐ* (粳米, *Oryza Sativa L.*) and *zhì gān cǎo* (炙甘草, *Radix et Rhizoma Glycyrrhizae Praeparata cum Melle*)

Zuǒ Jīn Wán (左金丸, "Left Metal Pill"), from *Teachings of [Zhu] Dan-xi* (*Dān Xī Xīn Fǎ*, 丹溪心法)

Ingredients: *Huáng lián* (黄连, *Rhizoma Coptidis*) and *wú zhū yú* (吴茱萸, *Fructus Evodiae*)

Index